Clinical Neurology

C. David Marsden FRS, DSc, FRCP, FRCPsych

The Institute of Neurology, The National Hospital for
Nervous Diseases, London

Timothy J. Fowler DM, FRCP

Consultant Neurologist, South-East Thames Region

Edward Arnold

A division of Hodder & Stoughton

LONDON   MELBOURNE   AUCKLAND

© 1989 C. David Marsden and Timothy J. Fowler

First published in Great Britain 1989

British Library Cataloguing in Publication Data

Marsden, C. David (Charles David)
   Clinical neurology
   1. Man. Nervous system. Diagnosis
   I. Title   II. Fowler, T. (Timothy)
   III. Series
   616.8'0475

   ISBN 0-7131-4432-7

Typeset in 10/11pt Baskerville by Colset Private Limited, Singapore. Printed and bound in Great Britain for Edward Arnold, the educational, academic and medical publishing division of Hodder and Stoughton Limited, 41 Bedford Square, London WC1B 3DQ by Butler & Tanner Ltd, Frome and London.

General preface to series

Student textbooks of medicine seek to present the subject of human diseases and their treatment in a manner that is not only informative, but interesting and readily assimilable. It is important, in a field where knowledge advances rapidly, that principles are emphasized rather than details, so that what is contained in the book remains valid for as long as possible.

These considerations favour an approach which concentrates on each disease as a disturbance of normal structure and function. Rational therapy follows logically from a knowledge of the disturbance, and it is in this field where some of the most rapid advances in Medicine have occurred.

A disturbance of normal structure without any disturbance of function may not be important to the patient except for cosmetic or psychological reasons. Therefore, it is disturbances in function that should be stressed. Preclinical students should aim at a comprehensive understanding of physiological principles so that when they arrive on the wards they will be able to appreciate the significance of disordered function in disease. Clinical students must be presented with descriptions of disease which stress the disturbances in normal physiological functions that are responsible for the symptoms and signs which they find in their patients. All students must be made aware of the growing points in physiology which, even though not immediately applicable to the practice of Medicine, will almost certainly become so during the course of their professional lives.

In this Series, the major physiological systems are each covered by a pair of books, one preclinical and the other clinical, in which the authors have attempted to meet the requirements discussed above. A particular feature is the provision of numerous cross-references between the two members of a pair of books to facilitate the blending of basic science and clinical expertise that is the goal of this Series. This coordination, which is initiated at the planning stage and continues throughout the writing of each pair of books, is achieved by frequent discussions between the preclinical and clinical authors concerned and between them and the editors of the Series.

MH
KBS
JTF

Preface

Few teaching programmes give their students adequate exposure to clinical neurology. The complaints of patients with disturbances of the brain, spinal cord and peripheral nervous system are often difficult to interpret, and the investigation and management of common neurological diseases may seem daunting. The student is often frightened by the complexities of the nervous system, but a sound understanding of its anatomy and physiology is the basis of good clinical practice.

Neurological symptoms are common: headache is the most frequent form of pain for which a patient consults the doctor. Many general medical conditions have neurological complications and these may be the presenting symptoms. There is also a considerable overlap of neurology with psychiatry. It is therefore very important that doctors in training have adequate exposure to neurology and this text covers these aspects.

This book is complementary to the neurophysiological work of Dr R. Carpenter and is written by a number of clinicians who are familiar with common neurological disorders, their symptoms and presentation. Emphasis is on the easy recognition of such disorders, their investigation, prognosis and management. This should enable the reader to use this as a practical guide to neurological diagnosis and treatment. Useful practical points about the neurological history and examination are described in the introductory chapters.

Exciting new diagnostic techniques have appeared in the last 10 years and these have greatly altered the investigation and understanding of a number of neurological conditions. Computerized tomographic and now magnetic resonance imaging scans have superseded many of the previously unpleasant invasive neuroradiological investigations. The practical application of these new techniques has been included. There is also discussion of the role of evoked potential studies, a more direct application of physiological techniques.

It is often said that neurology is an academic exercise in diagnosis but that treatment may be lacking. This is untrue, major advances have been and are being made in therapy. Such measures include the treatment of certain bacterial and now herpetic viral infections, the better control of epileptic seizures and the relief of certain movement disorders. From our increased understanding of the disordered immunology, myasthenia gravis can now be successfully treated in most patients. Modern neurosurgical techniques, aided by improved anaesthesia and the use of the operating microscope allows the removal of a number of spinal and cerebral tumours, the clipping of aneurysms and even the separation of small blood vessels in contact with nerves which may be producing neuralgic pains or muscle spasm. Interventional radiology is now useful in the treatment of some vascular disorders. These aspects are covered.

Appropriate attention is given to common neurological problems. These include the recognition of cerebrovascular disorders and their risk factors, and the management of head injuries with due regard for potential life-threatening complications. Inevitably some uncommon conditions are discussed. Doctors may meet these infrequently but if these are recognized, they will not be forgotten.

Neurology, in common with other branches of medicine, has a number of more chronic disorders where therapy is disappointing and progressive disability may occur, e.g. multiple sclerosis, motor neurone disease. The care and management of such patients and their families are important and attention is given to such aspects of treatment.

We are indebted to our many medical colleagues as well as the neurologists and neurosurgeons who have provided the patients and thus the stimulus to this volume. Informal discussions about clinical problems with specialists from all disciplines have helped to broaden our outlook and kept us up to date in many unrelated fields. To all these colleagues we add our thanks.

We should also like to thank Professor K. Saunders for his useful and constructive criticism, and our publishers, Edward Arnold, for all their invaluable help and support.

London, 1989   CDM
                                                                                                              TJF

Acknowledgements

We are grateful for all the help and inspiration provided by our medical and neurological colleagues in many disciplines, and in particular to the neuro-radiologists Dr C. Penney and Dr P. Butler who have provided many of the figures, and the MRI Centre at the National Hospital for Nervous Diseases where many of the MRI scans were performed. We should also like to thank Sir John Walton and the Oxford University Press for permission to use Figures 3.10 (a & b) and 3.11 (a & b) from *Brain's Diseases of the Nervous System*, and V. Hachinski and J. Norris and F.A. Davis Company for the use of Figure 19.6 from *The Acute Stroke*. We should like to thank Dr G. Holder for providing the pictures of evoked potentials (Figures 1.3 and 1.4), Dr M. Salmon for the photomicrographs (Figures 4.2 and 4.5) and Dr Testa for the SPET picture (Figure 10.5). Tables 11.1 and 5 are adapted from Dr D Chadwick's lecture at the ILAG meeting in 1987 with his kind permission. Some figures in chapter 19 have been previously published by Professor M Harrison and we thank the editors of Lancet (19.1) and Schattauer Publishers of Stuttgart (19.7, 15 & 16) for their kind permission to reproduce them. We should also like to acknowledge the help of a number of photographic departments but especially that of Greenwich District Hospital. We are also grateful to Mary Townsley and Sue Stratful for much of the hard work in typing the manuscript.

Contents

General preface to the series   v
Preface   vi
Contents of Neurophysiology by R.H.S. Carpenter   xiv
Contributors   xv

1 Introduction   1
Anatomical diagnosis   2
Pathological diagnosis   6
Special investigations   6

2 Symptoms of neurological disease   21
Headache   22
Pain in the face   26
Blackouts, fits and faints   28
Loss of vision   32
Giddiness   34
Pain in the arm   36
Pain in the leg   39
Difficulty in walking   41
Acute paraplegia   43
Acute quadriplegia   43
Chronic spastic paraparesis   44
Spastic weakness of one leg   44
Unsteadiness of gait   45
Movement disorders   45
Decline of memory, intellect and behaviour   47

3 Examination of the nervous system   50
The basic scheme of neurological examination   50
Specific abnormalities   63

4 Diseases of muscle and the neuromuscular junction   103
Diagnosis and investigation   103
Muscular dystrophy   104

Metabolic, endocrine and toxic myopathies   108
Inflammatory myopathies   112
Congenital myopathies   116
Myotonic syndromes   117
Myasthenia gravis   121
Carcinomatous neuromyopathy   124

5 **Peripheral neuropathy**   126
Pathogenesis   126
Symptoms and signs   127
Investigations   128
Guillain-Barré syndrome, acute polyradiculoneuropathy   129
Chronic inflammatory demyelinating neuropathies   131
Other causes of acute neuropathy   132
Diabetic neuropathies   132
Toxic neuropathies   134
Uraemia   135
Porphyria   135
Vitamin B12 deficiency   135
Vitamin E deficiency   136
Infective causes   136
Malignancy   137
Disorders of protein metabolism   137
Connective tissue disorders   137
Hereditary neuropathies   139
The unknown cause group   140

6 **Nerve and root lesions**   141
Pathogenesis of pressure palsies   141
Carpal tunnel syndrome   142
Ulnar nerve lesions   143
Sciatic nerve   145
Lateral popliteal nerve   146
Tarsal tunnel   148
Femoral nerve   148
Lateral cutaneous nerve of the thigh   148
Thoracic outlet compression   149
Brachial plexus damage   149
Cervical root problems   151
Lumbar root lesions   153

7 **Cranial nerve syndromes**   157
Cranial nerve I   157
Cranial nerve II   157
Cranial nerves III, IV and VI: oculomotor palsies 161
Cranial nerve V   164
Cranial nerve VII   166
Cranial nerve VIII   169
Cranial nerves IX, X, XI and XII   172

8 Spinal diseases   175
Symptoms and signs   175
Spinal compression   177
Investigations   179
Principles (benefits and hazards) of surgical treatment   186
Common causes of compression of the contents of the vertebral
canal   187
Disc rupture and degenerative diseases of the spine   192
Syringomyelia   196
Spinal injuries   197

9 Movement disorders   200
Parkinson's disease   200
Other akinetic-rigid syndromes   207
Wilson's disease   209
The dyskinesias   211
Benign essential (familial) tremor   214
Sydenham's chorea   216
Huntington's disease   217
Hemiballism   218
Generalized myoclonus   218
Focal myoclonus   219
Gilles de la Tourette syndrome   219
Torsion dystonia   220
Drug-induced movement disorders   221

10 Dementia   223
Problems of definition and classification   224
The epidemiology of dementia   226
The assessment of dementia   227
Investigation of dementia   229
Types of dementia   233
Dementia due to trauma and structural lesions   235
Subcortical.dementias   236
Dementia due to infections and inflammatory causes   236
Metabolic, nutritional and toxic causes   238
Miscellaneous conditions   239
Management of dementia   240

11 Epilepsy and sleep disorders   242
Epilepsy   242
Status epilepticus   256
Sleep disorders   259

12 Migraine   262
Classical migraine   262
Common migraine   263
Migraine variants   264
Migraine equivalents   265

Childhood migraine 265
Facial migraine and 'lower-half headache' 266
Migrainous neuralgia, cluster headache, periodic migrainous
neuralgia 266
Chronic paroxysmal hemicrania 267
Causes of migraine 267
Examination 268
Investigations 268
Treatment 269
Prevention of migraine 269

13 **Head injury** 272
Local effects of head injury 272
Injury to the brain 273
Intracranial pressure and head injury 275
Cerebral blood flow and head injury 278
Acute assessment and management 278
Special complications 288

14 **Raised intracranial pressure** 291
Symptoms and signs 291
Shifts and herniations 293
Hydrocephalus 295
Benign intracranial hypertension 297
Intracranial tumours 298
Posterior fossa tumours 310
Cerebellopontine angle tumours 313
Chordoma 317
Intracranial abscess 317
Parasitic cysts 320

15 **Infections of the central nervous system** 322
Meningitis 322
Encephalitis 333
CNS infection in the immunocompromised patient 337
Poliomyelitis 338
Tetanus 339
Syphilis 341

16 **Demyelinating disease of the central nervous system** 344
Multiple sclerosis (MS) 344
Acute disseminated encephalomyelitis 351
Diffuse cerebral sclerosis (Schilder's disease) 351
Transverse myelitis 351

17 **Degenerative diseases of the central nervous system** 353
Motor neurone disease 353
Spinal muscular atrophies 355
The hereditary ataxias and related disorders 356

Phakomatoses 359
Lipidoses 363
Mucopolysaccharidoses 363
Aminoacidurias 366

18 Developmental disorders of the central nervous system 367
Spina bifida 367
Hydrocephalus 370
Chiari malformation, Arnold-Chiari malformation 372
Basilar impression 374
Myelodysplasia 375
Prevention 375
Cerebral palsy 376

19 Cerebrovascular disease 378
Risk factors 378
Classification 379
Pathology 379
Clinical features 389
Unusual causes of stroke 402
Rehabilitation 405
Vascular disease of the spinal cord 406

20 Metabolic disorders 407
Vitamin deficiencies 407
Toxic effects—alcohol 409
Toxic effects of drugs 410
Heavy metals 411
Physical insults 412
Endocrine disturbances 414
Electrolyte disturbances 419
Calcium metabolism 420
Behçet's disease 421
Sarcoidosis 421

21 Psychiatric disorders 423
Psychiatric diagnoses 424
Neuroses and psychoses 431
The psychoses 432
Some other psychiatric disorders 443

Further reading and references 448
Addendum: proprietary drug names 451
Index 453

Contents of *Neurophysiology* by R.H.S. Carpenter

While reading this book you might find it helpful to refer to the companion volume, *Neurophysiology*. The following list of contents will enable you to look up the physiological background to the material contained in this book.

 1 Studying the brain
 2 Nerves
 3 Receptors and synapses
 4 Skin sense
 5 Proprioception
 6 Hearing
 7 Vision
 8 Smell and taste
 9 Types of motor control
10 The spinal level
11 The control of posture
12 Higher levels of motor control
13 Analysis and storage of information by the cerebral cortex
14 The higher levels of control

Contributors

John R. Bartlett FRCS
  Consultant Neurosurgeon, The Brook Hospital
  Chapter 8   Spinal diseases

Paul Bridges PhD, MD, FRCPsych
  Consultant Psychiatrist, Guy's and the Brook Hospitals
  Senior Lecturer, United Medical and Dental Schools, Guy's Hospital
  Chapter 21   Psychiatric disorders

Timothy J. Fowler DM, FRCP
  Consultant Neurologist, South-East Thames Region
  Chapters 5, 6, 7, 12, 16, 17, 18, and 20 – Peripheral neuropathy, Nerve and
  root lesions, Cranial nerve syndromes, Migraine, Demyelinating disease of
  the central nervous system, Degenerative disease of the central nervous
  system, Developmental disorders of the central nervous system, Metabolic
  disorders

Michael J.G. Harrison DM, FRCP
  Professor of Neurology, The Middlesex Hospital and The National Hospital
  for Nervous Diseases
  Chapter 19   Cerebrovascular disease

George Harwood FRCP
  Consultant Neurologist, South East Thames Region
  Chapter 11   Epilepsy and sleep disorders

C. David Marsden FRS, DSc, FRCP, FRCPsych
  Professor of Neurology, The Institute of Neurology, The National Hospital
  for Nervous Diseases
  Chapters 1, 2, 3, and 9 – Introduction, Symptoms of neurological disease,
  Examination of the nervous system, Movement disorders

Glen Neil-Dwyer MS, FRCS
  Consultant Neurosurgeon, The Wessex Neurological Centre
  Chapter 13   Head injury

Stephen S. Pollock MD, MRCP
Consultant Neurologist, South East Thames Region
Chapter 10   Dementia

Donald Riddoch FRCP
Consultant Neurologist, West Midlands Health Region
Chapter 4   Diseases of muscle and the neuromuscular junction

Michael M. Sharr MRCP, FRCS
Consultant Neurosurgeon, The Brook Hospital
Chapter 14   Raised intracranial pressure

Martin J. Wood MA, FRCP
Consultant Physician, Infectious Diseases, The East Birmingham Hospital
Chapter 15   Infections of the central nervous system

1

Introduction

Students have always found clinical neurology difficult. There are many reasons for this, quite apart from the failings of their teachers. Clinical diagnosis, at least the anatomical part of it, is heavily dependent upon an adequate if rudimentary knowledge of human neuroanatomy and neurophysiology, which is often learnt by rote and then forgotten by the time the student enters the neurological ward. Perhaps the greatest difficulty has been that neurology is full of irrelevant facts. Like the minutiae of gross anatomy, the neurological examination and a differential diagnosis can be drawn out to such an extent that the original aim is forgotten. The student becomes confused by a wealth of irrelevant detail, and so fails to grasp the main point. The problems of examination of sensory function illustrate the point. Armed with pin, cotton wool and tuning fork, the student approaches the patient to test sensation, but where to start? Human nature being what it is, many patients will try to help the doctor by attempting to perceive minor differences in the intensity of the pin or touch, and soon the hapless student is confronted with a mass of apparent abnormalities which he cannot decipher. He sees the experienced neurologist delicately mapping, with complete anatomical accuracy, an area of sensory loss, and wonders how he did it. The answer is simple; the experienced neurologist knows what he is looking for and has predicted what he will find on the basis of previous information. Sensory examination is the most difficult, so neurologists leave it till last when they have obtained as much information as they can concerning what they expect to find!

Here lies the clue to success in mastering clinical neurology. The student must learn to think on his feet at every moment of history taking and examination, building on a presumptive diagnosis as each new piece of information is collected, and predicting the outcome of the next series of questions or examinations. Thus, neurology employs a continuous process of deductive logic to arrive at a final conclusion.

The emphasis in this book is to simplify clinical neurology to manageable proportions. It is divided into three sections:

1. The patient's complaints.
2. The doctor's examination.
3. The individual neurological diseases and their treatment.

This is what happens in real life. The patient tells the doctor that he cannot walk, talk, see, hear, and so on. The doctor forms an opinion as to where the trouble lies (*the anatomical diagnosis*). Clinical examination confirms (or refutes) the hypothesis as to the anatomical site of damage. The combination of the tempo of the patient's complaint and the site of the lesion then provides the likely pathology (*pathological diagnosis*). Based upon this clinical evaluation, decisions as to further investigation will be made to confirm both anatomical and pathological diagnosis. The final conclusion will dictate treatment.

In practice, the emphasis in clinical neurology is on bedside evaluation of the patient's complaints and signs. The principles of anatomical and pathological diagnosis will be discussed briefly later in this Chapter. Special investigations are often not required at all for neurological diagnosis, and they can be misleading if not interpreted in the light of the history and clinical examination. The principles of use of the major investigative techniques employed in neurology will also be discussed briefly later in this Chapter.

A standard joke about neurologists has been that they are 'brilliant at finding out where the trouble is, but incapable of doing anything about it'! To some extent, such comments reflect a little bit of envy, but neurology remains one of the last bastions of clinical bedside medicine, being so dependent on the vagaries of the individual patient and the examiner's skill, rather than on inanimate figures on laboratory reports. In fact, there are few medical disciplines that can claim to have cures for all their major diseases, but many of the commonest neurological illnesses can be treated effectively. Thus, migraine, epilepsy, and Parkinson's disease are all amenable to drug therapy, while benign tumours in the head and spine can be removed successfully.

Quite apart from whether treatment exists, the doctor's role is also to relieve suffering. This is particularly important in clinical neurology, for many of its diseases produce severe physical disability. Part of the neurological apprenticeship is to learn the compassion and sensitivity to help disabled individuals to come to terms with, and surmount their problems.

Neurology thus provides a triple challenge. There is the intellectual exercise of defining the problem, the therapeutic challenge of treating it when treatment is available, and the humane responsibility of looking after those unfortunate enough to suffer from neurological diseases.

Anatomical diagnosis

The story of the patient's complaints as their history unfolds will direct attention to the part or parts of the nervous system involved. A few very simple rules will help to focus attention on the likely site of trouble.

Seizures (fits), disturbances of intellect and memory, and certain disorders of speech all point to disease of the cerebral cortex. Seizures are due to spontaneous discharges in cerebral cortical neurones, and do not occur with diseases of deep cerebral structures, the brainstem or cerebellum, unless the cerebral cortex also is involved. The faculties of intellectual prowess, reasoning and memory all depend upon the operations of the cerebral cortex, and any decline in these faculties points to damage in this zone of the brain. Disturbances of speech fall into three categories: (1) dysphasia, in which the content of speech is defective although articulation and phonation are intact; (2) dysarthria, in which the articulation of speech is abnormal due to damage to the neuromuscular mechanisms controlling the muscles concerned with speech production; and (3) dysphonia, in which the larynx, the sound-box, is damaged. Dysphasia points to a disorder of the cerebral cortex, particularly that of the dominant hemisphere.

Disturbances of vision are common neurological problems. Loss of visual acuity points to damage to the eye itself, or to the optic nerve. Lesions behind the optic chiasm produce loss of vision in the opposite half of the visual field (hemianopia), but leave intact at least the ipsilateral half of central macular vision, and this is sufficient to provide a normal visual acuity. Patients with hemianopias complain of difficulty in reading, or of bumping into objects in the blind half-field. Double vision (diplopia) occurs when the axes of the two eyes are out of alignment, i.e. not in parallel. This happens when one eyeball is displaced by some mass in the orbit, or if the ocular muscles are weak due either to primary muscle disease, or to damage to external ocular nerves.

Vertigo (a true sense of imbalance) is an illusion of movement and occurs with damage to the vestibular system, the vestibular nerve, or its brainstem connections. A combination of vertigo and diplopia suggests a lesion in the posterior fossa or brainstem, particularly when associated with bilateral motor or sensory disturbances.

Dysphagia and dysarthria are also usually due either to primary muscle disease, or to bilateral involvement of the neural mechanisms controlling the muscles of mastication and speech.

Weakness may be due to primary muscle disease or defective neuromuscular transmission, damage to the peripheral motor nerves or anterior horn cells in the spinal cord (lower motor neurone lesion), or to damage to the cortico-motoneurone pathways responsible for the cerebral control of movement (upper motor neurone lesion). Such weakness may affect all four limbs (quadriplegia), the arm and leg on one side (hemiplegia), or both legs sparing the arms (paraplegia). A quadriplegia in someone who is awake and can talk usually is due either to primary muscle disease, a generalized peripheral neuropathy, or a high cervical cord lesion. Hemiplegia suggests damage to the opposite cerebral hemisphere, particularly if the face is involved. Paraplegia most often is the result of spinal cord damage, particularly when there is also disturbance of sphincter control. Isolated weakness of one limb (monoplegia) frequently is caused by damage to its motor nerves, although sometimes a monoplegia may arise from lesions in the cerebral cortex.

The pattern of sensory symptoms usually follows that of motor disturbance. Thus, distal sensory loss in all four limbs suggests peripheral nerve disease. Sensory disturbance in a hemiplegic distribution suggests damage to the opposite cerebral hemisphere, particularly of the capsular sensory pathways, in which case the face often is involved. Hemiplegic sensory disturbance on one side of the body with involvement of the face on the opposite side suggests damage in the brainstem. If the cranial nerves are not involved, sensory disturbances on one side of the body, with motor disturbances on the opposite side of the body, suggest damage to the spinal cord. Sensory disturbance in both legs extending onto the trunk also points to a lesion of the spinal cord. Sensory loss affecting parts of one limb only is most often due to a local peripheral nerve or root lesion.

These simple rules for interpretation of symptoms usually give the first clue to the likely anatomical site of damage responsible for the patient's complaints. Of course, they are not infallible and many exceptions to such generalizations will be met in practice. However, they provide the easiest means of the first faltering steps in analysis of the anatomical site of the patient's lesion. The next stage in this exercise is the physical examination.

Neurological examination will be dictated by the patient's history, which helps to determine that aspect of the nervous system requiring most detailed attention. The methods employed will be described fully later in this book, but a certain number of simple principles will be stated here.

When the student approaches a neurological patient for the first time, armed with a standard textbook of neurological examination, he may well find that it takes him up to 2 h to complete the necessary bedside tests! When he sees the experienced neurologist completing the same task in under 10 min he may think that he faces an impossible apprenticeship. It cannot be stated too frequently that the secret of this art is to know what one is looking for. In fact, the neurologist divides his clinical examination conceptually into two halves. The first is a detailed evaluation of those parts of the nervous system to which his attention has been drawn in the course of taking the patient's history. The second is a general screen of other sections of the nervous system which, by history, do not seem likely to be involved, but which have to be examined in every patient to ensure that nothing is missed. To facilitate this method, the neurological trainee perfects a routine of clinical examination sufficient to act as a simple screen of the nervous system, onto which he grafts the extra detailed investigation of those sections to which his attention has been pointed. The routine screening examination, which can be undertaken very briefly in a matter of minutes, is learnt by repetition of the same sequence over and over again until it becomes second nature. For convenience, most start with a brief assessment of the mental faculties of the patient in the course of the interview, then move to the cranial nerves starting at the top and working down, then assess motor function of the limbs, which is much easier to examine and usually is much more informative than the sensory examination, which they leave to last. The details of this routine examination are discussed in Chapter 3.

One of the first problems that the neurological tyro encounters is the ease with which he detects apparent abnormalities on careful examination. Frequently it is difficult to decide on the significance of minor degrees of apparent weakness, fleeting and inconsistent sensory signs, slight asymmetry of the tendon reflexes, slightly less facility of repetitive movements of the left hand in a right-handed patient, or a few jerks of the eyes on extreme lateral gaze. To build a neurological diagnosis on minor deficits such as these is courting disaster. It is a useful exercise to classify each abnormality discovered as a 'hard' or 'soft' sign. 'Hard' signs are unequivocally abnormal – an absent ankle jerk even on reinforcement, a clear cut extensor plantar response, definite wasting of the small muscles of the hand, or absent vibration sense. Any final anatomical diagnosis must provide an explanation of such 'hard' signs. 'Soft' signs, on the other hand, such as those described above, are unreliable and best ignored when initially formulating a diagnosis. Base your conclusion on the 'hard' signs, and then see if any of the 'soft' signs that you have discovered may put that diagnosis into doubt. If so, go back and repeat that section of the examination and make up your mind again whether or not the 'soft' sign is real. Students will find that neurology becomes easier and easier the more confident they become in discarding unwanted 'soft' signs, as they become more experienced in determining the range of normal. This they will only achieve by constant repeated routine examination of the normal human nervous system.

The interpretation of physical signs found upon clinical examination of a neurological patient depends heavily upon a practical knowledge of neuro-anatomy. This is not the place to dwell upon this aspect of neuroscience, but it is worth emphasizing which parts of neuroanatomy are of greatest value to the clinical neurologist.

The visual system spans the whole of the head from front to back, so commonly is involved by intracranial lesions. The mechanisms controlling eye movements range from cortex through brainstem and external ocular nerves to the eye muscles themselves. Consequently, ocular motor function is frequently damaged by intracranial lesions. A careful anatomical knowledge of the visual and ocular motor pathways is essential to the trainee neurologist. So, too, is an understanding of the source of the individual cranial nerves in the brainstem, their course through the basal cisterns and exits through their appointed fora-mina in the skull, and their distribution to their extracranial target organs.

So far as the motor system is concerned, it is essential to be able to distinguish between the characteristics of primary muscle disease, a lower motor neurone lesion and an upper motor neurone lesion. Likewise, it is important to be able to detect the characteristic pattern of weakness in a patient with a hemiplegia, and to be able to distinguish this from the pattern of weakness that occurs with lesions affecting individual nerve roots or peripheral nerves. In the case of sensory findings, it is crucial to be able to recognize the pattern of sensory loss associated with damage to the spinal cord, or to individual nerve roots and peri-pheral nerves. The student should be thoroughly familiar with a cross-section of the spinal cord in order to be able to interpret the motor and sensory conse-quences of spinal cord damage. Likewise, they should know the segmental distribution of motor and sensory roots, and the characteristic motor and sensory consequences of damage to individual large peripheral nerves (*see* Fig. 3.11).

These are the minimum fundamentals of neuroanatomy required for neuro-logical practice. Without them students will be lost trying to interpret the results of their examinations. A short period spent refreshing the memory on these basic items prior to neurological training will be time well spent. It will allow the student to enjoy that period of neurological apprenticeship in learning about neurological disease, rather than being held back through ignorance of the essential first steps that must be mastered before any sensible discussion about neurological illness can be entertained.

From this brief introduction, it will be seen that the first stage of neurological diagnosis, the anatomical site of the lesion, is deduced initially from the history which points towards the likely parts of the nervous system to be involved and dictates which parts of the nervous system to examine in detail, and from the neurological examination itself which confirms and elaborates, or refutes, the initial impressions gained after hearing the patient's symptoms. At the end of history taking and clinical examination, the neurologist should, with confidence, be able to state what portions of the nervous system are affected. He can then pass to the second stage of defining the likely pathological cause.

Pathological diagnosis

The site of damage to the nervous system obviously will give some clue as to the possible pathological cause. For example, evidence of a lesion affecting the optic chiasm, indicated by the presence of a bitemporal hemianopia, suggests the possibility of a pituitary tumour. However, the course of the illness gives the greatest clue to the likely pathology responsible. Neurologists take great care to establish during history taking whether the onset of symptoms was sudden or gradual, and whether the subsequent course has been one of recovery, per-sistence with stable deficit, or progression of disability. Attention to these simple points provides the best guide to the likely pathology.

An illness of sudden, abrupt onset followed by subsequent gradual recovery is likely to be due to vascular disease.

An illness of gradual onset but relentless progression is likely to be due to a tumour or a degenerative condition.

An illness characterized by episodes of neurological deficit lasting days or weeks, followed by subsequent partial or complete recovery, is characteristic of multiple sclerosis.

An illness consisting of brief episodes of neurological disability lasting minutes or hours is typical of transient ischaemic attacks, migraine, or epilepsy.

Another factor that will help define the likely pathological cause of a neuro-logical disease is the age and sex of the patient. Thus, the sudden onset of a focal cerebral deficit lasting half an hour or so in an otherwise healthy 20-year-old woman taking the contraceptive pill almost certainly is migraine. A similar cerebral deficit of acute onset lasting an hour or so in a 65-year-old diabetic man, who is a heavy smoker, suggests the presence of primary cerebrovascular disease as the cause.

In general, attention to these three main categories of information, *the site of the lesion, its mode of onset and subsequent course,* and *the age and sex of the patient,* will point to the likely cause of the illness.

An important rule of thumb that is worth emphasizing at this point is that any neurological illness that is progressive must be considered to be due to a tumour until proven otherwise. One major task of neurology is to detect those benign tumours that can compress the brain, cranial nerves, or spinal cord to cause pro-gressive neurological deficit, which can be halted or reversed by appropriate neurosurgical treatment. Thus, progressive blindness not due to local eye disease, progressive unilateral deafness, a progressive hemiparesis, or a progressive spastic paraparesis all warrant full investigation to exclude a treatable tumour or other compressive lesion as the cause.

Special investigations

With the information obtained from the patient's history and examination, the neurologist will formulate a provisional anatomical and pathological diagnosis.

With many common neurological diseases no further investigation is required. For example, migraine is diagnosed solely on the basis of the history and the absence of any abnormal neurological signs on examination. Other patients, however, require special investigation to confirm, refute, or refine the provisional clinical diagnosis. The principles of special neurological tests will be described now, but detailed findings will be mentioned in connection with specific diseases to be described later. It is worth emphasizing at this point that most neurological tests require careful evaluation in the light of the individual clinical problem. Erroneous conclusions from radiological or electrophysiological investigation may arise if tests are interpreted in the absence of clinical information.

Unlike many other branches of medicine, it is difficult or impossible to obtain appropriate biopsy material to establish the diagnosis in many neurological patients. Biopsy of muscle or peripheral sensory nerve is used routinely, but for obvious reasons the spinal cord and brain are inaccessible. The special techniques that have been devised for examining these structures, which include those of neuroradiology, clinical neurophysiology, and examination of the cerebrospinal fluid (CSF), necessarily give indirect information.

Neuroradiology

The neuroradiologist has a range of techniques available for examining the brain and spinal cord. The most appropriate to employ in an individual problem can often only be decided by discussion between the neurologist and the neuroradiologist.

Simple X-rays of the skull often provide useful information and special tomographic studies of selected areas may be essential to specific diagnoses. Straight X-rays of the skull (lateral and posterior–anterior views) may pick up fractures, or the presence of bony destruction due to tumour or infection, and can detect evidence of raised intracranial pressure in the form of erosion of the lamina dura of the dorsum sellae, and even the existence of a supratentorial mass lesion which produces displacement of the calcified pineal shadow. Tomography of the pituitary fossa may be required to detect small pituitary tumours; of the internal auditory canals may reveal enlargement due to the presence of an acoustic neuroma; of the optic foramina may be required for the discovery of small meningiomas of the optic sheath or optic nerve gliomas; and of the foramen magnum may be necessary to demonstrate tumours or malformation in that region. Any patient suspected of having an intracranial lesion requires a chest X-ray to exclude the presence of a primary lung tumour or of secondary deposits in the lung.

The most powerful intracranial radiological investigation is the computerized tomography (CT) scan. In principle, CT scanning is a greatly extended version of tomography. The patient's head is secured in the centre of an arc which is traversed by X-ray equipment, to take hundreds of recordings of penetration of X-rays through a thin slice across the head, usually in the horizontal plane. The average density of penetration of X-rays for each of the many positions of the apparatus as it traverses the arc is automatically computed to provide the final radiological picture. By altering the focus of the arc relative to the head it is possible to scan horizontal slices each between 0.5–1 cm thick

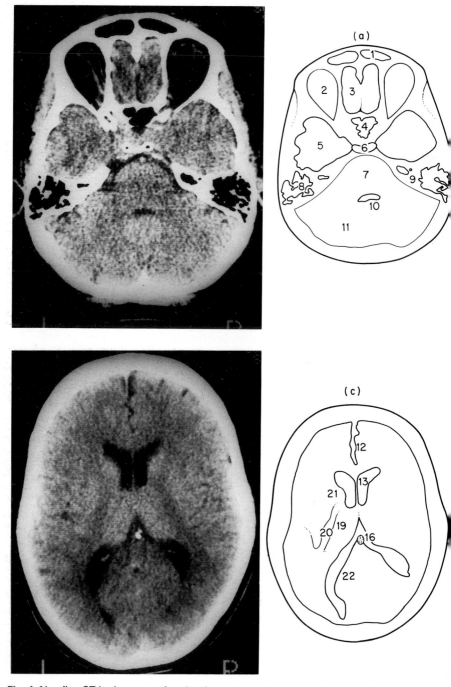

Fig. 1.1(a–d).   CT brain scan at four levels moving up from the orbitomeatal line.
1 Frontal sinus; 2 orbit; 3 ethmoid sinus and nasal cavity; 4 sphenoid sinus; 5 middle
fossa with temporal lobe; 6 dorsum sellae; 7 pons; 8 mastoid air cells; 9 petrous ridge;
10 fourth ventricle; 11 cerebellum, lateral lobe; 12 interhemispheric fissure; 13 lateral

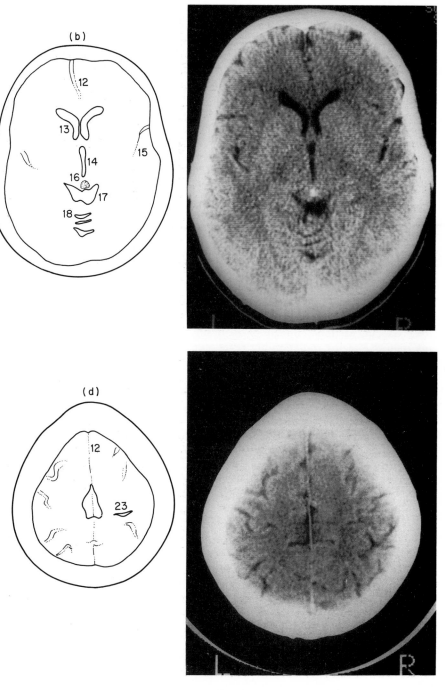

ventricles; 14 third ventricle; 15 sylvian fissure; 16 pineal; 17 quadrigeminal cistern;
18 vermis; 19 thalamus; 20 pathway of pyramidal tract; 21 caudate nucleus;
22 occipital horns; 23 surface sulci

working up from the foramen magnum to the vault.

Using this technique, the density of brain, CSF and bone differ, so can be easily distinguished. Indeed, the density of white matter is slightly different from that of grey matter allowing the two to be separated. Accordingly, the CT scan displays the position and size of the ventricular system, and the normal major landmarks of brain anatomy (Fig. 1.1). The presence of an intracranial lesion can be deduced from shifts of intracranial contents as well as by an abnormal density of the lesion itself. Thus, areas of infarction, oedema or tumour often appear hypodense, while haemorrhage is hyperdense. Further information can be obtained by repeated scanning after the intravenous injection of an iodine-containing contrast medium which may cause enhancement of lesions such as tumours or infarcts. The CT brain scan exposes the patient to a dose of X-rays no greater than that involved in a simple series of skull X-rays, so the investigation can be repeated as frequently as is necessary. It can be undertaken without anaesthesia or sedation in all but the most restless patients. It is quite painless and the only discomfort involved is that associated with the necessity to lie quite still for some minutes while the scan is executed. A few patients are allergic to iodine-containing contrast media and may show an acute sensitivity reaction. The development of CT scanning has revolutionized neurological and neurosurgical practice in recent years and its originator, Hounsfield, was justly awarded a Nobel prize for his achievements.

Magnetic resonance imaging (MRI) is the most recent technique introduced for producing sectioned images of the brain, spinal cord and body. This does not require ionizing radiation but relies on the fact that certain nuclei with an odd number of neutrons or protons, when placed in a magnetic field, align themselves with it. Hydrogen nuclei (with protons) are used and these give a high nuclear magnetic resonance signal. If such nuclei are placed in a magnetic field and stimulated by radiofrequency waves, the nuclei are displaced. When the radiofrequency waves cease, the nuclei return to their original position. Such changes can be detected by a receiver coil. The strengths of the magnets vary; usually 1.0 Tesla or more – over 20 000 times stronger than the earth's magnetic field. A number of variable images can be produced by different radiofrequency signals: two commonly used sequences are inversion recovery and spin echo. The rate of return may be indicated by two time constants T_1 (the longitudinal relaxation time) and T_2 (the transverse relaxation time).

The sectioned images may be produced in different planes, e.g. coronal, sagittal or transverse axial (the last like a CT scan). Because the hydrogen ion in bone cannot be resonated, bone artefact is not a problem, so MRI scans give greatly improved images of the posterior fossa, base of the skull and spinal canal (Fig. 1.2). MRI scans give good definition of lesions in white and grey matter. Their use in multiple sclerosis has shown that many more plaques can be detected than by CT scanning. They are also useful in giving details of posterior fossa pathology, particularly tumours and craniocervical junction abnormalities, e.g. a syrinx.

Unfortunately, MRI scanners are very expensive to install and run, so at present there is often limited access. Hopefully in the future this will improve. There is no danger of radiation damage but some patients find the procedure claustrophobic and the machine noisy.

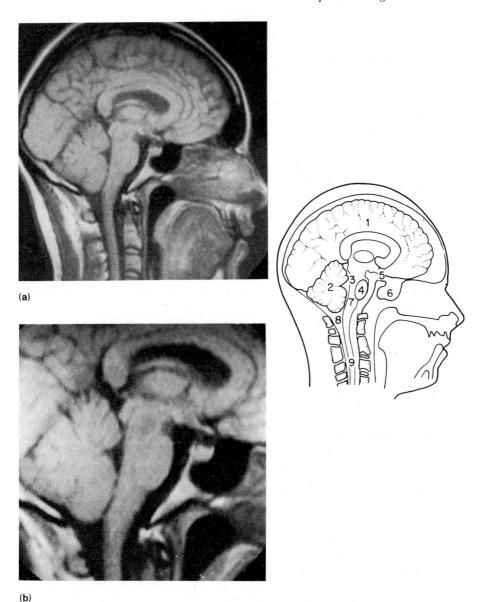

(a)

(b)

Fig. 1.2.   (a) MRI brain scan, Sagittal view. (b) Magnified view of posterior fossa.
1 Cerebral hemisphere; 2 cerebellum; 3 fourth ventricle; 4 pons; 5 pituitary stalk with
chiasm anteriorly; 6 sphenoid sinus; 7 medulla; 8 craniocervical junction; 9 cervical
spinal cord

Other neuroradiological investigations used to study the brain are now employed less frequently as a result of the widespread introduction of CT and MRI scanning into neurology and neurosurgery units. The older method of visualizing intracranial contents by the injection of air either into the CSF via a lumbar puncture (air encephalogram) or directly into the ventricles via a needle inserted through a burr-hole in the skull (air ventriculogram) has now virtually been superseded by CT scanning. In particular, air encephalography, which was an unpleasant and occasionally dangerous investigation, is now almost never undertaken.

Certain radioactive isotopes can be injected intravenously and the gamma radiation produced detected by a gamma camera. If there is damage to the blood–brain barrier, or the presence of certain types of pathology, e.g. certain tumours, abscesses or some vascular lesions, local areas of abnormal uptake in the brain may be detected. The usual isotope in brain scans is pertechnetate (technetium–99m). Vascular areas of the skull and head, e.g. the base of the skull and posterior fossa, are poorly shown because these are areas of high uptake. Most supratentorial meningiomas, cerebral abscesses, multiple metastases and subdural haematomas may be detected. However, only a proportion of primary brain tumours appear, and the detection of vascular lesions is dependent on their size and the timing of the scan. Radionuclide scans, however, are often readily available in district hospitals and play a useful role as a screening test to exclude or confirm the presence of metastases, and the presence of an abscess or meningioma. There may be a high risk (around 60%) of failure to detect some lesions at the base of the skull or in the posterior fossa. Small tumours, less than 1.5 cm in diameter, may be missed.

Cerebral angiography still retains an important place in the investigation of patients with stroke, subarachnoid haemorrhage, and some intracranial tumours. The extracranial and intracranial arterial and venous supply to the brain can be visualized by injection of contrast medium directly into the major cerebral blood vessels. This can be achieved by direct puncture into the common carotid or vertebral artery in the neck, or by the introduction of a catheter (usually via the femoral artery) which is then manoeuvred into the appropriate cranial vessel before injection of dye. Serial X-rays are then taken after each injection of contrast to outline the arterial filling, capillary and venous phases of the circulation. Cerebral arteriography in expert hands is relatively safe, but still carries a slight risk of causing damage to blood vessels or brain, particularly in those with pre-existing cerebrovascular disease. Nevertheless, cerebral arteriography is essential for demonstrating aneurysms responsible for subarachnoid bleeding, and for outlining the extracranial arterial system in those with strokes due to emboli from neck vessels. In addition, it is still widely employed in planning a neurosurgical approach to many intracranial tumours, particularly meningiomas.

The neuroradiological investigation of the spinal cord poses a different set of problems. Whole body CT scanning has entered routine practice: the CT pictures obtained of the spinal column and spinal cord are now increasingly used in neurological and neurosurgical investigation. However, tumours and other space-occupying lesions affecting the spinal cord are usually detected by a combination of straight X-rays to the spinal column and myelography using contrast media. Any patient with a spinal cord lesion requiring investigation needs good straight X-rays of the appropriate section of the spine, as indicated by the anatomical site of the lesion determined by clinical examination.

Such X-rays may demonstrate bony destruction due to tumour or infection, the presence of degenerative spinal disease, or of congenital malformation. Myelography is undertaken by the injection of contrast medium into the CSF surrounding the spinal cord, either by a lumbar puncture or through a lateral puncture in the neck into the upper cervical region. The contrast medium employed contains a radiopaque substance and can be manoeuvred into different parts of the spinal column by tilting the patient on a specially designed table. Originally the contrast medium used most commonly was Myodil containing iodine in an oil base. However, this substance occasionally provoked an inflammatory meningeal reaction with the late appearance of arachnoiditis. It has now been replaced by water-soluble media, e.g. metrizamide and iohexol, which can provide pictures of better definition with a much smaller risk of meningeal irritation. Such water-soluble media are routinely used for all investigations of the lumbosacral region, radiculography, and now have replaced Myodil for other spinal cord studies. Occasionally contrast may cause seizures if allowed to enter the head, or severe muscle cramps due to irritation of the spinal cord, but overall it is safe and its use is extending. The successful execution of a myelogram depends upon the neuroradiologist knowing what is being sought. After injection of the contrast material, the patient is manoeuvred in such a way to allow the area of interest to be displayed under direct vision by the neuroradiologist, who will then take X-rays of suitable views to display any lesion discovered.

MRI scanning of the spinal cord turns out to be a powerful method of detecting tumours and for certain problems (e.g. at the foramen magnum, for syringomyelia, and for intrinsic conditions), is the method of choice. CT scanning, at selected levels, is also a powerful way of examining local cord or vertebral disease.

Electroencephalography (EEG)

That the electrical activity of the brain could be recorded through the skull by surface electrodes applied to the scalp was a remarkable discovery. The technique of electroencephalography has now been refined into a routine method of examining brain function. Some 40 electrodes are secured to the scalp at standard positions, and the small electrical signals obtained between pairs of electrodes linked in standard arrays are amplified and displayed. Conventionally, eight or 16 channels are recorded. The individual signals are only a few microvolts in amplitude, so artefacts introduced by extraneous interference, eye movement, muscle contraction, or whole body movement must be scrupulously avoided or rejected.

The normal encephalogram is characterized by the presence of rhythmic alpha activity (at a frequency around 10 Hz) evident more in posterior channels and with the eyes shut. EEG abnormalities consist either of generalized changes in frequency of electrical activity, or focal abnormalities affecting specific regions. The background EEG activity may be generally slowed into the theta

(5–7 Hz) or delta (2–4 Hz) ranges by diffuse cerebral disease, such as that caused by inflammatory or metabolic encephalopathies, e.g. drug intoxication or liver failure. Local areas of cerebral abnormality due to infarction, trauma or tumour, may be indicated by a focal area of slowing of EEG activity. However, it is worth remembering that the EEG cannot explore all areas of the brain so that a normal electroencephalogram by no means excludes cerebral damage. The surface EEG reflects the electrical activity of the underlying cerebral cortex so that extensive lesions of the deeper structures such as thalamus and basal ganglia, and of posterior fossa regions may not cause any EEG abnormality. ·Even lesions of the temporal lobes may not be evident in the surface EEG; these structures are on the under-surface of the brain. Special techniques such as placement of electrodes in the nasopharynx or via sphenoidal needles inserted in front of the ears may be required to detect temporal lobe abnormalities. Another problem in interpreting the presence of an abnormality of brain function indicated by the EEG, is that it does not suggest the pathological cause. In general, neuroradiological studies, especially CT and MRI scanning, are more appropriate for investigation of patients suspected of having focal lesions of the brain, for they will give further information on the likely cause. In contrast, CT and MRI scanning and other neuroradiological techniques may reveal no abnormalities in patients with severe metabolic or inflammatory brain disease which produce profound changes in EEG activity.

The EEG finds its greatest use in the investigation of patients with epilepsy, in whom it can detect a wide range of abnormalities including frank seizure discharges. These may consist of either focal spike or sharp wave discharges arising in relation to an irritative lesion affecting the cerebral cortex, or of generalized spike and wave abnormalities that occur in primary generalized epilepsies such as petit mal. The details of such EEG changes will be discussed in Chapter 11, but it is important to note at this point that the EEG cannot diagnose epilepsy. A small proportion of those with undoubted seizures, particularly those arising in the temporal lobe, have normal surface EEG recordings, and a small proportion of the normal population who have never had a fit may show EEG abnormalities similar to those found in patients with epilepsy.

Evoked potential studies

Standard electroencephalographic recordings have been supplemented in recent years by the addition of evoked potential investigation. Early on it was discovered that abnormal discharges could be provoked in a proportion of patients suffering from epilepsy by repetitive photic stimulation with flash stimuli. The principle has been extended to computerized averaging of the electrical activity generated by individual sensory stimuli repeated hundreds of times to generate an averaged evoked potential signal. In the visual domain, the stimulus now used most widely is that of a black and white chequer-board which is moved in front of the eyes. Each movement of the chequer-board is used to trigger the recording of electrical activity from the surface of the scalp over the occipital cortex. The average of a series of several hundred such responses is computed after stimulation of each eye separately. The latency of this visual evoked response can be measured to, say, the first major positive peak following

PVEP

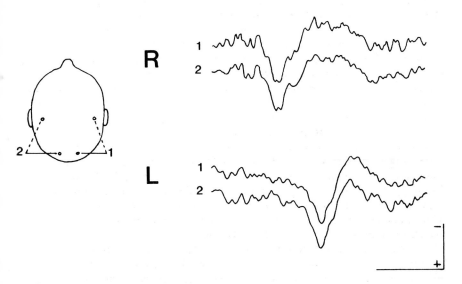

Fig. 1.3. Pattern visual evoked potential (PVEP). Patient with a left optic neuritis: visual acuity right 6/5, left 6/9. Traces (1) from right and (2) from left hemisphere. Upper pair of traces from right eye are normal showing a major positive component with a latency of 100 ms. Lower pair of traces from left eye showing gross delay with major positive component's latency 160 ms with preservation of amplitude. Calibration: amplitude 5 mv; latency 100 ms

the movement of the pattern, and the size of such a component of the visual evoked response can be recorded (Fig. 1.3). It has been found that demyelinating lesions of the optic nerve may reliably produce delays in such a visual evoked response, indicating the presence of an optic nerve lesion even in the absence of any clinical symptoms or signs of such damage. This technique now is widely used in the investigation of patients suspected of having multiple sclerosis. The method of evoking visual responses to pattern stimulation can be adapted for half-field or even quarter-field stimulation in patients suspected of hemianopic or other visual disturbances.

Similar principles underlie the use of auditory evoked potentials (BSAEP) to investigate the auditory pathways. The electrical activity recorded from the lateral surface of the scalp, usually in relation to the ear in response to a standard click stimulus delivered through headphones to one or other ear, is averaged for a few hundred responses (Fig. 1.4). The resulting auditory evoked response consists of a whole series of components, each one of which has been carefully established by neurophysiological experiment to arise from activity in different segments of the auditory pathway. Thus, cochlear activity can be

BSAEP

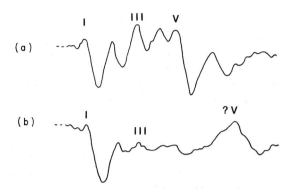

Fig. 1.4. Brainstem auditory evoked potential (BSAEP). **(a)** Normal trace: Wave I probably arises from the cochlear nerve, i.e. peripheral function; Wave III probably arises from the superior olive, i.e. in the lower pons; Wave V probably arises from the inferior colliculus, i.e. more centrally. **(b)** Patient with multiple sclerosis showing grossly increased central conduction and loss of waveform (note the different latencies from I–V **(a)** and **(b)**). Calibration: amplitude 0.3 mv; latency 2 ms

distinguished from that of a number of brainstem nuclei and fibre tracts, which can be distinguished from activity in the auditory cortex.

Averaged somatosensory evoked potentials (SSEP) can be recorded from electrodes placed over the sensory cortex in response to electrical stimulation of the contralateral digits or peripheral nerves of arms or legs.

The details of these various electrophysiological techniques are beyond the scope of this book and the techniques themselves are constantly being refined and developed at the present time. Specific abnormalities encountered in various neurological diseases will be mentioned where appropriate in later sections.

Electromyography (EMG) and nerve conduction studies

In the same way that electrical activity of the brain can be recorded by the electroencephalogram, the electrical activity of contracting muscles can be recorded either by surface electrodes or through needles inserted directly into the muscle itself. Surface recordings pick up and average the activity from many individual motor units, while needle recordings can detect the activity from single motor units or even from single muscle fibres if the recording surface is made small enough. Needle recordings of the electromyographic activity in weak muscles may be used to decide upon the cause of muscle weakness. Motor unit action potentials in primary muscle disease (myopathies) characteristically are reduced in size and shortened in duration. Spontaneous activity in the form of fibrillation potentials occurs in muscles denervated by damage to peripheral nerves, nerve roots, or anterior horn cells. Muscle action potentials become abnormally large due to collateral re-innervation in anterior horn cell disease. The normal picture of EMG activity that occurs on muscle contraction when recorded with needle electrodes (the interference pattern) is distorted in upper motor neurone disease in a manner distinctive from that seen in denervation or primary muscle disease. Single fibre recording may reveal instability of neuro-muscular transmission in a variety of conditions, but particularly in myasthenia gravis. In the latter condition, the muscle is incapable of responding to repetitive nerve stimulation, showing characteristic electrical and contractile fatigue.

The function of peripheral nerves may also be assessed by electrical techniques. Motor nerve conduction can be studied by stimulating a mixed nerve containing motor fibres, and recording the resulting compound action potential from the muscle activated by surface or needle electrodes. Motor nerve conduction velocity can be calculated by stimulating the motor nerve at two different sites proximally and distally, measuring the difference in latency to the onset of the muscle action potential, and the distance between the two sites of stimulation. Motor conduction through a particular region, e.g. in the ulnar nerve across the elbow, may be calculated by measuring conduction velocity in response to stimulating above and below the site of interest. Sensory nerve conduction can be studied by stimulating pure sensory nerves, such as those of the digits with ring electrodes, and recording the nerve action potential with surface or needle electrodes applied close to the appropriate nerve trunk. For sensory studies, it is usually necessary to average many responses to obtain a reproducible wave form. Sensory nerve conduction also may be measured by recording somatosensory cortical evoked potentials in response to stimulation of peripheral nerves at different proximal and distal sites, calculating the difference in latency and the distance between the two sites in the usual manner.

Most nerve conduction studies are undertaken on peripheral segments of nerves, and it is more difficult to study proximal nerve roots. However, certain electrical reflexes may be employed to investigate their function, including the H reflex which is elicited on stimulation of a mixed nerve with low intensity electrical shocks which selectively activate spindle afferent fibres to produce an electrical analogue of the tendon jerk. Likewise, the activity in proximal segments of motor nerves may be assessed by recording the F wave which results from retrograde stimulation of motor nerve fibres invading the anterior horn cell to produce a descending volley which is subsequently detected from the surface or needle electromyogram.

As in the case of evoked potential studies, electromyographic and nerve conduction investigations are continuously being refined and improved to add greater sensitivity and specificity. A recent example is the use of magnetic stimulation of the motor cortex through the scalp to study the corticomotorneurone pathway.

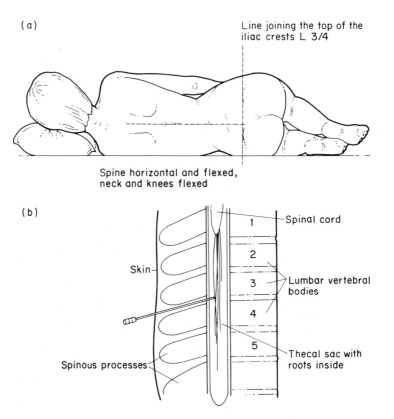

(a)

Line joining the top of the
iliac crests L 3/4

Spine horizontal and flexed,
neck and knees flexed

(b)

Skin—

Spinous processes

1 — Spinal cord

2

3 — Lumbar vertebral
bodies

4

5

Thecal sac with
roots inside

Fig. 1.5.   (a) Position of patient for lumbar puncture. (b) Diagram to show correctly
positioned needle within the subarachnoid space

Cerebrospinal fluid (CSF)

Samples of CSF may be obtained with relative ease at the bedside by lumbar
puncture. The technique requires some practice, but once mastered is simple
and usually painless. However, when there is an intracranial or intraspinal
mass lesion, lumbar puncture carries some risk of causing rapid deterioration in
function as a result of shifts of intracranial or intraspinal contents. Accordingly,
lumbar puncture is not an investigation to be considered if a patient is suspected
of harbouring an intracranial or intraspinal tumour. Lumbar puncture is also
contraindicated in the presence of local skin sepsis or breakdown in the lumbar
region. It is dangerous in patients with any intracranial tumour whether this is a
neoplasm or abscess as this may precipitate a pressure cone (p. 95). Lumbar
puncture is essential to the diagnosis of meningitis and subarachnoid
haemorrhage, and is a valuable adjunct to the diagnosis of a number of
inflammatory conditions such as multiple sclerosis or encephalitis.

For lumbar puncture the patient is best positioned lying on the side, flexed
and with the spine horizontal (Fig. 1.5). The needle is usually introduced at the
L3/4 interspace which is indicated by a line drawn joining the tips of the iliac
crests (Fig. 1.5). It is worth recalling in adults that the spinal cord usually ends
at the lower border of L1 so a needle inserted into the subarachnoid space below

this level will enter the sac containing the cauda equina floating in CSF. Local anaesthetic is used for the skin and immediate tissues. After allowing time for this to be effective, a sharp disposable fine lumbar puncture needle (22 gauge) with stilette in position is introduced through the skin and advanced through the space between the two spinous processes. The needle point usually needs to be directed slightly forwards (anteriorly). At a depth of about 4–7 cm more firm resistance may be encountered as the ligamentum flavum is reached. Beyond this there is a slight 'give' as the needle punctures the dura. The stilette is then removed and clear CSF will drip out of the needle if this has been correctly positioned. If no fluid appears or bone is encountered, it is probable that the needle is not in the correct place. The stilette should be re-inserted, the needle partially withdrawn and then advanced with a slightly different angle. The commonest causes of failure are that the needle is not in the midline, or is at too great an angle with the skin (Fig. 1.5).

The CSF findings characteristic of specific conditions will be discussed later in this book, but a few general principles will be mentioned now. It is crucial always to obtain the maximum information from examining the CSF (Table 1.1). If the presence of blood is suspected, three sequential tubes of CSF should be collected to establish whether the fluid is uniformly and consistently blood-stained, or whether the initial bloody CSF gradually clears as occurs as a result of a traumatic tap. Likewise, when haemorrhage is suspected, the sample should be centrifuged and the supernatant examined for the presence of xanthochromia which indicates pathological bleeding rather than the consequences of trauma at the time of lumbar puncture. If infection is suspected, the CSF sugar may be an invaluable guide to the presence of bacterial or fungal inflammation. However, the CSF glucose can only be interpreted in the light of the blood level obtained at the same time. Thus, bacterial or fungal meningitis is suggested if the CSF contains an excess of cells in the presence of a glucose concentration of 2 mmol/litre or less than 40 per cent of the blood glucose concentration. Bacterial infections will also raise the CSF lactate (greater than 3.3. mmol/litre). If there are red cells in significant numbers resulting from a traumatic tap, a rough guide suggests that about 10 white cells may be allowed for every 7000 red cells.

Specific abnormalities of CSF protein content may be invaluable in diagnosis, particularly the excess gamma globulin present in many patients with multiple sclerosis, who also commonly exhibit the presence of oligoclonal bands of gamma globulin on electrophoresis. Examination of CSF for specific bacteria or fungi, such as the tubercle bacillus or cryptococcus, or for malignant

Table 1.1 Normal cerebrospinal fluid (CSF) values

Clear colourless fluid	
Pressure	40–180 mm
Cells	0–5 lymphocytes/mm^3
Sugar	2.5–4.4 mmol/l (60% of blood glucose)
Lactate	Less than 2.8 mmol/l
Protein	0.2–0.5 g/l
IgG	Less than 14% of total protein (70% of serum globulin)
Volume (adult)	150 ml

cells requires considerable care and expertise. It will be apparent that thought must be taken before lumbar puncture as to what information is to be sought from the material obtained, and care must be exercised in ensuring that the samples are delivered to the appropriate laboratories and individuals. Finally, lumbar puncture provides an opportunity to record CSF pressure using simple manometry, which should be undertaken routinely.

Muscle and nerve biopsy

Muscle biopsy is undertaken routinely in most patients suspected of primary muscle disease, the sample being removed from a weak muscle that has not previously been subjected to electromyographic needling. Routine histology is supplemented nowadays by histochemistry to type muscle fibre populations, and by biochemical investigation of muscle energy metabolism. Muscle biopsy also gives the opportunity to examine small blood vessels in patients suspected of inflammatory diseases such as polyarteritis nodosa. In patients thought to have generalized giant cell arteritis, however, it is usual to biopsy the temporal artery directly.

Nerve biopsy is used less frequently, but it is simple and safe to remove the cutaneous branch of the sural nerve at the ankle, which leaves no motor deficit and only a slight insignificant patch of sensory loss. Examination of nerve biopsy in patients with peripheral nerve disease may reveal the evidence of arteritis, or of infiltration with substances such as amyloid. In addition, the spectrum of nerve fibres, their diameter and myelin content, may be quantified and compared with normal, and teased preparations may be examined for the presence of segmental or generalized demyelination.

Other investigations

Many other investigations are employed in individual patients with neurological disease. For instance, liver, rectal, or marrow biopsy may be required for diagnosis of a number of storage diseases causing progressive encephalopathy in childhood. Biopsy of skin, e.g. Kveim test, may help in the diagnosis of sarcoidosis. Occasionally, even biopsy of the brain itself is required to establish the diagnosis in progressive obscure cerebral disorders.

Many metabolic and hormonal diseases may affect the nervous system, so that the full range of examination of serum electrolytes, liver, renal and bone function may be required, as will tests of thyroid, parathyroid, pancreas, and pituitary function. Neurosyphilis, and now AIDS are the great mimics of neurological disorders so that serological tests such as a *Treponema pallidum* haemagglutination test (TPHA) and human immunodeficiency virus (HIV) titres are essential to exclude these disorders.

2

Symptoms of neurological disease

In this Chapter I will discuss the common symptoms with which patients with neurological disorders present in the clinic. The first step in unravelling the neurological problem is to decide on the basic category of disorder the patient is trying to describe. The discovery that the patient's complaint is one of headache, a black-out, difficulty in walking, or a disturbance in memory, immediately sets in train an established thought process that includes the likely differential diagnosis of the causes of such a complaint, and the questions necessary to ask at some stage in the interview to establish which diagnosis is likely to be correct. In other words, specific complaints act as triggers to the neurologist's diagnostic process, selecting programmes of enquiry and differential diagnosis for each complaint.

The commonest symptoms encountered in neurological practice are shown in Table 2.1. This is by no means exhaustive, but it does account for the majority of complaints encountered.

In addition to the patient's presenting complaint, it is important to obtain the answers to a series of routine questions, the purpose of which is to disclose the possibility of disease in other parts of the nervous system. A suitable range of ten routine neurological questions is:

1. Have you noticed any change in your mood, memory or powers of concentration?
2. Have you ever lost consciousness or had a fit or seizure?
3. Do you suffer unduly from headaches?
4. Have you noticed any change in your senses: i) smell, ii) taste, iii) sight, iv) hearing?
5. Do you have any difficulty in talking, chewing or swallowing?
6. Have you experienced any numbness, tightness, pins and needles, tingling or burning sensation in the face, limbs or trunk?
7. Have you noticed weakness, stiffness, heaviness or dragging of arms or legs?
8. Do you have any difficulty in using your hands for skilled tasks, such as writing, typing or dressing?
9. Do you have any unsteadiness or difficulty in walking?
10. Do you ever have any difficulty controlling your water-works or bowels?

Table 2.1   Common symptoms in neurological disorders

Pain
  Headache
  Facial pain
  Spinal pain – cervical, lumbar
  Limb pain – often accompanied by weakness and tingling
Loss of consciousness
  Epileptic seizures
  Syncope
Disturbances of the senses
  Visual upsets – impaired acuity, blurred, double vision
  Deafness
  Giddiness
  Impaired smell, taste
Motor
  Weakness
    limbs – often with pain and tingling
    bulbar muscles – swallowing, speech
    respiratory muscles – breathless
  Clumsiness – incoordination
  Ataxia – unsteady
  Tremor
  Involuntary movements
Sensory
  Loss of feeling – numbness
  Distorted – tingling, paraesthesiae, bizarre sensations, hyperaesthesiae
  Loss of position sense – sensory ataxia
Autonomic
  Disturbances of bowel, bladder, sexual function
  Faintness – postural hypotension
Disturbances of higher functions
  Memory impairment – dementia
  Confusion
  Changes in mood, behaviour
  Changes in speech – aphasia
  Disordered thinking – psychiatric

It is not our purpose here to describe in detail the individual diseases causing the various symptoms discussed. Rather, I will concentrate on the approach to the differential diagnosis of each symptom, and upon the practical management of such patients.

Headache

Headache is one of the commonest symptoms encountered in general practice, and certainly is the commonest complaint of patients attending the neurologist. It is estimated that approximately one in five of the general population may suffer from headache of sufficient severity to consult a doctor. The majority of these patients will have no abnormal physical signs on examination, and diagnosis depends entirely on the history. The most important distinction is how long the patient has suffered headache. The diagnosis and management of someone with the acute onset of their first severe headache is entirely different from that of someone who has suffered from chronic headache for a matter of many years.

Acute sudden headache

The sudden, acute onset of severe headache over a matter of minutes or hours often poses a medical emergency, for this may be the presenting symptom of intracranial haemorrhage or infection. Most patients with *subarachnoid haemorrhage* from aneurysm or angioma present with a sudden, dramatic, and explosive onset of devastating headache, which rapidly becomes generalized and is accompanied by neck stiffness. 'It was as if I had been kicked by a mule.' Many patients with subarachnoid haemorrhage lose consciousness and some may develop mild focal neurological signs. Patients with *primary intracerebral haemorrhage* often complain of headache and vomiting, and then rapidly lose consciousness. Commonly they are hypertensive. They also exhibit dense neurological deficit due to brain destruction, and often do not have a stiff neck. If subarachnoid haemorrhage is suspected, lumbar puncture or CT scan must be undertaken as soon as is convenient to establish the diagnosis. Patients who have bled from an intracranial aneurysm, which is the commonest cause of subarachnoid haemorrhage, are at serious risk of a second bleed in the next few weeks which often is lethal. Surgical clipping of the aneurysm can prevent rebleeding, so those in whom subarachnoid haemorrhage is confirmed by lumbar puncture or CT scan require referral to neurosurgical centres for further treatment.

The commonest condition which may be confused with subarachnoid haemorrhage is the acute onset of a *migraine* headache. Migraine usually builds up over a matter of some time, but on occasion may apparently start sufficiently abruptly to suggest a subarachnoid bleed. Such patients also may have mild neck stiffness and photophobia as part of their severe migraine, but examination of the cerebrospinal fluid reveals no blood.

The headache of *meningitis and encephalitis* does not start with dramatic suddeness, but builds up over a matter of some hours. Such patients also are likely to have fever and, in the case of meningitis, severe neck stiffness. In the case of encephalitis, neck stiffness is less conspicuous, but early coma and seizures are characteristic. Any patient suspected of meningitis or encephalitis requires lumbar puncture to establish the diagnosis and the cause.

Subacute headache

Headache that has been present for a few weeks or months in an individual not previously prone to this complaint must always be taken seriously. In fact, such a complaint usually turns out not to be sinister, but to be the beginning of a more chronic problem such as tension headache or migraine. However, the possibility of other, more serious, conditions should always be considered in those with the recent onset of disabling headache.

In the elderly patient, or in anyone aged over about 55 years, *cranial or giant cell arteritis* should be considered. Such patients are usually unwell with systemic symptoms of malaise, weight loss, and generalized aches and pains. Their main symptom, however, is persistent headache with tenderness of the scalp, as when brushing the hair. The cranial arteries, particularly the superficial temporal arteries, may be visibly enlarged, tortuous, and tender to the touch, and there may be obvious reddening of the overlying skin. Patients with giant cell arteritis are at risk of losing vision due to ischaemic damage to the optic nerves, so suspicion of the condition should lead to urgent action. The erythrocyte sedimentation rate (ESR) almost invariably is raised above 40 mm/h and a biopsy of the temporal artery is frequently diagnostic. Such patients should be urgently started on steroids to suppress further complications of the illness, particularly sudden visual loss.

The headache of *raised intracranial pressure*, of whatever cause be it tumour, subdural haematoma, or obstructive hydrocephalus, characteristically has been present for a matter of some weeks or months. Frequently it may wake the patient from sleep and is made much worse by coughing, sneezing, bending or straining at stool, all of which increase intracranial pressure. The headache of raised intracranial pressure may be accompanied by effortless vomiting. Frequently, papilloedema is evident on examination and there may be signs suggesting a focal intracranial mass lesion. However, patients with intracranial space-occupying lesions producing severe headache may not have papilloedema and may exhibit no focal neurological signs, yet the history may be sufficient to warrant further investigation. The majority of patients with isolated cough headache, or isolated headache at the peak of sexual excitement (orgasmic headache or coital cephalgia), do not have brain tumours. The mechanisms responsible for these benign conditions are not known.

Persistent headache after minor concussive head injuries is a common complaint, often accompanied by other symptoms such as postural dizziness, fatigue and depression. This *post-traumatic syndrome* is well-recognized in the law courts as one of the commonest sources of claims for compensation for injury. Once settlement occurs, which unfortunately may take many years, such symptoms frequently disappear. However, a true post-concussional syndrome, with all the symptoms mentioned, may occur in otherwise stable individuals in whom no thought of compensation exists. It is now apparent that minor head injuries may cause cerebral damage and, also, lesions of the vestibular system, which may be responsible for the persistent symptoms that occur in a proportion of patients in such circumstances.

Chronic headache

The commonest causes of chronic headache are migraine and tension headache. It is a useful working rule to realize that patients who have been complaining of headache for 3 years or more without any other sinister symptoms or physical signs on examination nearly always turn out to have one of these two conditions.

Migraine is exceedingly common and approximately 20 per cent of the population are likely to suffer one or more migrainous episodes in their life. Characteristic of migraine is that it is a periodic disorder, with episodes of headache separated by periods in which the subject is entirely normal. Classical migraine is instantly recognizable because of the presence of characteristic prodromal symptoms in the half hour or so prior to the onset of headache. The commonest of these are visual, in the form of the flashing lights or zig-zags due to ischaemia or spreading depression in the occipital cortex. Other prodromal symptoms of migraine are hemisensory disturbances, alarming dysphasia, and diplopia with dysarthria and ataxia. These prodromal symptoms of migraine may occur in the absence of subsequent headache. When headache does occur, it may be hemicranial, but more frequently it is generalized. During the period of headache, the patient feels ill, nauseated, anorectic, photophobic and drowsy. Frequently they vomit, following which the headache often subsides and the patient sleeps. The headache itself usually lasts several hours, but may persist for 2 or more days. Once the headache disappears, the patient soon returns to normal and remains so until a further episode occurs. Migraines usually appear at intervals of a few weeks or even months, and some luckier sufferers may experience only one or two attacks in their lifetime.

The intermittency of migraine contrasts with the persistent, continuous headache characteristic of *tension/muscle contraction headache*. Such patients complain that they are never free of pain, day in and day out for months or years. Nothing appears to help the pain which commonly is blamed for causing disturbance of sleep and depression. In fact, tension headache is a common symptom of an underlying depressive illness, the latter being responsible for early morning waking, loss of appetite, and malaise. In other patients, tension headache appears to be a symptom of long-standing anxiety states, often preci-pitated by marital discord, other family tensions, or job dissatisfaction. The patient usually describes tension headache as a constant aching or pressure sensation, which may be generalized or confined to the vertex or acting like a band around the head. Prodromal symptoms do not occur and vomiting is not a feature. The pain may be exacerbated, or may occur only at times of obvious stress, and few of us have not experienced the typical tightening sensation in the scalp when under considerable external pressure. In fact, tension headache is associated with excessive sustained contraction of the muscles of the scalp and neck.

Uncommon causes of headache

Typical tension headache frequently is blamed on other common conditions such as constipation, dental caries, hypertension, sinusitis, cervical spondylosis, and eye strain. Few of these conditions cause headache, and the majority of patients suffering from them do not complain of this symptom.

Headache does occur in patients with malignant hypertension, or during paroxysmal hypertension provoked by phaeochromocytoma, but is not a symptom of lesser degrees of high blood pressure. Constipation never causes headache, and dental caries-causes pain in the face rather than in the head. There is no doubt that straining to read with defective vision in a poor light may cause muscle contraction headache, eased by appropriate prescription of spectacles, but such patients are aware of the cause of their head pain. Acute sinusitis undoubtedly causes intense pain and local tenderness over the affected sinus, made worse by lying flat, coughing or sneezing. In contrast, chronic sinusitis is not a cause of headache, unless there is intermittent obstruction to drainage from the affected sinus, which then causes the typical features of acute sinus disturbance. Cervical spondylosis causes pain in the neck, which may radiate up to the occiput, and typically is made worse by neck movement. A rare cause of occipital pain, accompanied by paraesthesiae in the side of the tongue, is sudden trapping of the upper cervical roots on neck movement.

Pain in the face

As in headache, patients complaining of pain in the face frequently exhibit no neurological signs and the diagnosis must be made solely on the history. When confronted with a patient complaining of pain in the face, it is useful to keep in mind that this may arise from local structures such as eyes, sinuses, teeth or jaw; referred pain due to fifth nerve involvement, in which case there are likely to be signs of sensory loss in trigeminal territory; and disorders with no abnormal physical signs such as trigeminal neuralgia, post-herpetic neuralgia, migrainous neuralgia, migraine variant (lower-half headache), and atypical facial pain.

Local causes

Disease of teeth, sinuses, the parotid glands, and the eyes can, of course, cause pain in the face, but nearly always also cause obvious symptoms due to damage to these structures. Pain due to dental caries is precipitated by extremes of temperature and sweets, as is familiar to everyone. A dental abscess causes throbbing pain and marked local tenderness, particularly to percussion of the affected tooth. Acute maxillary sinusitis causes a severe, explosive, throbbing pain in the cheek, increased by lying flat, coughing or sneezing, and accompanied by considerable local tenderness. Eye disease, such as acute glaucoma or iritis, causes intense local pain and tenderness in the affected eye, with disturbance of vision and evident reddening of the eye itself. Salivary calculi cause pain in the appropriate salivary gland on eating or anticipation of good food. Arthritis involving the temporomandibular joint may cause pain in the face and neck, provoked by chewing or opening of the mouth. Pain on chewing also may occur in giant cell arteritis, due to claudication in ischaemic jaw muscles.

Referred pain

Pain referred into the face may be provoked by compression or infiltration of the trigeminal nerve by posterior fossa tumours, tumours invading the base of the skull, or extracranial tumours involving the sinuses or salivary glands. Such referred pain typically is constant, sometimes with superimposed spontaneous jabs of discomfort, and is accompanied by signs of sensory loss in the distribution of the affected nerves. The acute onset of pain in the forehead and eye, associated with a third nerve palsy involving the pupil, is a not uncommon presentation of an aneurysm of the internal carotid at the origin of the posterior communicating artery. Acute third nerve palsies due to arteritis or vascular disease in hypertension and diabetes mellitus also may cause pain in and around the eye.

Facial pain with no signs

Trigeminal neuralgia is a common cause of intermittent pain in the face in the second half of life. Pain, which is unilateral, is usually confined to the second or third division of the fifth nerve, and possesses two absolute characteristics. First, the individual spasms of pain are extremely brief, like a knife jabbing into the cheek or jaw. Second, these spasms are triggered by at least two of the following events: talking, eating, washing the face, brushing the teeth, blowing the nose, touching the face, cold wind on the face, or attempting to put on make-up. The paroxysm triggered by these stimuli lasts a few seconds to several minutes, during which time the patient may clutch the side of the face in agony. Commonly, the pain shoots from a characteristic site of onset, in the cheek or side of the nose or gums, to another part of the face, e.g. to the ear or jaw. The illness characteristically is intermittent with bouts lasting days or weeks, followed by long periods of freedom which tend to become shorter as the patient ages.

Glossopharyngeal neuralgia is analogous to trigeminal neuralgia in that the pain is paroxysmal and extremely severe. It is felt in the back of the throat or tongue, or deep in the ear, and is triggered by swallowing.

The ophthalmic division of the trigeminal nerve is a common site for involvement by herpes zoster, and a proportion of such patients, usually the elderly, are left with the distressing aftermath of *post-herpetic neuralgia*. Such pain is felt in the eye and forehead, where typical scarring and sensory loss is evident. The pain is continuous and often has a burning quality, superimposed on which are occasional jabs of pain which may be triggered by light touch to the affected area.

Some patients with otherwise typical migraine may also experience pain of similar calibre and character in the face (facial migraine). As with migraine headache, the pain lasts for a few hours to a day or so, is often accompanied by nausea, vomiting and prostration, and is intermittent leaving the patient normal between attacks. A variant of migraine, *migrainous neuralgia*, produces a different history. The sufferer is usually a young man who, during a bout, is attacked regularly at the same time of day or night by the onset of a continuous pain in one eye, building up over a matter of an hour or so to a maximum and lasting then for a period of a few hours. At the height of the pain, the eye frequently reddens and waters, the nostril may become blocked and the eyelid may droop. Such pain occurs daily for a matter of some weeks and then disappears for long periods until another bout starts. These features of migrainous neuralgia are quite different from those of migraine, but the condition may respond to prophylactic ergot treatment. A similar continuous pain in the eye accompanied by a progressive ptosis rarely may be due to a structural lesion, sometimes malignant, or granulomatous, at the base of the skull involving the paratrigeminal region (Raeder's neuralgia).

Finally, there is a collection of patients complaining of pain in the face whose description accords with none of the entities outlined above, and who have no abnormal physical signs on examination. Such patients are said to suffer *atypical facial pain*. Most complain of a continuous pain in the face unrelieved by any medication and present unaltered for months or years. These features have much in common with those of tension headache, and a proportion of those with atypical facial pain also have clinical symptoms of depressive illness, including sleep disturbance, diurnal mood fluctuation, anorexia and weight loss. Others, however, are not depressed, although they may exhibit a long-standing anxiety state. Frequently, the intensity of their atypical facial pain is related to the stresses of everyday living, in the same way as occurs in patients with tension headache. This latter group of patients are sometimes said to suffer psychogenic facial pain.

Blackouts, fits and faints

Patients commonly use the word blackout to describe loss of consciousness, when it really means loss of vision. In a faint, due to a drop in systemic blood pressure, vision goes black before consciousness is lost; the retinal circulation is also compressed by intraocular pressure, so fails before that to the brain. The reverse, a red-out, sometimes happens to fighter pilots in supersonic aircraft who take corners too tightly, causing blood to be thrown into the eyes.

The doctor rarely has the opportunity to be present when a patient has an attack of loss of consciousness, and the diagnosis nearly always has to be established on the basis of the history. Naturally, if the patient passes out with no warning whatsoever, they will be unaware of the circumstances or what happened during the attack. Accordingly, a description of events from an independent witness is absolutely essential in coming to the correct conclusion about the cause of many such episodes. The circumstances in which the attack occurred must be determined, and details of exactly what happened during the attack, and afterwards, must be obtained. Eye-witnesses often describe what they think they saw, e.g. by concluding that the patient had a fit, but are not trained to distinguish between epilepsy and hysteria.

Epilepsy

The majority of patients presenting with sudden, unexplained episodes of loss of consciousness will turn out to have epilepsy, but many other causes can provoke such events. Epilepsy itself takes many forms, some of which do not cause loss of consciousness. *Focal or partial epileptic seizures* arising in one temporal lobe, or in some other cortical area, may not cause unconsciousness until the abnormal seizure discharge propagates to involve both hemispheres to become generalized. Then the patient will go into a typical *grand mal seizure*. Such a major seizure consists of a period of tonic muscle contraction, during which the subject becomes anoxic, followed by repetitive generalized whole body jerking in the clonic phase. The whole event lasts less than about 5 min, when the subject stops fitting and either drifts into sleep or recovers.

If such grand mal fits are due to secondary generalization from some primary focal cortical source, then they may be prefaced by an aura the patient remembers. The aura is appropriate to the focal source of the seizure, e.g. a discharge arising in the sensorimotor cortex will provoke contralateral motor and sensory phenomena for a short period prior to the loss of consciousness and the commencement of the generalized fit. Details of the characteristics of focal or partial seizures occurring in different parts of the cerebral cortex will be found in Chapter 11. However, many patients with idiopathic epilepsy develop major grand mal seizures without any focal onset or aura. They are said to have primary generalized epilepsy of grand mal type.

Another form of epilepsy that causes temporary loss of consciousness, occurring in children, is also a form of primary generalized seizure discharge causing a brief absence attack, called *petit mal*. For a few seconds or so, the child ceases to speak or move, appears stunned with open flickering eyes, and then rapidly recovers back to normal. Similar absence attacks also may occur during brief focal seizures arising in temporal lobe structures, often accompanied by purposeless movements of chewing or fumbling with clothing. Such temporal lobe attacks frequently are accompanied by highly complex distortions of thought, sensation and emotion to produce a typical psychomotor seizure (*complex partial seizures*).

Sometimes, following grand mal seizures, particularly those due to generalization from temporal lobe foci, the patient may enter into a period of automatic behaviour for up to about an hour or so. During this phase of *post-epileptic automatism*, the patient may undertake relatively coordinated action, for which they subsequently have no memory (amnesia). In such a state, the epileptic patient may travel long distances and arrive at a destination with no idea as to how he got there.

The criteria that contribute to a confident diagnosis of epilepsy are:

1. The sudden, unexpected onset in an otherwise apparently healthy individual of a brief period of loss of consciousness not exceeding 5 min.
2. The episode of loss of consciousness may be prefaced by a characteristic aura in which the same events occur in every attack.
3. If the seizure is of grand mal type, witnesses will say that the patient fell, went stiff and blue, and shook. The patients may find afterwards that they have injured themselves, bitten their tongue, or been incontinent.
4. If it was an absence seizure, due either to petit mal or temporal lobe epilepsy, witnesses will remark that the patient suddenly lost contact with the world and was inaccessible for a short period, during which they may have undertaken simple crude motor automatisms.
5. The attacks are always brief (unless the patient goes into repeated attacks as in status epilepticus), and the patient returns to normal between the episodes.

Finally, it should be noted that many patients complaining of 'blackouts' may be suspected of suffering from epilepsy, but the evidence initially is insufficient to be certain of that diagnosis. As already has been stated, the electroencephalogram cannot be used to establish a certain diagnosis of epilepsy. In this situation, it is usually best to avoid any firm diagnosis and to await subsequent events. To label someone as an epileptic on insufficient evidence may be catastrophic for the patient's livelihood and there is little risk in seeing what happens.

If the patient's attack of loss of consciousness is confidently diagnosed as due to epilepsy, the next stage is to determine its cause.

A simple but important principle is that the aetiology of epilepsy changes with age. Epilepsy in the infant indicates some serious metabolic or structural cause. Epilepsy in the child usually is of unknown cause (idiopathic) or due to some static cerebral pathology, such as that produced by birth injury or head trauma. Epilepsy beginning in the younger adult often is the first sign of a cerebral tumour. Epilepsy commencing for the first time in the elderly frequently is due to vascular or other degenerative disease. A second useful simple principle is that focal epilepsy commonly is due to some identifiable structural lesion, while primary generalized grand mal or petit mal frequently appears idiopathic in origin. These principles guide the subsequent management of the patient whose episodes of loss of consciousness are diagnosed as being due to epilepsy, which is discussed in greater detail in Chapter 11.

Epilepsy must be distinguished from other causes of loss of consciousness, in particular from fainting (syncope), sleep attacks of narcolepsy, hypoglycaemia, cerebrovascular disease, and psychogenic illness.

Syncope

Syncope is defined as transient loss of consciousness caused by an acute decrease in cerebral blood flow. Fainting provoked by the sight of blood, needles, prolonged standing in church or on parade, or intense emotion and pain (*reflex or vasovagal syncope*) is commonplace. The term vasovagal indicates two components of reflex fainting, vagal slowing of the heart and peripheral vasodilatation. Such patients 'come over queer', feel dizzy and swimmy, their eyesight dims and hearing recedes, their face goes pale, and they slump forward or fall to the ground. Provided they are laid flat, consciousness soon returns, although the patient feels sick and breaks out into a heavy sweat.

This sequence of events is precipitated by a profound drop in systemic systolic blood pressure, below about 60 mmHg, due to a combination of sudden bradycardia and peripheral vasodilatation in skeletal muscle and internal organs. A similar sequence of events may be triggered by straining to pass water in elderly men with prostatic problems (*micturition syncope*), or pressure over the cartoid bifurcation in the occasional patient with excessive sensitivity of the carotid sinus (*carotid sinus syndrome*). Repeated coughing in those with chronic lung disease also may provoke fainting by causing obstruction of venous return to the heart (*cough syncope*). A similar mechanism is responsible for syncope during trumpet playing and weight-lifting.

Another cause of fainting is damage to peripheral or central autonomic pathways (*areflexic or paralytic syncope*). In this situation, patients faint when they stand upright, because they are unable to adjust heart rate and the resistance of peripheral blood vessels to cope with the rapid shift of blood to the legs and viscera that occurs when suddenly standing up. Such postural syncope occurs in any type of peripheral neuropathy affecting the autonomic system, but particularly in those with diabetes. In addition, drugs such as hypotensive agents, alcohol, barbiturates and phenothiazines may all interfere with the operation of normal baroreceptor reflexes to cause postural faintness. Ageing itself leads to some loss of efficiency of baroreceptor reflexes, and many elderly patients experience transient dizziness on rising quickly from bed or a chair. Such patients are particularly sensitive to relative small doses of hypotensive agents.

Fainting due to cardiac disease (*cardiac syncope*) is also relatively common in the elderly. Symptoms typical of a faint may occur in those with cardiac dysrhythmias, aortic stenosis or congenital heart disease. However, many patients with heart block lose consciousness abruptly (*Stokes-Adams attack*) probably as a result of cardiac arrest.

In general, a careful history will distinguish syncope from epilepsy, but a complication arises if failure of cerebral perfusion during a syncopal attack persists for longer than a minute, for in these circumstances the patient who faints may go on to have a fit. This situation may occur if someone faints in a position where they are unable to lie with the head below the heart, as may happen on the stairs or in the lavatory; if unconsciousness lasts longer than 20 s convulsive features may occur. In addition, if the bladder is full during a faint incontinence may occur.

Other causes of episodic loss of consciousness

Other conditions that may be confused with epilepsy, or with syncope, are much less common. *Spontaneous hypoglycaemia* certainly can lead to loss of consciousness and many patients with this condition do not recall the premonitory symptoms of anxiety, palpitations and sweating. The only definitive way of making the diagnosis is to obtain a blood sugar estimation during an attack: a value of < 2 mmol/litre is diagnostic. Any patient found unconscious for no apparent reason must have blood withdrawn for estimation of sugar content, and 50 g of glucose should be given intravenously; it can do no harm but may save life. Fortunately, spontaneous hypoglycaemia (which usually is due to an islet cell pancreatic tumour) is rare, but should be considered in any patient with episodes of altered behaviour or loss of consciousness for which there is no other ready explanation.

Cerebrovascular disease also can cause episodic loss of consciousness without other obvious neurological symptoms, particularly when transient ischaemia occurs in the distribution of the vertebrobasilar arterial system. However, such patients usually suffer other symptoms such as diplopia, dysarthria and ataxia, indicating brainstem ischaemia. Some patients with cerebrovascular disease affecting the posterior cerebral arterial territory, which supplies the medial portions of the cerebral hemispheres, may experience prolonged periods of loss of awareness. Such *transient global amnesia* may last minutes to hours. During such an episode the patients are disorientated, unable to recall what they are doing, where they are; or when it is, but can undertake simple automatic tasks, such as washing, dressing, or cooking. Subsequently they have no memory for the event, i.e. they are amnesic. Likewise, patients with *migraine* in whom there is profound ischaemia in the vertebrobasilar territory (basilar artery migraine) occasionally may also complain of episodes of loss of awareness for up to 30 min although they too usually describe other symptoms of brainstem ischaemia and severe occipital headache. Patients with intense *vertigo* also may complain of loss of consciousness. The diagnosis of vertigo will be considered in a later chapter, but it should be noted here that some patients with epilepsy have a vertiginous aura to their epileptic seizure, while other patients with intense vertigo due to labyrinthine disease may complain of loss of consciousness at the height of an attack. The sleep attacks characteristic of *narcolepsy* should not be confused with either epilepsy or syncope. Such sufferers describe lapsing into otherwise typical sleep, from which they can be awoken, at quite inappropriate moments.

Occasionally, patients with *obstructive hydrocephalus* may suddenly lose consciousness, often at the height of a bout of severe headache. *Head injuries* sometimes may present with a complaint of loss of consciousness, if the blow was unexpected and there is residual amnesia for the events surrounding the incident.

Prolonged overbreathing, *hyperventilation*, may produce a respiratory alkalosis with symptoms of paroxysmal tingling in the extremities and around the mouth. These are usually accompanied by giddiness, and rarely loss of consciousness. If the attack persists, carpopedal spasm and muscular twitching may appear. A proportion of these patients complain of headache and visual upset. Many are young women and a trial with overbreathing may provoke similar symptoms.

Finally, it will rapidly become apparent to the student attending neurological outpatients that many patients complaining of blackouts cannot be easily allocated to one of the diagnostic categories described above. Frequently this is because there is insufficient information on the circumstances of the attack, particularly if a witness is not available. However, many of these patients describe attacks of altered awareness occurring in relation to *emotional provocation*. As usual, marital discord, family tensions, job dissatisfaction, and other such stresses may provoke acute episodes of phobic anxiety in which the subject is distraught, breathless, and incoherent, a state of affairs for which they claim subsequent amnesia. Often it is obvious that such patients have an underlying severe anxiety state, and careful enquiry may unearth the usual precipitating circumstances. Other patients may actually feign epileptic attacks or faints to attract attention. Such patients, frequently adolescent females, exhibit other hysterical features and careful enquiry into the circumstances and character of their attack will indicate their hysterical origin. Unfortunately, some such individuals who also suffer from epilepsy may be prone to hysterical attacks as well (hystero-epilepsy). In such individuals, it may take prolonged observation and careful searching through every facet of the history to establish the true situation. As a general principle, it is best not to commit oneself to a certain diagnosis in those with bizarre attacks of uncertain origin.

Loss of vision

The patient complaining of disturbance of vision either may have disease of the eye, or may have damage to the optic nerve or posterior parts of the visual pathways. Local eye disease is common, and it is necessary to exclude refractive error, corneal damage, cataract, glaucoma, and obvious retinal lesions by appropriate ophthalmological techniques. These will not be considered in detail here, but most refractive errors are due to short-sightedness (myopia), which can be corrected with a pin-hole. This simple test should be employed in all complaining of visual loss, before considering other causes. A neurological cause of visual failure can only be assumed if vision cannot be improved to normal by correction of refractive error, the ocular media are clear, and there is no gross retinal abnormality.

Visual sensitivity or acuity depends upon intact central or macular vision. Lesions of the optic nerve cause loss of central macular vision (scotoma) and reduced visual acuity. However, lesions placed further back in the visual pathways, in the optic chiasm or radiations, or in the occipital cortex, only produce loss of vision in one half of the visual field (hemianopia) (*see* later). Visual acuity is normal in patients with such posteriorly placed lesions because, although they have lost vision in the opposite half-field, the remaining intact half of central macular vision is sufficient to preserve normal visual acuity. As a consequence, patients with visual failure due to anteriorly placed lesions of the optic nerve complain of loss of visual sensitivity of perception of detail of distant objects or of reading print, and can be demonstrated to have reduced visual acuity, which cannot be improved by correcting refractive error. In contrast, patients with posteriorly placed visual pathway damage complain of difficulty in perceiving objects in the affected opposite field of vision, but retain sensitivity in the remaining intact visual field so that they can still make out detail and read print, and show a normal visual acuity on formal testing. Patients with posteriorly placed lesions do complain of difficulties with reading, but they are of a different character. Those with loss of the right half of vision have difficulty seeing the next word in a sentence, while those with loss of the left half of vision have difficulty in moving from one line to the next. The significance of such hemianopic field defects will be discussed later. Here I will consider the problem of visual failure due to reduced visual acuity that cannot be attributed to local disease of the eye.

The most valuable aid in distinguishing different causes of neurological visual failure is the tempo of the illness. Visual deficit may be: present from early life and static (amblyopia); sudden and transient; sudden but persistent; or progressive. Usually it is possible to distinguish between these patterns of visual loss, but one problem is that of the patient who discovers visual impairment in one eye accidentally when rubbing the other, whereupon the onset is thought to be acute. In fact, many patients with progressive unilateral visual failure are not aware of their problem until, for some reason or another, they occlude vision of the opposite intact eye.

Amblyopia

Ocular deficits in early life, particularly muscle imbalance, cause suppression of visual acuity in one eye to prevent continuing double vision. Such visual suppression is known as amblyopia, which is not progressive after about 6–8 years of age, and which does not affect perception of colour or pupillary responses. Amblyopia as a cause of reduced visual acuity is suggested by visual loss since early childhood, evidence of a squint, or obvious refractive error.

Sudden transient visual loss

Sudden, but temporary loss of vision occurs in a number of circumstances. *Obscurations* of vision, due to raised intracranial pressure, consist of episodic visual loss affecting one or both eyes and lasting for a few seconds to one-quarter of a minute. Obscurations may be provoked by any manoeuvre that increases intracranial pressure, such as straining, coughing, sneezing, or bending. Examination will reveal swollen optic discs and further investigation and treatment are a matter of some urgency, for obscurations threaten impending permanent visual loss. *Amaurosis fugax* refers to episodic unilateral visual loss due to vascular disturbance in ophthalmic artery territory. The patient commonly describes a curtain ascending or descending to occlude the lower or upper half of vision, due to involvement of the superior or inferior branches of the ophthalmic artery. Such episodes may last for minutes to hours, but sooner or later the curtain gradually disappears and vision returns to normal. Amaurosis fugax thus is a transient ischaemic attack in ophthalmic artery distribution and, in the middle-aged or elderly subject, is likely to indicate the existence of cerebrovascular disease. *Uhthoff's phenomenon* describes dimness or loss of vision provoked by a rise in body temperature, such as occurs when taking a hot bath or on vigorous physical exercise, and is a feature of optic nerve demyelination produced by multiple sclerosis.

Sudden persistent visual loss

Sudden persistent visual loss is nearly always a result either of *acute optic neuritis* (most commonly due to multiple sclerosis) in the younger subject, or a vascular cause (*ischaemic optic neuropathy*) in the middle-aged or elderly. Occasionally a tumour or cyst compressing the optic nerve expands suddenly to cause abrupt visual failure.

Progressive visual loss

In the absence of any ocular pathology, a history of progressive loss of vision in one or both eyes must be taken to suggest compression of the anterior optic pathways until proven otherwise by appropriate investigations. Many such compressive lesions turn out to be *benign tumours*, such as pituitary adenomas or suprasellar meningiomas, which can be surgically removed with restoration of sight. *Toxic damage* to the optic nerve by drugs and alcohol/tobacco, and *hereditary optic neuropathies*, are less common than compressive lesions, which always must be excluded in a patient with progressive visual failure.

In practice, patients complaining of visual loss must be assessed by an ophthalmologist and, if the eyes are found to be normal, by a neurologist. Acute loss of vision must be treated as an emergency, and progressive loss of vision must always be investigated fully to establish the cause.

Giddiness

Patients use the words 'giddiness', 'dizziness', 'light-headedness' and 'unsteadiness' to describe a great variety of sensations due to many causes. Thus, the patient with postural syncope will say that he goes giddy when standing up, while the patient with cerebellar ataxia of gait may say that he is dizzy and unsteady. Vertigo refers to a sensation of unsteadiness or disequilibrium that is felt in the head. The patient with a cerebellar ataxia knows that he is unsteady when he tries to walk, but the sensation of disequilibrium is not felt in the head so it is not vertigo.

The sensation of vertigo is one of disequilibrium whatever its nature; it may be a sensation of rotation, a sensation of falling, a sensation as if on a pitching boat moving up and down, or a sensation of swaying. All are sensations of disequilibrium which, if felt in the head, may be described as vertiginous. Defined thus, vertigo implies a defect in function of the vestibular system, either of the labyrinthine end-organ or of its central connections, particularly those in the brainstem. Thus, vertigo commonly arises from damage to the ear, the vestibular nerve or brainstem. Lesions of the cerebral hemispheres rarely cause vertigo, although it may form an uncommon symptom in occasional patients with temporal lobe epilepsy.

The first step in diagnosis of a patient with vertigo is to decide whether the cause lies *peripherally in the labyrinthine mechanisms*, or *centrally in the brainstem*. Peripheral lesions causing vertigo also commonly cause intense nausea, vomiting, sweating and prostration. Because of the proximity of auditory to vestibular fibres in the VIIIth cranial nerve, deafness often accompanies vertigo. Conductive deafness due to middle ear disease suggests a peripheral lesion, but perceptive deafness, due to damage to the cochlear end-organ or vestibular nerve may be due to peripheral or central lesions. If peripheral, perceptive deafness is often less severe with loud sounds (loudness recruitment), and also causes severe speech distortion. Central lesions of the VIIIth nerve rarely show loudness recruitment, but exhibit auditory fatigue in that the intensity of sound has to be increased progressively to maintain the constant noise level. Vertigo due to vestibular damage is also often accompanied by evidence of nystagmus on examination, which consists of to-and-fro movements of the eyes due to interrupted visual fixation. Different types of nystagmus will be described later. Suffice to say here that peripheral vestibular lesions causing vertigo are usually accompanied by horizontal jerk nystagmus in one direction which gets worse with loss of visual fixation, while central lesions produce nystagmus that changes direction depending upon the patient's gaze and which often is rotatory and vertical as well as horizontal.

The differential diagnosis of the cause of vertigo is aided by considering the time course of the symptoms. Some diseases produce an acute single episode of vertigo, others produce recurrent attacks (and, of course, any single episode may be the first of such attacks), while others produce persistent disequilibrium.

Acute single attack of vertigo

An acute episode of vertigo may be provoked by sudden loss of unilateral labyrinthine function, or by sudden brainstem damage. Either may cause the sudden onset of acute severe vertigo, nausea, vomiting, and great distress because the patient is unable to move without provoking further severe vertigo. The patient will lie with the affected ear uppermost. The acute episode commonly lasts a matter of some days and then gradually recovers because adaptation to vestibular failure occurs. During the recovery phase, which may last 3 or 4 weeks, any sudden head movement may cause brief vertigo and unsteadiness. Acute vestibular failure due to sudden unilateral labyrinthine damage may develop in the course of *middle ear disease* when infection gains access to the labyrinth. Such a course of events must be treated as an emergency. If the middle ear is normal, acute peripheral vestibular failure may be attributed to virus infection (*vestibular neuronitis*) or to *ischaemia* in the distribution of the internal auditory arteries. However, in many such cases, the cause is uncertain. *Acute brainsteam lesions* that may provoke an attack of vertigo include a plaque of demyelination due to multiple sclerosis, or a vascular lesion such as infarction or haemorrhage of the brainstem.

Recurrent attacks of vertigo

If the patient describes repeated attacks of acute vertigo with recovery between episodes, they may be suffering from peripheral vestibular disease such as *Ménière's syndrome*, or from repeated *brainstem ischaemia*. The latter occurs as basilar artery migraine in the younger subject, or as vertebrobasilar transient ischaemic attacks in the middle-aged and elderly. Very rarely such recurrent episodes of vertigo may indicate *epilepsy*. Other patients may describe recurrent fleeting episodes of vertigo provoked by some critical position. This is usually most striking when lying down at night, or when moving the head suddenly. Such positional vertigo may be due to damage peripherally to the utricle (*benign positional vertigo*) as occurs quite frequently after trauma to the head, or occasionally may be due to brainstem disturbance.

Persistent vertigo

Chronic persistent vertigo actually is uncommon, due to the rapid compensation that occurs for vestibular deficits. Those patients complaining of persistent dizziness are not really describing vertigo proper, but are drawing attention to minor degrees of true instability or a sense of insecurity. However, drug damage to the vestibular nerves, brainstem demyelination or infarction, and occasionally posterior fossa tumours, all may cause mild persistent vertigo.

Pain in the arm

The painful, tingling or weak arm

Acute pain in the arm, of course, is most commonly caused by trauma or local disease of muscle, joint or bone. Only after these are excluded can neurological causes be considered. Damage to the peripheral nerves, brachial plexus, or cervical roots causes sensory disturbance and muscle wasting with weakness in a characteristic distribution, which must be learnt (*see* later) in order to diagnose the site of damage to these structures. Pain due to lesions of peripheral nerves, plexus, or spinal roots, however, often does not follow exact anatomical distribution. For example, pain due to compression of the median nerve at the wrist (carpal tunnel syndrome) often spreads up to the elbow or even to the shoulder. The pain due to damage to a spinal root is felt in the myotome and not in the dermatome, e.g. a lesion of C7 causes pain in the triceps, forearm extensors, and pectoralis, while paraesthesiae occur in the middle finger. Pain in the arm also may be felt occasionally by patients with cerebral disease. For example, pain and clumsiness in one arm may be the first signs of Parkinson's disease.

Paraesthesiae, which describes positive sensory symptoms such as pins and needles or tingling, may be due to damage to peripheral sensory neurones from the peripheral nerve itself to the spinal root, or due to lesions of the central sensory pathways in spinal cord, brainstem or internal capsule. Cortical lesions generally do not produce positive paraesthesiae. Sensory disturbances, whether paraesthesiae or sensory loss, are often difficult to put into words, and terms such as pins and needles, tingling, numbness, stiffness, constriction, wrapped in bandages, or like going to the dentist, all may be used to describe sensory deficit.

Weakness of the arm may be due to primary muscle diseases (rarely), lesions of peripheral nerves, brachial plexus or cervical roots, or to damage to central motor pathways. The latter causes the signs typical of upper motor neurone lesions (weakness without wasting, spasticity, and enhanced tendon reflexes). Lesions of peripheral nerves, plexus or roots cause the signs of a lower motor neurone lesion (weakness with wasting, normal or diminished tone, reduced or absent tendon reflexes).

Acute pain in the arm

Acute disease of the shoulder joints or adjacent structures is a common cause of pain in the arm. A variety of conditions is responsible for the clinical syndrome of *'frozen shoulder'* which causes acute severe pain, restriction of joint movement, and later wasting of the surrounding shoulder muscles. The frozen shoulder sometimes is accompanied by a curious sympathetic disturbance of the hand, which becomes swollen, painful, shiny and weak, for reasons that are not understood. This shoulder–hand syndrome occurs in some patients with a hemiplegia due to stroke and, occasionally, after myocardial infarction.

Primary muscle disease confined to the arm is very unusual, but giant cell arteritis may affect the muscles around the shoulder girdles to cause the syndrome of *polymyalgia rheumatica*. This illness affects middle-aged or elderly patients who develop increasing pain and stiffness symmetrically in the muscles of both shoulder girdles, which become tender to palpation and painful to move. The ESR is high, as in cranial arteritis which may coexist in a few patients with polymyalgia rheumatica.

Neuralgic amyotrophy is another mysterious condition which presents as acute, very severe pain affecting one upper limb and shoulder girdle, and accompanied by subsequent rapid wasting of the muscles of the arm, usually of those around the shoulder. Sensory disturbance is minimal, but there often is a patch of altered sensation over the deltoid corresponding to the circumflex nerve distribution.

A *cervical disc prolapse* may present with acute pain and stiffness of the neck, with referred pain in the distribution of the cervical root involved, usually C5, 6 or 7. In addition, there may be paraesthesiae and weakness of the arm in the distribution of the affected nerve root. The neck is fixed or extremely painful to move and coughing and sneezing also frequently provoke impulse pain referred into the arm.

Herpes zoster may cause pain in the arm, even before the appearance of the characteristic skin rash, if the cervical roots are affected.

The acute pain of neuralgic amyotrophy, cervical disc prolapse, and herpes zoster usually resolves in a matter of weeks or months.

Chronic pain in the arm

A number of entrapment neuropathies affecting peripheral nerves in the arm are common causes of chronic pain.

The *carpal tunnel syndrome* is by far the commonest cause of chronic arm pain, particularly in women. A complaint of pain at night accompanied by paraesthesiae in the fingers, particularly the thumb and index finger, relieved by flapping the hands or hanging them out of bed is quite characteristic. Signs often are minimal. Occasionally, the carpal tunnel syndrome may occur in patients with acromegaly, myxoedema or rheumatoid arthritis.

In men, it is usually the *ulnar nerve* that is affected, particularly at the elbow. Previous damage to the elbow joint causing osteoarthritis, or entrapment of the ulnar nerve in the cubital tunnel cause local pain, paraesthesiae in the little and ring fingers, and weakness and wasting of the muscles of the hand.

The *lower cord of the brachial plexus* may be compressed by a cervical rib, or infiltrated by malignant disease extending from an apical lung carcinoma (Pancoast's syndrome), or by local spread from breast carcinoma. Such lesions cause pain referred down the inner side of the arm, paraesthesiae on the medial aspect of the forearm, and weakness of the small muscles of the hand. Cervical ribs compressing the brachial plexus often may compress the subclavian artery to cause vascular disturbances in the arm.

Cervical spondylosis, degenerative disease of the cervical spine, is very common with advancing years and sometimes causes chronic pain in the arm, accompanied by paraesthesiae and weakness in the distribution of affected root or roots. Such chronic pain may follow acute cervical disc protrusions or, more commonly, may be due to compression of cervical roots by osteophytes narrowing the spinal exit foramina through which the roots enter the neck. C5, 6 and 7, most commonly are involved.

Spinal tumours may present with pain in the arm. Malignant disease of the cervical vertebrae, usually from breast or lung, may lead to compression of cervical roots. Benign neurofibromas and occasional intrinsic cervical cord tumours such as gliomas may present with chronic arm pain. So, too, may *syringomyelia*, which also causes characteristic dissociated sensory loss, loss of tendon jerks and wasting of the hand.

The wasted hand

Wasting of the small muscles of the hand either with or without pain, is a common clinical problem. These muscles are innervated predominantly by the ulnar nerve (the median nerve only supplies muscles of the thenar eminence), the inner cord of the brachial plexus, the T1 spinal root, or the equivalent group of anterior horn cells. Obviously, lesions of the ulnar nerve, the inner cord of the brachial plexus, the T1 root or that part of the spinal cord may all produce wasting of small hand muscles. However, wasting of the hand is also one of the commonest presenting features of motor neurone disease, which also causes fasciculation and signs of upper motor neurone damage, but no sensory loss.

Wasting of the muscles around the shoulder occurs in the frozen shoulder syndrome, neuralgic amyotrophy, cervical spondylosis affecting the C5 roots, and motor neurone disease. Symmetrical wasting around the shoulder may also be a sign of primary muscle disease, including thyrotoxicosis.

Pain in the leg

The painful, tingling or weak leg

As in the arm, the commonest cause of pain in the leg is local bone or joint disease. The speed with which quadriceps muscle wastes after a knee injury may amaze the young sportsman, while the commonest cause of pain in the thigh and wasting of the quadriceps in later life is osteoarthritis of the knee. The commonest neurological cause of acute leg pain is sciatica, but a number of conditions may cause chronic pain in the lower limb.

Acute sciatica

Traditional terms such as lumbago and sciatica describe syndromes of acute pain in the back and acute pain radiation into the leg respectively. Acute lumbago probably has many causes including tear of paraspinal muscles, or spinal ligaments, acute damage to hypophyseal joints of the spine, and acute central ruptures of lumbar discs. Radiation of the pain into the leg may be due to hip disease, however, when it extends below the knee it is most usually due to irritation of the corresponding lumbosacral nerve root by a lateral disc protrusion. Sciatica is commonly accompanied by lumbago, but may occur by itself; lumbago often occurs without sciatica. Typically, the onset is sudden during physical activity, particularly when lifting weights with the back flexed. Excruciating pain in the back, with or without radiation into the leg, is accompanied by spasm of the back muscles so that the spine 'locks', and any slight movement causes exquisite agony. Coughing, sneezing, or straining at stool all cause impulse pain. The sciatica is in the distribution of the nerve root involved, down the back of the leg to the heel in the case of S1, or down the lateral surface of the leg to the instep in the case of L5, these being the two roots most commonly affected by disc degeneration at the L4/5 (L5 root) and L5/S1 (S1 root) disc spaces respectively. Root compression also gives rise to typical sensory symptoms of numbness or paraesthesiae and motor weakness in the appropriate distribution. When the onset is acute in the setting of physical exercise, the diagnosis of acute sciatica is rarely in doubt. However, disc protrusions not uncommonly may cause a more gradual onset of pain without any obvious precipitating cause. In this situation, alternative diagnoses have to be considered.

Chronic leg pain

Pain referred into the leg may be due to *pelvic carcinoma* spreading from uterus, cervix, prostate or rectum to infiltrate the lumbar or sacral plexus. Such pain is insidious in onset and gradually becomes more severe and constant. A rectal examination, which is essential in all patients with unexplained persistent leg pain, will usually reveal the cause.

Meralgia paraesthetica is due to an entrapment neuropathy of the lateral cutaneous nerve of thigh as it passes through the lateral end of the inguinal ligament. This causes pain, often of burning quality, and tingling or numbness on the lateral aspect of the thigh down to, but not below, the knee.

Diabetic amyotrophy is another common cause of pain in the leg. This complication of diabetes presents as subacute severe pain in the thigh accompanied by wasting of the quadriceps and minor or minimal sensory changes in the distribution of the femoral nerve. It is usually due to an acute vascular lesion affecting the femoral nerve. The femoral nerve also may be compressed acutely by haemorrhage into the iliopsoas muscle in those with a bleeding diathesis or on anticoagulant therapy.

The *tarsal tunnel syndrome* is a rare cause of pain in the foot. It is directly analagous to the carpal tunnel syndrome in the arm, being due to an entrapment neuropathy of the tibial nerve beneath the flexor retinaculum of the ankle. This causes pain, numbness and tingling of the medial plantar surface of the foot, aggravated by standing and walking, and often worse at night.

Foot drop

Paralysis of the dorsiflexors of the ankle may be due to lesions of the common peroneal nerve, the sciatic nerve, the L5 root, or occasionally the motor cortex.

The common peroneal nerve is extremely vulnerable as it travels the neck of the fibula, where it may be compressed by external pressure, or stretched by prolonged bending or sitting with the knees fully flexed. Apart from the foot drop, such patients also exhibit numbness on the dorsum of the foot, but the ankle jerk is preserved. The sciatic nerve is vulnerable to misplaced injections into the buttocks or thigh, which leave not only a foot drop, but also weakness of plantar flexion of the foot, sensory loss extending onto the sole of the foot, and loss of the ankle jerk. L5 root lesions are difficult to distinguish from common peroneal palsies, but presence of lumbago and extension of weakness to involve the knee flexors will point to this proximal lesion. Motor cortex lesions affecting the foot area may present with a foot drop, but the plantar response will be found to be extensor.

Cramps in the legs

Many patients use the word cramp to describe pain in the legs due to vascular insufficiency, or nerve damage. However, genuine cramp consists not only of pain but also intense and involuntary muscle contraction affecting particularly the calf muscles. Such cramps are the plague of the untrained athlete, and are well known to occur in hot climates due to salt depletion. Muscle cramps occur in those recovering from sciatica and in motor neurone disease, but other findings will point to these diagnoses. Occasionally, isolated muscle cramps may be found to be due to primary metabolic muscle disease, but in the majority of such patients no obvious cause can be discovered and they are extremely difficult to treat.

True muscle cramps are electrically silent on electromyographic (EMG) study. In contrast, flexor spasms of leg muscles that occur in those with damage to corticospinal pathways are associated with intense electromyographic activity and, of course, with the signs of an upper motor neurone lesion (weakness without wasting, spasticity, and exaggerated tendon reflexes).

Restless legs

Some patients will complain of discomfort in the legs that is not due to pain, cramp, or paraesthesiae. They find it impossible to put into words the quality of the intense discomfort that they feel, but describe relief from movement. Such patients cannot sit still because of the discomfort, and may be forced to get out of bed at night to walk around to gain relief from this distressing complaint. The cause of this bizarre symptom, known as Ekbom's syndrome, is not known, although some patients are found to have an iron deficient anaemia or uraemia.

Intermittent claudication

Pain in the calves or buttocks on exercise, relieved rapidly by rest, is, of course, the characteristic feature of arterial insufficiency in the legs. However, this syndrome of intermittent claudication occasionally may be mimicked by disease of the lumbar spine, particularly in those with congenital spinal canal stenosis and degenerative lumbar spondylosis. Such patients also complain of pain in the legs on exercise, but the pain is in the distribution of one of the spinal roots, and is accompanied by neurological symptoms including foot drop or paraesthesiae. Rest relieves the pain, but usually after a longer period of time than is required in the case of vascular intermittent claudication. This neurological syndrome, because it mimics vascular claudication, has been called intermittent claudication of the cauda equina.

Difficulty in walking

This is one of the commonest neurological complaints. The first step is to distinguish the different anatomical causes that may provoke difficulty in walking. It is convenient to work mentally from muscles up to cerebral cortex.

Difficulty with walking with wasted legs

Primary muscle disease (*myopathy*) often presents with an abnormality of gait, because it affects proximal muscles of the hip girdle symmetrically at an early stage. Similar symmetrical proximal weakness around the shoulder girdle usually occurs later. Characteristically the gait is waddling due to failure to stabilize the pelvis on the femur when the opposite leg is lifted from the ground.

In addition, patients with primary muscle disease frequently complain of difficulty in getting out of a low chair, and of climbing stairs or getting onto the platform of a bus, because of weakness around the hips. When the arms are affected, an early symptom often is difficulty raising the hand above the head to brush the hair. Other characteristics of primary muscle disease are that sensation is normal and sphincter function is not affected. There are many causes for myopathy including hereditary muscular dystrophy, inflammatory myositis, thyrotoxicosis, steroid therapy and metabolic myopathies. A family history suggests muscular dystrophy, which causes painless progressive wasting of muscles in characteristic distribution. Pain and systemic disturbance suggest polymyositis. Many endocrine and electrolyte disturbances may cause metabolic myopathies. The physical signs of primary muscle disease are those of muscle wasting and weakness, symmetrical and proximal, with normal or reduced tendon jerks, and no evidence of sensory deficit.

Defects of neurotransmission due to *myasthenia gravis*, or to the much rarer myasthenic (Lambert Eaton) syndrome often associated with carcinoma, may also present with difficulty in walking due to proximal leg weakness. However, the legs are not wasted in myasthenia. As in primary muscle disease, sensation is not affected. The characteristic feature of myasthenia is muscle fatigue. The patient does not complain of feeling tired, but of weakness of muscle action on exercise. Thus, they may start the day walking strongly, but as time goes on and as exercise continues, they become weaker and weaker. Rest restores strength, but further exercise leads to further weakness.

Peripheral nerve disease may also cause difficulty in walking. This may arise either as a result of damage to an isolated peripheral nerve (*a mononeuropathy*) such as a common peroneal palsy or femoral nerve palsy, or to a number of peripheral nerves but sparing others (*mononeuritis multiplex*), or to generalized peripheral nerve disease (*peripheral neuropathy*). In all such conditions, the signs will be those of a lower motor neurone lesion (wasting with weakness, normal or reduced tone, and normal or depressed tendon reflexes). In addition, there will be appropriate sensory disturbance in the distribution of the affected peripheral nerves. In the case of a generalized peripheral neuropathy, symptoms commence in the feet symmetrically, with paraesthesiae and numbness which spreads upwards into the legs, and bilateral foot drop due to distal weakness. Generalized peripheral neuropathies usually affect the legs before the arms, because long axons are affected first. Sphincter function, however, is normal. Subacute peripheral neuropathy, with onset and progression rapidly over a matter of a few days or weeks, most commonly is due to the acute idiopathic inflammatory polyneuritis known as the Guillain-Barré syndrome. More rarely, similar subacute generalized peripheral neuropathy may occur in infectious mononucleosis, acute intermittent porphyria, or from toxic heavy metals and industrial agents. Diphtheria now is exceedingly rare, but the early palatal palsy and paralysis of accommodation is characteristic. There are many causes for chronic peripheral neuropathy, but the commonest in the UK would be diabetes, with alcohol and malignancy close behind.

Proximal lesions of the lumbosacral nerve roots (*cauda equina lesions*) may present with difficulty in walking due to weakness of the legs, associated with sensory disturbance which characteristically is focused around the perineum (the patient sits on his signs), and early disturbance of sphincter function. Motor neurone disease, too, may present with painless wasting, weakness and fasciculation of leg muscles, usually asymmetrically, and without sensory or sphincter disturbance.

Difficulty in walking with spastic legs

Lesions of the corticomotoneurone pathways bilaterally will cause a spastic paraplegia, which manifests as a characteristic disturbance of gait. The patients walk with stiff straight legs, scuffing the toes and outer border of the feet along the ground. Physical examination will confirm the signs of an upper motor neurone lesion (weakness without wasting, spasticity, exaggerated tendon reflexes and extensor plantar responses). The next stage is to decide on the cause of such a spastic paraplegia.

Acute paraplegia

Acute damage to the spinal cord by *trauma*, inflammatory disease (*acute transverse myelitis*), or *vascular lesion* as may occur with spinal angioma, all produce an acute paraplegia, but initially the signs are not those characteristic of spasticity. Immediately after such an acute insult the segment of spinal cord below the lesion is in a state of shock, when it is unresponsive to peripheral input. Accordingly, the legs are flaccid, the tendon reflexes absent, and the plantar responses often unobtainable. Spasticity, exaggerated tendon reflexes, and extensor plantar responses gradually emerge over a matter of some weeks following the acute insult. An acute flaccid paraplegia, or quadriplegia if the arms also are affected, therefore may be difficult to distinguish from a subacute peripheral neuropathy or even from severe acute metabolic myopathies such as that due to hypokalemia, at least in the early stages. The presence of sensory loss obviously will exclude primary muscle disease, and urinary retention points to spinal cord damage rather than a peripheral neuropathy. In those with an acute paraplegia thought to be due to spinal cord damage, it is crucial to exclude *spinal cord compression*, e.g. by dorsal disc protrusion or extradural abscess, for the longer the delay before surgery the less the chance of useful recovery. All such patients demand immediate neurological assessment and myelography if spinal cord compression is thought to be a possible diagnosis.

Acute quadriplegia

Sudden or rapid paralysis of all four limbs may be a medical emergency if breathing is threatened. Respiratory failure occurs when arterial oxygen tension falls below 8.0 kPa (60 mmHg), or if arterial carbon dioxide tension rises above 6.6 kPa (50 mmHg). However, patients with neurological disease causing respiratory distress may be in severe difficulty long before blood gases are compromised. A rising respiratory rate and breathlessness indicate impending respiratory failure which may require assisted respiration. The best index of respiratory reserve is the vital capacity (VC), which is the volume of maximal expiration following a maximal inspiration. In an adult, a falling VC with a value of less than 50 per cent of the predicted normal is a warning of impending crisis, and action is undoubtedly required if the VC falls to 1.0 litre or less.

The common causes of acute or subacute (with onset over days) quadriplegia are polymyositis, myasthenia gravis, acute inflammatory polyneuritis (Guillain-Barré syndrome), and high cervical cord lesions due to trauma or vascular damage. Rarer conditions include hypokalaemic paralysis, acute porphyria, poliomyelitis, tetanus, and other causes of high cervical cord damage such as subluxation of the odontoid peg (as occurs in rheumatoid arthritis) or cord tumours. Brainstem lesions may also cause a quadriplegia, but bulbar muscles also are involved to cause diplopia, dysphagia and dysarthria.

Chronic spastic paraparesis

The commonest cause of a prolonged spastic paraparesis in the young adult is *multiple sclerosis*, and in the middle-aged or elderly individual it is *cervical spondylosis*. However, it is crucial to exclude other treatable causes of spinal cord disease in both age groups before accepting either diagnosis. In particular, any patient with a chronic progressive spastic paraparesis requires myelography to exclude *spinal cord tumour*, unless there are obvious signs or symptoms of multiple sclerosis elsewhere, or some other clear evidence to establish an alternative diagnosis. To undertake a few unnecessary myelograms is much better than to miss treatable benign spinal cord tumours, such as neurofibromas or meningiomas, until the damage is too severe to remedy by surgical treatment. Unfortunately, in the older age group metastatic deposits in the spine, usually from breast, lung or prostate, are more often than not the cause of spinal cord compression. Rarer causes include dorsal disc prolapse, arachnoiditis, intramedullary cord tumours, and syringomyelia. It is also essential to exclude *subacute combined degeneration* due to pernicious anaemia and vitamin B12 deficiency, and *neurosyphilis* as causes of chronic spastic paraparesis. Subacute combined degeneration nearly always presents with paraesthesiae first in the feet, due to the associated peripheral neuropathy, and the ankle jerks will be found to be absent. The picture of a spastic paraplegia but with absent ankle jerks also may be seen in patients with *hereditary spinocerebellar degenerations*, and as a *remote complication of a primary neoplasm*. *Motor neurone disease* also may present as a spastic paraparesis before evidence of lower motor neurone damage with wasting and fasciculation is evident.

Spastic weakness of one leg

Stiffness and dragging of one leg also is a common presenting complaint in neurology. The difficulty is always to decide whether the lesion lies in the spinal cord or in the brain. Full investigation would include X-rays of the spine and a CT scan, but if the latter is normal then myelography may be required. Progression to involve the arm does not necessarily help to decide between spinal cord or brain, while spread to involve the opposite leg does not always indicate that the lesion is in the spinal cord. The notorious parasagittal meningioma may produce upper motor neurone signs in both legs.

Unsteadiness of gait

An unsteady, uncertain gait may be caused by sensory loss (sensory ataxia), cerebellar disease (cerebellar ataxia), hydrocephalus or extrapyramidal disease such as Parkinson's disease or chorea.

In *sensory ataxia* the patient characteristically walks unsteadily with feet wide apart and lifted high off the ground to slap onto the floor. In addition, the patient with sensory ataxia is much worse in the dark when vision cannot be used to compensate. The patient with *cerebellar ataxia* again walks with feet wide apart and reels from side to side as if drunk. The patient with *Parkinson's disease* slowly shuffles with small steps and a bent posture. The patient with *chorea* unexpectedly dances and lurches as the balance is disturbed by unpredictable involuntary movements.

Extensive sensory loss in the legs may be due to profound sensory peripheral neuropathy or to degeneration of the posterior columns as in tabes dorsalis. In both conditions the tendon jerks are absent, in peripheral neuropathy there are likely to be distal motor signs, while in tabes dorsalis there is likely to be urinary retention with overflow and abnormal pupils.

Progressive cerebellar ataxia occurs in diffuse diseases of the central nervous system, e.g. multiple sclerosis, when it is often accompanied by a spastic paraplegia to produce a typical spastic–ataxic gait. Isolated progressive cerebellar ataxia may be due to cerebellar tumour, hereditary spinocerebellar degenerations, alcohol, endocrine disturbance such as myxoedema, or as a remote effect of a primary neoplasm elsewhere. A cerebellar syndrome in childhood most frequently is due to a posterior fossa tumour, which may present without symptoms suggesting raised intracranial pressure. In adults this is seldom so, and most isolated progressive cerebellar ataxias without headache and vomiting are found to be degenerative in origin.

Extrapyramidal diseases are discussed in the next section.

Movement disorders

The term 'movement disorders' has come to be applied to those diseases of the nervous system, mostly of the basal ganglia, which cause disturbances of movement which cannot be attributed to sensory loss, weakness or spasticity, or obvious cerebellar ataxia. Such movement disorders fall into two main categories: (1) those characterized by a poverty (hypokinesia) and slowness (bradykinesia) of movement, the so-called *akinetic-rigid or parkinsonian syndrome*; and (2) those characterized by excess abnormal and uncontrollable involuntary movements, otherwise known as *dyskinesias*.

Idiopathic *Parkinson's disease*, associated with a characteristic pathology including the presence of Lewy bodies in affected pigmented nerve cells, is the commonest cause of an akinetic syndrome in middle or late life. A similar condition could be produced as an aftermath of encephalitis lethargica (post-encephalitic parkinsonism), and occurs commonly nowadays as a result of intake of neuroleptic drugs such as phenothiazines or butyrophenone (drug-induced parkinsonism). Rarer causes include multiple system atrophy and progressive supranuclear palsy in the older age group, while in juveniles or young adults Wilson's disease and the rigid form of Huntington's disease have to be considered. An important distinction is between Parkinson's disease, or the other conditions mentioned which may cause parkinsonism, and the akinetic-rigid features that occur in patients with many diffuse cerebral degenerations. In the latter conditions, which include diffuse cerebrovascular disease and Alzheimer's disease, the akinetic-rigid features are only part of a much greater disorder of higher mental function which produces profound disturbances of memory, intellect and cognitive function.

Abnormal involuntary movements (*dyskinesias*) are a feature of many diseases of the nervous system, but most can be included within five main categories – tremor, chorea, myoclonus, tics and torsion dystonia. These are not diseases, but clinically identifiable syndromes with many causes. In some patients such dyskinesias are accompanied by other neurological deficits, but in others the involuntary movements occur in isolation and constitute the illness.

Tremor is a rhythmic sinusoidal movement which may occur at rest (rest tremor), or on action (action tremor), when it may be present while maintaining a posture (postural tremor), or on executing a movement (kinetic or intention tremor). Rest tremor is characteristic of Parkinson's disease. Postural tremor often is no more than an exaggeration of physiological tremor by anxiety, drugs, alcohol, or thyrotoxicosis. Intention tremor is a distinctive sign of cerebellar disease.

Chorea is characterized by continuous, randomly distributed and irregularly timed muscle jerks. The limbs, trunk and facial features are continually disturbed by brief, unpredictable movements. Walking is interrupted by lurches, stops and starts (the dancing gait), hand movements and fine manipulations are distorted by similar unpredictable jerks and twitches, while speech and respiration also deteriorate. Strength is usually normal, but the patient is unable to maintain a consistent force of contraction so that the grips waxes and wanes (milkmaid's grip), while the protruded tongue pops in and out of the mouth (fly-catcher tongue). The limbs are hypotonic and tendon jerks brisk and often repetitive. The chief diseases causing chorea are shown in Table 9.5 (*see* p. 212). Sydenham's chorea and Huntington's disease are the commonest causes of generalized chorea, but this may be the presenting feature of a number of general medical illnesses or may occur as a side-effect of drug therapy. Hemichorea or hemiballism describes unilateral chorea most apparent in proximal muscles, so that the arm and leg are thrown widely in all directions.

Myoclonus consists of brief, shock-like muscle jerks, similar to those provoked by stimulating the muscle's nerve with a single electrical shock. Myoclonic jerks may occur irregularly or rhythmically, and they often appear repetitively in the same muscles. In this respect myoclonus differs from chorea, which is random in time and distribution. The chief diseases causing myoclonus are shown in Table 9.6 (*see* p. 213).

Tics resemble myoclonus for they too consist of brief muscle contractions, but they differ in a number of respects. The movements themselves are repetitive and stereotyped, can be micked by the observer, and usually can be controlled through an effort of will by the patient, often at the expense of mounting inner tension. Tics typically involve the face, e.g. with blinking, sniffing, lip smacking or pouting, and the upper arms, e.g. with shoulder shrugging. In fact, tics occur in at least one-quarter of normal children, but disappear with maturity. A number of normal adults also display persistent motor tics as part of their personality. The chief causes of pathological tics are shown in Table 9.7 (*see* p. 214).

Torsion dystonia differs from the other movements that are mentioned in that it is caused by sustained, irregular spasms of muscle contraction which distort the body into characteristic postures for prolonged periods of time. The neck may be twisted to one side (torticollis) or extended (retrocollis); the trunk may be forced into excessive lordosis or scoliosis; the arm is commonly extended and hyperpronated with the wrist flexed and the fingers extended; the leg is commonly extended with the foot plantar flexed and in-turned. Initially these muscle spasms may occur only on certain actions (action dystonia), so that the patient walks on his toes or develops the characteristic arm posture on writing. In progressive dystonia, however, such abnormal muscle spasm and postures soon become apparent at rest and cause increasing dystonic movements and deformity. The term athetosis is also used to describe similar dystonic movements, although originally it was employed to describe wavering movements of the fingers and toes. The chief causes of torsion dystonia are shown in Table 9.8 (*see* p. 215).

Decline of memory, intellect and behaviour

A global loss of all higher intellectual function, memory and cognitive function, accompanied by disintegration of personality and behaviour forms the clinical syndrome known as *dementia*, which usually is due to diffuse cerebral cortical disease. The syndrome of dementia may occur acutely, as after head injury or cerebral anoxia due to cardiac arrest, or may commence insidiously and be progressive, as in the various presenile and senile dementing illnesses of which Alzheimer's disease is the commonest. However, there are other causes of a progressive dementia which are reversible, including certain treatable brain tumours, and metabolic diseases such as myxoedema or vitamin B12 deficiency. When faced with a patient, or their relatives, complaining of memory difficulty, intellectual decline, or changes in personality, three questions have to be answered:

1. Is this really due to a true dementia as a result of organic brain disease, or are these symptoms those of a pseudodementia due to psychiatric illnesses such as depression.
2. Are these symptoms those of a true global dementing illness, or are they due to a focal cortical syndrome as the result of damage to one part of the cerebral cortex, rather than to a diffuse disease.
3. If they are due to a true global dementia, then is there any treatable cause for the condition?

Pseudodementia

Impairment of memory with change in personality and behaviour, of course, are typical symptoms of *depression*, which also produces sadness, sleep disturbance, diurnal mood swing, loss of libido, anorexia and weight loss. Difficulty arises because a considerable proportion of patients with true organic dementing illnesses experience a reactive depression in the early stages of their illness. Accordingly, in a patient who exhibits decline of memory and intellect with alteration in personality and behaviour accompanied by depression, it can be exceedingly difficult to distinguish a primary depressive illness from a dementing process with reactive depression. Careful assessment by experienced psychologists may assist, but often does not resolve the matter. If in doubt, it is prudent to treat the illness as a depression and to await events. Other psychiatric conditions that may produce a pseudodementia include *hysteria* and even *malingering*, but these are rare.

Focal cortical syndromes

Bilateral damage to the temporal lobes, particularly to their medial structures including the hippocampus, or to the hypothalamus may produce a pure *amnesic syndrome*, consisting of dense loss of memory for recent events with inability to retain new information, but with preserved intelligence and personality. Such amnesic syndromes are seen most commonly in Korsakoff's psychosis as a result of thiamine deficiency in alcoholics, but occasionally may occur as a result of parapituitary tumours, or bilateral temporal lobe damage secondary to head injury or encephalitis. A transient global amnesia also occurs as one of the manifestations of transient cerebral ischaemia in posterior cerebral territory. An amnesic syndrome may persist for some time after head injury (post-traumatic amnesia), or after an epileptic seizure (post-epileptic amnesia).

Dysphasia (*see* p. 64) may be mistaken for dementia. The severe disturbance of the content of spoken speech that occurs in a Wernicke's dysphasia due to damage to the posterior temporal region of the dominant hemisphere may consist of such nonsensical language and jargon that the inexperienced observer may mistake the behaviour for that of dementia.

Damage to the frontal lobes, by tumour which is often a benign meningioma, by syphilis as in general paralysis of the insane, or in myxoedema, may produce a remarkable change in personality and behaviour, without deterioration of intellect or memory. Such a focal *frontal lobe syndrome* is often mistaken either for primary psychiatric illness or global dementing disease.

Causes of dementia (Table 2.2)

If the conclusion is that the patient's symptoms are those of a diffuse global dementing illness, the next stage is to decide on its cause. In about 10 per cent of patients, some potentially treatable condition will be discovered on careful examination and full investigation, the yield being greatest in those under the age of 70. The commonest cause of dementia is *Alzheimer's disease* which becomes increasingly frequent with age. (Previously the term 'presenile dementia' was used for the syndrome with onset prior to the age of 65, while 'senile dementia' was applied when the illness commenced after the age of 65. Senile dementia became equated with Alzheimer's disease which, in fact, can occur at any age, and accounts for over 80 per cent of those dementing in later life.) *Cerebrovascular*

Table 2.2   Common causes of dementia

Reversible or arrestable
  Vitamin B12 deficiency
  Hypothyroidism
  Neurosyphilis
  Normal pressure hydrocephalus
  Benign intracranial tumours e.g frontal meningioma, obstructive hydrocephalus
  Drug intoxication
  Calcium metabolic upsets
Degenerative, progressive
  Alzheimer's disease
  Pick's disease
  Huntington's chorea
  Multi-infarct dementia
  Spongiform encephalopathy (Creutzfeldt-Jakob disease)

---

disease is a less common cause of dementia, and usually is suggested by the presence of established hypertension and a history of previous repeated stroke-like episodes (multi-infarct dementia). Rarer degenerative causes of dementia include *Pick's disease* which is difficult to differentiate from Alzheimer's disease on clinical grounds, *Huntington's disease* which is suggested by the typical chorea and family history, and *Creutzfeldt-Jakob disease* which is a slow viral encephalopathy producing subacute rapidly progressive dementia often with characteristic myoclonus and EEG findings.

Treatable causes of dementia include not only unexpected *cerebral tumours* and other mass lesions such as giant aneurysms, but also obstructive or communicating *hydrocephalus, neurosyphilis*, and various metabolic conditions such as *vitamin B12 deficiency, chronic drug intoxication, myxoedema*, and disturbances of *calcium* metabolism. Full investigation is required to exclude such treatable causes and should be undertaken in every patient under the age of 70, and in all those over that age in whom the cause of dementia is not established.

3

Examination of the nervous system

A fully comprehensive clinical examination of the nervous system could occupy a whole day but, in practice, it must be completed in half-an-hour or less. A routine screening examination has to be undertaken in 5–10 min. Accordingly, the neurological examination has to be highly selective. What actually is carried out on each individual patient will be determined by their history, which will focus attention on that aspect of the nervous system which needs the most detailed investigation.

When approaching each neurological patient, it is helpful to have in one's mind two simple plans:

1. The routine basic scheme of examination that is to be conducted in every neurological patient – *the screening examination.*
2. Those special tests required in this patient because of the history of their complaint – *the specific examination.*

This plan will be followed here. First, the basic routine screening examination will be described. Details of individual tests will not be elaborated, since they are best learned at the bedside. Second, more specific detailed examinations required in patients with certain problems will be discussed.

The basic scheme of neurological examination

The basic scheme for neurological examination should consist of:

1. Assess higher mental function
   (a) intellect, memory, personality and mood
   (b) speech and cognitive function.
2. Test the cranial nerves.
3. Test motor functions.
4. Test sensory functions.
5. Test autonomic functions.
6. Examine related structures.

Higher mental function

Intellect, memory, personality and mood

The clarity with which the patient presents his story and answers questions, and his cooperation during examination, will convey a picture of his intellectual capacity and of his personality and mood. Compare your own estimate with what might be expected from the patient's type of work and scholastic record. The patient's mood and insight may be further demonstrated by his reaction to the illness, while his power of memory may be indicated by the coherence and ease with which the symptoms and past history are recalled and dated. Whenever there is doubt about a patient's higher mental function, it is crucial to obtain the story and observations of an independent witness who can testify to the patient's intellectual competence.

If history taking does not suggest any defect of higher cerebral function, then no further testing is required. However, if a decline in higher mental function is suspected, more extensive examination is necessary (*see* later).

Speech and cognitive function

The content and articulation of speech will be evident while taking the history. Always note whether the patient is right or left-handed, and if speech difficulty is apparent it also is worth checking which eye and which leg are dominant. Abnormalities of speech may include the following.

1. *Dysphonia*, in which the content of the speech is normal and articulation preserved but basic voice production is disturbed by mechanical abnormality of the organs of speech including vocal cords and resonating sound boxes. The hoarse voice of laryngitis and the nasal speech of the common cold are examples of dysphonia.

2. *Dysarthria*, which describes abnormal articulation due to damage to the nervous pathways or muscles responsible for speech production, with intact language content. Lower motor neurone paralysis of the soft palate produces nasal escape of air and the characteristic nasal speech of a *paralytic dysarthria*; spasticity of the tongue, palate and mouth produces a monotonous, stiff, slurred type of speech known as a *spastic dysarthria*, which sounds as if the patient is talking with a plum in his mouth; incoordination of muscular action responsible for speech due to cerebellar disease results in irregular, staccato, and explosive speech known as *scanning* or *cerebellar dysarthria*; the akinetic-rigid syndrome of parkinsonism produces a characteristic slow, soft, monotonous speech known as an *extrapyramidal dysarthria*.

3. *Dysphasia*, which describes impairment of language, either of under-standing the spoken or written word, or of speaking or writing itself. The various types of dysphasia that may be encountered with lesions affecting the dominant hemisphere are described later.

Cognition refers to the capacity to know and perceive one's surroundings and one's self in relationship to those surroundings. The inability to recognize objects in space, colours, faces or even one's own body parts is known as *agnosia*. Inability to undertake a skilled motor act despite intact power, sensation and coordination is known as *apraxia*. (Different types of agnosia and apraxia will be described later.)

Provided history taking does not suggest any defect of speech or any abnormality of perceptual or motor skills, further testing of higher cerebral function will not be necessary. However, if aphasia, agnosia or apraxia are suspected further investigation will be necessary (*see* later).

Cranial nerves

I Olfactory nerve

The sense of smell should always be tested if there are complaints of disturbance of taste or smell, suspicion of a lesion involving the anterior fossa, or of dementia. It should be tested after any head injury. It is important to realize that a patient complaining of loss of taste is usually describing the effects of damage to the olfactory nerve, which results in loss of appreciation of subtleties of good food or wine. Such patients can still recognize the elementary tastes of sweet, sour and salt but are unable to appreciate flavour. Sense of smell may be tested by the ability to identify and distinguish the odours of common objects such as coffee, tobacco or orange peel, with each nostril in turn. Unilateral anosmia suggests a lesion of the olfactory nerve, but bilateral anosmia is usually due to local nasal disease such as often follows the common cold.

II Optic nerve

The function of the optic nerve can be tested by examining visual acuity, visual fields, and the optic fundus.

Visual acuity tests the integrity of central macular vision. Distance acuity is recorded in each eye using the standard Snellen chart at 6 m using spectacles to correct for refractive error. If spectacles are not available, a refractive error can usually be excluded by getting the patient to read the chart through a pinhole aperture. Normal distance acuity is recorded 6/6, the numerator representing the distance of the patient from the chart (6m) and the denominator the distance in metres at which a normal person is able to read that line. Decreasing acuity is recorded as 6/9, 6/12, 6/18, 6/24, 6/36, 6/60, and then as the ability to count fingers, perceive hand movements or finally distinguish light. Near acuity may be tested by asking the subject to read standard test type, after correction of refractive error. Near acuity does not necessarily correlate with distance acuity. Most patients with 6/18 distance vision are capable of reading the normal N5 size test type. For driving in the UK it is necessary to recognize a number plate at 75 feet (22.9 m) which is equivalent to a Snellen value of 6/10, i.e. an acuity between 6/9 and 6/12. Colour vision is often affected by optic nerve or anterior visual pathway damage earlier than other visual function, and can be tested by asking the subject to read the standard Ishihara plates.

The *visual fields* may be tested at the bedside by the method of confrontation, in which the patient's field is compared with the observer's. It is important to know what question is being asked by visual field testing in order to employ the correct technique. Lesions of the anterior visual pathways cause damage to the optic nerve leading to reduced visual acuity and central defects in the visual field (*central scotomas*). Lesions of the posterior visual pathways cause defects in visual appreciation in the opposite half of the space (*hemianopias*) which may be detected as abnormalities in the peripheral visual field. The patient faces the examiner, who ensures steady fixation by the patient on the examiner's eye. Peripheral fields may be tested by recognition of finger movements or the gradual introduction of a white or coloured pinhead into each of the four quadrants of peripheral vision. Each eye should be tested separately, and then both together to exclude an *inattention hemianopia* (*see* later). The best object for testing central vision is a small bright red target some 2–5 mm in diameter. Within the scotomatous defect, the colour appears pale or even white, and the normal blind spots can regularly be charted by this technique. Visual fields are recorded in the notes with the right eye field on the right and the left eye field on the left. Defects may be indicated by shading (Fig. 3.1). Central macular vision can be assessed with ease using an Amsler chart. This is a 'grid' printed on paper and the patient is asked to look at this and point out any fault. It tests the central 20° of the field.

Examination of the *optic fundi* with an ophthalmoscope is an art that can only be learnt by practice. Good illumination is essential and the surest way of not being able to see the optic discs is to allow dust to accumulate on your ophthalmoscope. It is helpful to pursue a routine in fundus examination, concentrating initially on the optic disc, looking for swelling (papilloedema) or optic atrophy when a disc is unusually pale, then exploring the four quadrants of the retina looking for haemorrhages or exudates and examining the retinal arteries, which should be about two-thirds of the diameter of the veins, the latter often being pulsatile at least as they emerge from the optic disc. Visible venous pulsations in the vessels entering the optic cup in the disc indicate there is no papilloedema. It is important to distinguish between swelling of the optic nerve and local disease (optic neuritis) and papilloedema resulting from raised intracranial pressure. In optic neuritis, there will be an obvious and often profound drop in visual acuity accompanied by a central scotoma, while in papilloedema due to raised intracranial pressure the visual acuity remains normal, and the only field defect initially is an enlarged blind spot. Later effects of damage to the optic nerve or chiasm lead to a pale clearly demarcated disc, optic atrophy.

III, IV and VI Oculomotor, trochlear and abducens nerves

Examination of the three nerves innervating the muscles of the eyes involves assessment of pupillary function and of eye movement. The size, shape and equality of the pupils should be recorded. Their reaction to a bright light should be tested both directly, by shining the light into the eye under observation, and consensually, by shining the light into the opposite eye, both of which should produce brisk pupillary constriction. The pupillary response to accommodation should be tested by asking the subject to focus upon a finger or object which is carried towards the nose; again, the pupils will constrict on convergence. The position of the upper eyelid should be noted, looking particularly for the presence of drooping (ptosis). Defects of pupillary function are described later (*see* p. 69).

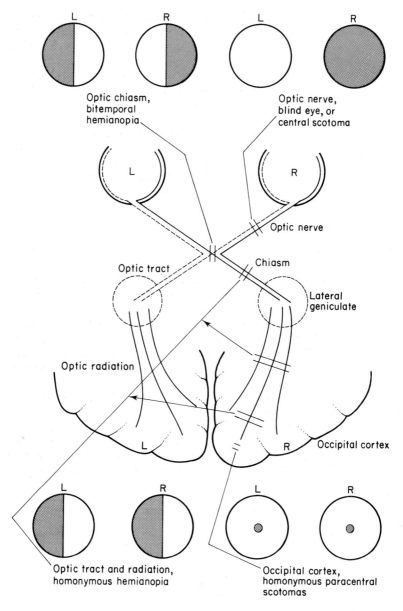

Fig. 3.1. Common visual field defects

Eye movements should be tested in two ways. The *saccadic* system is examined by asking the patient to look voluntarily to right and left, and up and down. The *pursuit* system is examined by asking the patient to follow an object moved to right and left, and up and down. Note the range of movement of each eye in all directions, and whether the movements of the two eyes are yoked together (conjugate eye movements). Note whether saccadic movements are carried out rapidly to the extremes of gaze in each direction, and whether pursuit movements are carried out smoothly without interruption.

Look for nystagmus, which is a repetitive drift of the eyeball away from the point of fixation, followed by a fast corrective movement towards it. Ask whether the patient sees double at any point (diplopia); this is the most sensitive index of defective ocular movement and may be evident to the patient even when the examiner can see no abnormality of gaze.

V Trigeminal nerve

Both the sensory and motor divisions of the trigeminal nerve should be examined.

The most sensitive index of impairment of sensation in the trigeminal nerve is usually loss of the corneal reflex. The corneal reflex is elicited by touching the cornea with a wisp of cotton wool, which evokes an afferent volley in the ophthalmic division of the trigeminal nerve, to cause a blink, which is mediated by motor impulses in the facial nerve. Sensation in all three divisions of the trigeminal nerve should be examined with pin and cotton wool to test pain and light touch respectively. Remember the anatomical confines of trigeminal territory, which extends back to meet the zone innervated by the C2 sensory division well past the crown of the head behind the ears (Fig. 3.2). Also, the mandibular division of the trigeminal nerve supplies the skin over the jaw, but spares that portion over the angle of the jaw, which again is supplied by C2. These landmarks are of value in distinguishing true trigeminal sensory loss from false claims of facial numbness. Another useful point is that the fibres of the trigeminal nerve supplying the cornea travel with the nasociliary branch of

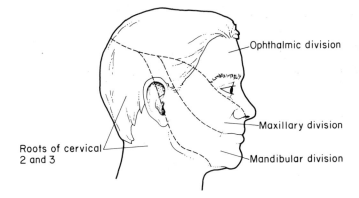

Fig. 3.2. Trigeminal sensory innervation

the ophthalmic division so that depression of the corneal reflex is almost always accompanied by impairment of pinprick sensation at the root of the nose next to the eye.

The motor functions of the trigeminal nerve are examined by comparing the size of masseter and temporalis muscles on each side by palpation while the teeth are clenched. Look for unilateral wasting of these muscles on the side of a trigeminal nerve lesion. Then ask the patient to open his mouth; normally the jaw does not deviate from the midline on mouth opening. In a unilateral trigeminal nerve lesion, the jaw will deviate towards the side of damage, because of weakness of the pterygoid muscles which normally protrude the jaw. However, a common cause of jaw deviation is subluxation of one temporo-mandibular joint, so before diagnosing a trigeminal nerve lesion, always check, by palpation, that the mandibular condyle has not flipped out of its socket. Finally, test the jaw jerk by a brisk tap applied to a finger placed on the point of the half open jaw.

VII Facial nerve

Test facial movements by asking the patient to wrinkle the forehead, screw up the eyes, show the teeth and whistle. Asking a patient to whistle often makes them laugh, which will give you the opportunity to assess facial weakness around the mouth. Lesions of the facial nerve, or of its nucleus, produce weakness of the whole side of the face including the forehead. In contrast, a unilateral lesion of the supranuclear corticobulbar pathway for facial movement (an upper motor neurone lesion) only affects the lower half of the face, sparing the forehead.

The facial nerve itself has no important sensory component. However, fibres originating in the lingual nerve, which carry a sensation of taste from the anterior two-thirds of the tongue, join the facial nerve via the chorda tympani branch in the petrous temporal bone. Rarely, it is necessary to test the sensation of taste. To do so, ask the subject to protrude the tongue, and keep it out, while a test substance is applied to the side of the front of the tongue. There are four tastes – salt, sweet, bitter and acid (or sour).

VIII Auditory nerves

The auditory nerve has two divisions, one conveying impulses from the cochlea subserving hearing, and the other conveying impulses from the labyrinth responsible for vestibular function.

Hearing can be tested quickly by asking the patient to repeat whispered words or numbers with the eyes shut and one ear occluded by the examiner's forefinger. Alternatively, a wrist watch may be brought towards the ear and the distance at which the subject hears the ticking is noted for each side. A watch ticking is a high frequency sound and useful for detecting nerve deafness. If deafness is detected, define whether it is due to middle ear disease (conductive deafness) or to a nerve lesion (perceptive deafness). To do this, compare the noise of a tuning fork held close to the ear (air conduction) with that when the fork is placed on the mastoid (bone conduction); this is called Rinne's test. In normal subjects, and in those with perceptive deafness, air conduction is better than bone conduction. In patients with conductive deafness the reverse is true. Weber's test also may help to distinguish between unilateral conductive and perceptive deafness. A tuning fork is placed on the centre of the forehead; in the normal subject this is heard equally well in both ears. In conductive deafness it is usually heard loudest in the deaf ear, whereas in perceptive deafness it is heard loudest in the normal ear. These bedside tests, however, are crude. Deafness is more accurately assessed by formal audiometric investigation, which will provide a quantitative measure of auditory acuity at different frequencies of sound.

It is not necessary to test vestibular function routinely. In those with vertigo or imbalance, special tests are required which will be described later.

IX and X Glossopharyngeal and vagus nerves

The glossopharyngeal nerve supplies sensation to the posterior pharyngeal wall and tonsillar regions. The vagus nerve, apart from supplying autonomic fibres to thoracic and abdominal contents, supplies motor fibres to the muscles of the soft palate. Interference with glossopharyngeal and vagus nerve function causes difficulty with talking and swallowing.

Vagus function can be examined easily by watching the uvula rise in the midline when the patient says 'Aah'. A unilateral palatal palsy causes drooping of the affected side, and on phonation the palate deviates to the opposite side, pulled in that directed by the intact muscles. A unilateral vagal lesion will also paralyse the ipsilateral vocal cord to cause a typical hoarse voice and 'bovine' cough.

It is not necessary to test glossopharyngeal sensation routinely, because this involves eliciting the 'gag' reflex, which is unpleasant. When required, the 'gag' reflex is obtained by touching the posterior wall of the pharynx with an orange stick which causes the patient to 'gag'; both sides of the pharynx should be tested.

XI Accessory nerve

The accessory nerve innervates the sternomastoid and trapezius muscles. Its fibres are derived both from the lower brainstem and the upper cervical cord segments. The sternomastoid turns the head to the opposite side, while the trapezius is activated by shrugging the shoulders.

If a patient sustains a stroke then it is the sternomastoid muscle contralateral to the hemiparesis that is affected. This will result in weakness of head turning towards the side of the hemiparesis.

XII Hypoglossal nerve

The hypoglossal nerve innervates the muscle moving the tongue. Normally the tongue is held in the floor of the mouth by activity in the tongue retractors. A unilateral hypoglossal lesion therefore will cause the tip of the tongue to deviate away from the affected side when lying in the floor of the mouth. On protrusion, the tip of the tongue will deviate towards the affected side. Wasting of the tongue can be appreciated in lower motor neurone lesions, sometimes accompanied by fasciculation. In bilateral upper motor neurone lesions, the tongue may be small and spastic. Spasticity is elicited by asking the subject to attempt rapidly to protrude the tongue in and out, or move it from side to side.

Motor functions

It is most convenient to screen for motor deficits by examining *coordination* first. Any type of motor abnormality will impair the capacity to execute rapid fine arm and finger movements, or the ability to walk normally. Ask the patient to hold the arms outstretched, fingers spread, with the eyes shut. Look for a tendency for the arm to drop which suggests weakness of the shoulder, for the forearm to pronate, which suggests mild upper motor neurone deficit or dystonia, for the fingers to waver uncertainly (pseudoathetosis) which suggests sensory loss, or for abnormal movements to develop such as tremor. Then ask the patient rapidly to touch his nose with the point of his forefinger and then the examiner's finger, going to and fro as fast and accurately as possible. Such 'finger-nose testing' examines the skill of large proximal arm movements. Look particularly for kinetic or intention tremor, an oscillation that appears during movement and becomes worse as the point of aim is reached. Also note if the finger over- or undershoots its target (dysmetria). Then test the capacity for rapid fine finger movement by asking the patient to approximate the pulp of the thumb to the pad of each finger in succession rapidly and accurately. This 'five finger exercise' directly tests the integrity of the 'true pyramidal' pathway which controls fine manual skills. Gait should always be examined, either as the patient walks into the consulting room, or before he undresses to lie on the couch. The patient already in bed should always be asked to get up and walk at some stage during the examination to examine gait. Many defects of motor control of the legs can be rapidly deduced from watching the patient walk. For example, a footdrop due to a lateral popliteal nerve palsy or L5 root lesion will cause the patient to lift the foot high to help the toes clear the ground, and then the affected foot 'slaps' onto the floor as it is returned to the ground. Spastic legs drag as they are moved, with the foot plantar flexed and inverted, the toes scuffing the ground. The small-stepped, shuffling gait of parkinsonism is unmistakable. The wide based unsteady reeling gait of someone with cerebellar disease or sensory ataxia is also diagnostic. Ataxia of gait can be exaggerated by asking the subject to walk heel-to-toe along a straight line. If ataxia is due to sensory loss, it becomes much worse with the eyes closed (Romberg's sign). Incoordination of the legs is best detected by watching the patient walk, but also may be brought out on the bed by asking him to run the heel carefully up and down the opposite shin, or by asking the patient to touch the examiner's finger with the big toe.

During the examination for coordination of arms and legs, observe the limbs for the presence of *wasting* and *involuntary movements*. The presence of muscle wasting implies either primary muscle disease (myopathy) or a lower motor neurone lesion. It can be difficult, particularly in the elderly or in those with joint disease, to decide whether apparent thinning of muscle bulk is merely due to disuse or indicates neurological deficit. Muscle wasting is only of significance if it is accompanied by definite muscle weakness. The characteristics of the typical abnormal movements of tremor, chorea, myoclonus, tics and dystonia have been described earlier (*see* p. 46). Other abnormal movements that may be observed include fasciculation, which is a random and involuntary twitching of large motor units that occurs as a result of denervation and re-innervation. The characteristic of pathological fasciculation is that the twitches of muscle fascicles occur randomly in time and site.

Rapidly test muscle tone by noting the resistance of the limbs to passive movement. In the arms, this can be studied by shaking the shoulders with the subject standing, looking for the ease with which the limp arms swing from side to side, or by pronation/supination movements of the forearm. In the legs, tone can be assessed by rolling the thigh to and fro, or by passive flexion of the leg onto the abdomen. Muscle tone must be assessed with the subject attempting to relax. Resistance to passive movement may take one of three forms. *Spasticity* is a resistance to attempted stretch of the muscle which increases with applied force, until there is a sudden give at a certain tension, the 'clasp-knife' or 'lengthening' reaction. *Rigidity* is a resistance to passive movement that continues unaltered throughout the range of movements, and so has a plastic or 'lead pipe' quality. *Gegenhalten* describes a curious intermittent resistance to movement in which the patient seems to be unknowingly attempting to oppose your efforts to displace the limb.

Muscle power is tested by asking the patient to exert force against resistance imposed by the examiner. In a simple screening examination of the nervous system, all that is necessary is to test the strength of two critical muscles, one proximal and one distal, in both arms and legs. The reason for choosing a proximal and a distal muscle to examine is that primary muscle disease will be detected by proximal muscle weakness, while the impact of peripheral nerve disease will be apparent in distal muscle weakness. The proximal and distal muscles chosen to test can be selected also to detect weakness due to an upper motor neurone lesion. The latter has a quite distinctive distribution, which can be remembered by recalling the posture of a patient rendered hemiplegic by a stroke. The stroke victim carries the arm held to the side, the elbow flexed and the fingers and wrist flexed onto the chest. The leg is held extended at both hip and knee, with the foot plantar flexed and inverted. This characteristic posture is the result of a selective distribution of spasticity, working against a selective distribution of weakness. Hemiplegic weakness in the arm affects the shoulder abductors, elbow extensors, wrist and finger extensors, and small hand muscles. Hemiplegic weakness in the leg affects hip flexors, knee flexors, and dorsiflexors and evertors of the foot. Accordingly, the critical muscles to test in a screening motor examination are, in the arm, proximally the shoulder abductors and distally the small muscles of the hand which spread the fingers, and in the leg, proximally the hip flexors and distally the dorsiflexors and evertors of the ankle.

The reflexes

Elicit the following reflexes

The deep tendon reflexes of biceps, triceps, supinator, and finger flexors in the arm; and of the knee and ankle in the legs (Table 3.1). When eliciting such 'tendon jerks' always compare the two sides, taking care to have the limbs in comparable positions. When hyper-reflexia is present, try to elicit clonus (a repetitive self-sustaining reflex contraction) by rapid passive dorsiflexion of the ankle, and by downward thrust of the patella. Also routinely elicit the superficial reflexes known as the plantar responses, by firmly stroking the outer border of the whole of each foot. This normally produces plantar flexion of the big toe (a flexor plantar response). The abnormal response consists of upward movement of the big toe, often accompanied by fanning of the toes; this is known as an extensor plantar response or Babinski's sign. If there is doubt as to the presence of hyper-reflexia or Babinski's sign, elicit the abdominal reflexes by gently stroking the skin of the abdomen in each quadrant in turn. This normally causes a twitch contraction of the appropriate quadrant of the underlying muscles, tending to pull the umbilicus in that direction. The abdominal reflexes are lost in an upper motor neurone lesion. They may also be absent after extensive abdominal surgery or with very lax stretched muscles.

Table 3.1   Reflexes

Arm	
Supinator	C5/6
Biceps	C5/6
Triceps	C7
Finger flexors	C8
Abdominal	
Upper	T8–10
Lower	T10–12
Cremasteric	L1/2
Anal	S4/5
Leg	
Knee	L3/4
Ankle	S1

Sensory functions

The student will soon learn that testing sensation is difficult and frustrating. It is crucial to have some clear idea of what is being looked for, before embarking on this part of the neurological examination. In a routine screening of the nervous system, sensory examination may be brief, provided the patient has no sensory complaint and there is no other good reason for extensive sensory testing.

Test appreciation of pinprick and light touch on the tips of the fingers and the toes. Examine the ability to appreciate joint movement in the fingers and toes. Remember that joint position sense is extremely sensitive, such that movements of a digit of only a few degrees may be perceived accurately and rapidly by the normal subject. Finally, examine appreciation of vibration by applying a standard tuning fork to the tips of the fingers and the medial malleoli. Some estimate of quantitative sensory appreciation of vibration may be obtained by employing a standard tuning fork set into motion by a standard 'tweek' of the fingers, the subjects being asked how long they perceive the vibration for. You will have to learn the normal for your own vibration fork, but most individuals can detect vibration at the ankles for 12 or more seconds and at the fingers for even longer.

Autonomic functions

The autonomic nerves innervate the viscera, bowel, bladder and sexual organs and are responsible for control of the circulatory reflexes, sweating and pupillary reactions. Symptoms of autonomic failure may include constipation with impaired bowel motility, incomplete bladder emptying from a hypotonic bladder which may lead to urinary incontinence, and impotence in the male. Failure of the circulatory reflexes may cause postural hypotension with feelings of faintness or dizziness on standing, sometimes syncope, and often a fixed relatively rapid heart rate. There may be impaired sweating with difficulties in temperature regulation, occasionally patchy hyperhidrosis, dry eyes and oral mucus membranes. The pupils may become non-reactive.

The easiest simple tests of autonomic function include measurement of the blood pressure (BP) standing and lying, and the measurement of the pulse rate at rest, during the Valsalva manoeuvre, to deep breathing and on standing up. With autonomic failure the BP will fall by more than 30 mmHg on standing. With a Valsalva manoeuvre during the strain the BP normally falls and the pulse rate rises. With release the BP rises and the pulse rate falls. With autonomic failure there is no change in pulse rate. On standing the pulse rate normally rises: in autonomic failure this may not occur. Normally the pulse rate varies with deep breathing, but again with autonomic failure this may not occur. Measuring the R-R interval on an ECG during such tests is a useful way of measuring such heart rate changes. More detailed tests of urodynamic function, penile plethysmography, and pharmacological tests for sweating and pupillary reactions may also be used.

Examination of related structures

The neurological examination is completed by looking at:

1. The skeletal structures enclosing the central nervous system.
2. The extracranial blood vessels.
3. The skin.

Observe the shape and size of the skull; palpate the head, feeling for bony defects and lumps. Listen with a stethoscope over both eyes and mastoid processes for bruits, which suggest narrowing of an artery or an intracranial vascular malformation. Palpate the carotid artery and listen for a murmur in the neck; the presence of such a bruit suggests narrowing of one of the extra-cranial arteries. Look for meningism by flexing the head and neck. In the normal subject the chin will reach the chest without pain, but when there is irritation of the meninges by blood or by infection, movement is limited by painful spasm of the extensor muscles of the neck. Similar meningeal irritation in the lumbar spine causes spasms of the hamstring muscles so that when the thigh is at 90° to the trunk, the knee cannot be straightened (Kernig's sign). In the case of spinal lesions, examine the spine for local tenderness or deformity, and test spinal movements. Throughout the examination, observe the skin for vascular malformations, for nerve tumours (neurofibromas) and for 'café-au-lait' spots.

Of course, a general physical examination will also be undertaken in every patient. In particular, the blood pressure should be recorded because of the frequency with which hypertension affects the central nervous system. Likewise, the heart must be examined with care as a possible source of damage to the brain. The lungs and abdomen should be examined as possible sources for clues for neurological complications of systemic diseases.

Interpretation of abnormal findings

As discussed in the introduction, the first object of history taking and clinical examination is to find the anatomical site of damage to the nervous system. Every abnormality discovered on physical examination suggests that a particular group of neurones is damaged. By defining the pathways involved, the likely site or sites of the disease may be deduced.

This exercise in applied neuroanatomy is hampered by the ease with which minor insignificant abnormalities may be discovered on examination. Even normal findings sometimes may be misinterpreted as indicating a disease process. For instance, the helpful patient will manufacture sensory abnormalities as fast as you suggest to him that they may be present! To overcome this problem, it is a useful exercise to classify each abnormality discovered as a 'hard' or 'soft' sign. 'Hard' signs are unequivocally abnormal! – an absent ankle jerk, even on reinforcement, a clear cut extensor plantar response, definite wasting of the small muscles of the hand. Any final anatomical diagnosis must provide an explanation for such 'hard' signs. 'Soft' signs are found frequently in the absence of any definite abnormality and are, therefore, unreliable. Examples of such 'soft' signs are a slight asymmetry of the tendon reflexes, slightly less facility of repetitive movements of the left hand in a right-handed person, and a few jerks of nystagmus of the eyes on extreme lateral gaze. When in doubt, it is best to ignore such findings in the initial assessment of the case. Base your first attempt at diagnosis on the 'hard' signs only. Having taken each of these into account in your final conclusion, then review the 'soft' signs that you discovered on the way, and just make certain that none of them raises doubts about your conclusion.

Another point of neurological examination must be emphasized. The speed and precision with which the site of the lesion may be established depends upon continual deduction throughout the process of history taking at examination. Throughout these first few chapters, emphasis has been laid on the way the findings obtained at one stage in the diagnostic process determine the pattern of the succeeding phases of history taking or examination. Whenever an abnormality has been detected, either in the history or on physical examination, its implications must be followed up to the full. For example, the discovery of a bitemporal hemianopia demands a careful search for evidence of pituitary dysfunction. If a patient with headache is discovered to have such a physical sign, then immediately the examiner may return to ask more questions on this history, e.g. whether a man still shaves regularly or whether a woman's menstrual periods remain regular. This is the true art of neurology. Each clue that emerges during history taking or examination should prompt new thought. Previous provisional conclusions should be re-examined and new questions or physical tests considered. In other words, to arrive at the correct final conclusion requires a constant alert mental processing of every scrap of information that is available.

Specific abnormalities

Having described briefly a basic scheme for examination of the nervous system, one to be undertaken in every neurological patient, we will now turn to the more detailed examinations that may be required when certain abnormalities are discovered. The topics chosen by no means cover all the abnormalities that may be found on clinical examination, but they represent the commonest problems which will require further exploration.

Dementia

If the patient's complaint is one of memory difficulty or impairment of intellectual processes, or if a relative or acquaintance suggests that this may be the case, then extensive investigation of higher mental function will be required. Likewise, a detailed examination of the mental state is necessary if, in the course of history-taking and physical testing, the patient's intellectual processes seem impaired. Detailed analysis of intellect, reasoning and powers of memory can be a very time-consuming business, requiring the expertise of trained clinical psychologists. They will undertake a formal psychometric assessment of the patient's current level of intellectual performance, using tools such as the Wechsler Adult Intelligence Scale (WAIS), Raven's progressive matrices, and other standardized test batteries. The WAIS test is used most widely, and consists of a number of subtests which assess both 'verbal' and 'performance' abilities. Details of such complex investigations are beyond the scope of this book. Here we are concerned with simple bedside testing of mental powers. However, once the need for formal examination of the mental state has been decided upon, it is best to proceed to gather information in a standard fashion.

An appropriate, standardized, bedside tool for evaluating higher mental function is the Mini-Mental State Examination (MMS) (Table 3.2). The tests included in the MMS have been devised to examine most aspects of mental activity briefly but reproducibly. The whole test takes no longer than 5 min to complete, and will be a reliable index of intellectual function.

Table 3.2   The Mini-Mental State examination

---

1. *Orientation*
   Ask the date, the day, the month, the year and the time: score one point for
      each correct answer   (5)
   Ask the name of the ward, the hospital, the district, the town, the country:
      again score one point each   (5)
2. *Registration and calculation*
   Name three objects and ask the patient to repeat these: score 3 for all correct,
      2 if only two   (3)
   Ask the patient to subtract 7 from 100 and repeat this five times (93, 86, 79,
      72, 65)   (5)
   Recall: ask for the three objects to be named again   (3)
3. *Language*
   Name two objects shown to the patient (e.g. pen, watch)   (2)
   Score one point if they can repeat 'No, ifs, ands or buts'   (1)
   Ask the patient to carry out a three stage command e.g. 'Take a piece of
      paper in your right hand, fold it in half, and put it on the table'   (3)
   Reading: write in large letters 'Close your eyes' and ask the patient to read
      and follow this   (1)
   Write: ask the patient to write a short sentence: it should contain a subject, a
      verb and make sense   (1)
   Copying: draw two intersecting pentagons, each side about one inch and ask
      the patient to copy this   (1)

Total   (30)

Aphasia

Once a defect of the use of language has been detected, either on history-taking or examination, a more extensive evaluation of speech function is required. A great deal of detailed information is available on the way in which human speech and the use of language can break down in neurological disease, but much of this is irrelevant to routine neurological practice.

Disorders of language with faulty speech may arise from damage to the dominant hemisphere and are important localizing signs. The left hemisphere is dominant in right-handed subjects, but also in some 70 per cent of left handers. Much of our understanding of language disorders results from the study of patients who have sustained dominant hemisphere damage. More recently, CT scanning has added to our understanding of the anatomical localization of certain faults. Strictly, aphasia implies a severe or total loss of speech; dysphasia being a milder deficit.

A global aphasia describes impairment of all functions – comprehension, expression, problems in reading, writing and in repetition. These should all be tested. A global aphasia arises from extensive damage.

Two particular speech areas are recognized. Broca's area lies in the posterior frontal region (Fig. 3.3) which is close to the motor cells concerned with articulation. Broca's aphasia causes expressive difficulties with non-fluent speech with telegrammatic utterances. Short connecting words may be missing and there may be difficulty with 'ifs, ands or buts'. Sometimes there is perseveration and there may be writing difficulties. Comprehension is good.

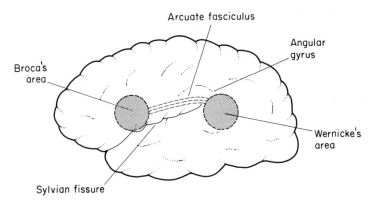

Fig. 3.3. Speech areas of the brain

The second area lies in the posterior part of the superior temporal gyrus, Wernicke's area, which is close to the region of the brain concerned with auditory input. In Wernicke's aphasia there are comprehensive difficulties with fluent speech which lacks content. Phrases may be incorrect and often repeated – paraphasia. Writing is abnormal and commonly there is difficulty understanding the written word, dyslexia.

The speech areas are connected by the arcuate fasciculus (Fig. 3.3). A lesion in this pathway may separate the two sites allowing fluent paraphasic speech with preserved comprehension. In some aphasic patients the deficit appears to be one of naming, word finding, anomic aphasia. This may occur with lesions in the angular gyrus, but can also arise from more diffuse upsets, e.g. metabolic disorders. In general, cortical lesions in the dominant hemisphere disrupt spontaneous speech and repetition. Subcortical lesions (transcortical aphasia) leave repetition intact (Table 3.3).

Table 3.3 Aphasia

Broca's aphasia	Wernicke's aphasia	Conduction aphasia (arcuate fasciculus)	Anomic aphasia
Speech non-fluent telegrammatic	Fluent speech poor content	Fluent speech	Fluent speech
	Paraphasic errors	Paraphasic errors	
Comprehension good	Comprehension poor, both verbal and written	Comprehension good	Comprehension good
Repetition good	Repetition poor	Repetition very poor	Repetition normal
Object naming poor	Object naming poor	Object naming poor	Object naming poor
Often hemiparesis arm > leg	Absent or mild hemiparesis ± hemianopia	Cortical sensory loss	Usually no hemiparesis
Global aphasia – large lesions affect all functions			

Although strict divisions are made, in nearly 60% of aphasic patients there appears to be a mixture of problems

Agnosia

This is the failure to recognize objects when the pathways of sensory input from touch, sight and sound are intact. This sensory input cannot be combined with the ability to recall a similar object from the memory areas of the brain, i.e. a sort of 'mind-blindness'. Such deficits can be tested by asking patients to feel, name and describe the use of certain objects.

Tactile agnosia, astereognosis, is the inability to recognize objects placed in the hands. There must be no sensory loss in the fingers and sufficient motor function and coordination for the patient's fingers to explore the object. Such defects usually reflect parietal lobe damage.

Visual agnosia is the inability to recognize what is seen when the eye, optic nerve and main visual pathway to the occipital cortex are preserved. Affected patients can often describe the shape, colour or size of an object without recognizing it. Prosopagnosia is the inability to recognize a familiar face. Parieto-occipital lesions are responsible.

Anosognosia is a term used to describe the lack of awareness or realization that the limbs on one side are paralysed, weak or have impaired sensation. It is most often seen in patients with right-sided parietal damage who may seem to be unaware of their faulty left limbs.

Apraxia

This is the inability to perform purposeful willed movements in the absence of motor paralysis, severe incoordination or sensory loss. It is the motor equivalent of agnosia. Patients should also be able to understand the command, although it is quite common for some dysphasia to be present. To test this patients may be asked to perform a number of tasks, e.g. to make a fist, to pretend to comb their hair, lick their lips, to pretend to light a cigarette or to construct a square with four matches. Gait apraxias create problems walking, although patients may show good leg movements when tested on the bed.

In dressing apraxias, patients cannot put their clothes on correctly. In ideomotor apraxia patients cannot perform a movement on command, although they may do this automatically, e.g. lick their lips. In ideational apraxias there is difficulty in carrying out a complex series of movements, e.g. to take a match from a box to light a cigarette. Constructional apraxias produce problems in copying designs or arranging patterns on blocks.

In most instances apraxias are caused by dominant parietal lobe damage with breakdown in the connections via callosal fibres with the opposite hemisphere and in the links between the parietal lobes and the motor cortex.

Visual field defects

Light from an object on the left-hand side of the body falls on the right-hand half of each retina after passing through the narrow pupillary aperture. The temporal or outer half of each retina eventually is connected to the cerebral cortex on that side by nerve fibres which never cross the midline. The inner, or basal, half of the retina is connected to the cortex on the opposite side by fibres which cross the midline of the optic chiasm. It follows that the right-hand halves of both retinae are connected to the right occipital cortex, which view objects on the left side of the body. Analysis of visual field defects follows from these simple anatomical principles.

The visual field defect may be due to a lesion affecting the eye, the optic nerve, the optic chiasm, the optic tract between chiasm and lateral geniculate bodies, the optic radiation, or the occipital cortex. The resulting patterns of visual field defect are illustrated in Fig. 3.1.

A lesion of the optic nerve usually damages fibres from the macula first, for these are most sensitive to pressure or ischaemia. Accordingly, the initial symptoms of an optic nerve lesion are a loss of visual acuity accompanying a central visual field defect (a central scotoma). Degeneration of optic nerve fibres can be seen with the ophthalmoscope as optic atrophy, in which the disc becomes unnaturally white. As an optic nerve lesion progresses, visual acuity falls further and the size of the central scotoma enlarges. Eventually, a complete optic nerve lesion will lead to blindness in that eye (*see* Fig. 3.1). However, the patient will still be able to see clearly and to either side with the remaining opposite intact eye. The pupil of the blind eye will not react to light shone directly into it, but will react briskly when the light is shone in the opposite eye to evoke the consensual reaction. This principle is also employed to detect minor optic nerve lesions by the swinging light test. If a light is flashed from one eye to another, the direct response on the side of the affected optic nerve will be less powerful than the consensual response evoked from the normal eye. As a result, when the light is shone into the affected eye the pupil will dilate, the so-called *afferent pupillary defect* or *Marcus-Gunn phenomenon*.

The optic chiasm contains both non-crossing fibres from the outer halves of the retina, which lie laterally, and decussating fibres from the inner halves of the retinae. The decussating fibres are arranged with those from the upper part of the retina posteriorly, and those from the lower part anteriorly. Macular fibres also lie in the posterior part of the chiasm.

Another anatomical peculiarity is that the fibres from the lower part of the nasal retina, having passed in the chiasm, may loop anteriorly into the optic nerve before passing posteriorly into the optic tract. Accordingly, a posteriorly placed lesion of the optic nerve will cause not only a central scotoma on that side, but also an upper temporal quadrantic defect in the visual field of the opposite eye, the so-called 'junctional scotoma'.

A lesion dividing the optic chiasm in the midline interrupts fibres from the inner half of each retina and results in the loss of the temporal field of vision in each eye, the bitemporal hemianopia (*see* Fig. 3.1). It is important to realize that the visual fields of the two eyes overlap binocularly when they are both open. The extent of overlap is almost complete except for a few degrees at each temporal crescent. Accordingly, it is possible to miss entirely a total bitemporal hemianopia when examining the visual fields to confrontation, unless each eye is tested separately. The details of the anatomical arrangement within the optic chiasm dictate the pattern of visual defects caused by different lesions in this region.

Pressure on the chiasm from behind and below, e.g. by a pituitary tumour, often affects the decussating macular fibres first to produce bitemporal para-central scotomas. As such a tumour enlarges, the scotomas extend out to the periphery to cause the characteristic bitemporal hemianopia. Pressure on the chiasm from one side first affects the non-crossing fibres from the outer half of the retina to cause a unilateral nasal hemianopia.

Lesions of the optic tract will damage all fibres conveying vision from the opposite side of the patient to cause a homonymous hemianopia, in which the field defects of the left and right eyes will be the same (*see* Fig. 3.1). However, such lesions also often impinge upon the posterior part of the chiasm thereby damaging fibres from the upper inner quadrant of the ipsilateral retina before they cross to the opposite side. This results in the addition of an ipsilateral lower temporal field defect to the contralateral hemianopia, so that optic tract lesions commonly are incongruous.

Lesions in the region of the optic nerve, optic chiasm and optic tract lie close to and may arise from the pituitary, and to the adjacent hypothalamus above. Accordingly, such parapituitary lesions often produce disturbances other than visual field defects including abnormalities of eye movement, hypopituitarism and diabetes insipidus. The effect of damage to the optic nerve on the pupillary reaction to light was described above, and any lesion in this region causing damage to central vision may produce an afferent pupillary defect. However, if the field defect is a hemianopia, sufficient vision remains in the intact half of the macular region to preserve visual acuity as normal, and the pupillary reaction likewise will be normal.

The fibres of the *optic radiation* leave the lateral geniculate body to pass via the posterior limb of the internal capsule to the visual cortex. In their course, fibres carrying impulses from the homonymous upper portions of the retinae pass via the parietal lobe to the supracalcarine cortex. Fibres representing the lower portions of the retinae pass over the temporal horn of the lateral ventricle, where they lie in the posterior portion of the temporal lobe before reaching the infra-calcarine cortex. Destruction of the whole optic radiation produces a con-tralateral homonymous hemianopia (*see* Fig. 3.1) without loss of visual acuity, without optic atrophy (because optic nerve fibres have synapsed in the lateral geniculate body), and without alteration of the pupillary light reflex. Partial lesions of the radiation are common. Parietal lobe lesions will produce pre-dominantly an inferior homonymous quadrantic field defect, while temporal lobe lesions produce superior homonymous quadrantic defects.

When dealing with hemianopic field defects, it is important to test both eyes simultaneously to confrontation. The earliest sign of a hemianopia may be the inability to perceive an object in the affected field of vision when the corres-ponding portion of the normal field is tested at the same time; this is called an inattention hemianopia.

The characteristic field defect due to a lesion of the *occipital cortex* is a contra-lateral homonymous hemianopia (*see* Fig. 3.1) without loss of visual acuity and with preserved pupillary responses. However, local anatomical arrangements of visual representation in the occipital cortex and of blood supply to this area may cause a variety of other field defects. The macula is extensively represented in the cortex of the tip of the occipital pole, an area sometimes supplied by the middle cerebral artery. Compressive lesions at this site, or middle cerebral arterial insufficiency, may produce contralateral homonymous paracentral scotomas (*see* Fig. 3.1). The remainder of the occipital cortex is supplied by the posterior cerebral arteries which, because they derived from a common stem, the basilar artery, often are occluded simultaneously. If the occipital tip is supplied by the middle cerebral artery in such patients, then bilateral occlusion of posterior cerebral artery flow will cause grossly constricted visual fields with preservation of small tunnels of central vision. These central 'pinholes', the size of which will depend upon the extent of middle cerebral supply to the occipital cortex, may be sufficient to preserve normal visual acuity. It is important to distinguish such constrictive visual fields from those seen in some patients with hysterical visual loss. It is a physical fact that the size of the central pinhole must increase the further away from the patient one moves. In contrast, hysterical 'tunnel' vision commonly takes the form of preservation of a central area of vision the size of which remains the same whether one is one foot (0.31 m) or 10 feet (3.1 m) from the patient's face – this is physically impossible. Finally, if the whole of the occipital cortex is supplied by the posterior cerebral arteries, and both are occluded, then the patient will develop cortical blindness in which the patient can perceive nothing, yet pupillary responses are preserved and the optic discs appear normal. Because damage often also involves adjacent areas of cortex in some patients, many of them may exhibit other cognitive deficits including even denial of blindness – *Anton's syndrome*.

Pupillary abnormalities

The size of the pupil is controlled by the influence of two divisions of the autonomic nervous system, which act in response to the level of illumination and the distance of focus. The sphincter muscle makes the pupil smaller (miosis), and is innervated by cholinergic parasympathetic nerves; the dilator makes it large (mydriasis), and is innervated by noradrenergic sympathetic fibres.

The parasympathetic fibres, which control both pupillary constriction and contraction of the ciliary muscle to produce accommodation, arise from the Edinger-Westphal nucleus. They travel by the IIIrd nerve to the ciliary ganglion in the orbit; post-ganglionic fibres from the ciliary ganglion are distributed by the ciliary nerve. A lesion of the parasympathetic nerves produces a dilated pupil which is unreactive to light or accommodation. The parasympathetic fibres to the eye are nearly always damaged by lesions affecting the IIIrd nerve, which also produce ptosis and a characteristic loss of ipsilateral eye movement (*see* later). A rarer cause is the result of damage to the parasympathetic fibres within the ciliary ganglion itself to produce *Adie's tonic pupil* (Fig. 3.4). This condition commonly presents in young women with the sudden appreciation that one pupil is much larger than the other. The dilated pupil does not react immediately to light, but prolonged exposure in a dark room may cause slow and irregular contraction of the iris. Likewise, accommodation on convergence is very slow to take place. With time, the dilated tonic pupil gradually constricts and may end up eventually smaller than its opposite number. The diagnosis can be established by demonstrating denervation hypersensitivity of the affected iris. Weak pilocarpine (0.125 per cent) or methacholine (2.5 per cent) eyedrops, will cause the tonic pupil to constrict but have no effect on the normal pupil. Some patients with a tonic pupil, or tonic pupils, also lose their tendon jerks in the so-called *Holmes-Adie syndrome*.

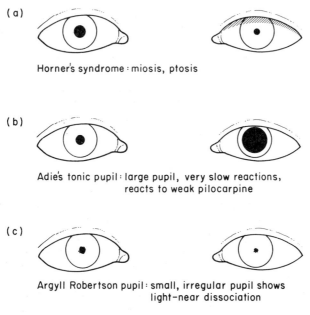

(a)

Horner's syndrome : miosis, ptosis

(b)

Adie's tonic pupil : large pupil, very slow reactions,
reacts to weak pilocarpine

(c)

Argyll Robertson pupil : small, irregular pupil shows
light-near dissociation

Fig. 3.4.   Abnormal pupils

The pupillary response to light also depends on the integrity of the afferent pathways. As described above, the direct light response is impaired with damage to the retina or optic nerve, and an afferent-pupillary defect detected by the swinging light test (Marcus-Gunn) is a sensitive means of confirming an optic nerve lesion. The relevant optic nerve fibres responsible for the light reaction leave those responsible for perception of light to terminate in the pretectal region of the midbrain, from whence a further relay passes to the Edinger-Westphal nucleus. Damage to this pretectal region is believed to be responsible for the *Argyll Robertson* pupil classically seen in neurosyphilis. The characteristics of the Argyll Robertson pupils are that they are small, irregular and unequal, and exhibit light-near dissociation (Fig. 3.4). Light-near disso-ciation refers to the loss of pupillary reaction to light, with preservation of that to accommodation. Pupils resembling those of Argyll Robertson also occur occa-sionally in diabetes and other conditions with autonomic neuropathy. Large pupils exhibiting light-near dissociation are characteristic of damage in the region of the superior colliculi, as may be produced by tumours of the pineal gland. These cause *Parinaud's syndrome* in which there is pupillary light-near dissociation, with paralysis of upgaze and convergence.

The sympathetic fibres supplying the eye arise from the eighth cervical and the first two thoracic segments of the spinal cord. They synapse in the cervical ganglia and pass via the carotid plexus to the orbit. The activity of these fibres is controlled by hypothalamic centres, from which central sympathetic pathways pass to the spinal cord. A lesion of the ocular sympathetic pathways anywhere along this route will produce a *Horner's syndrome* (*see* Fig. 3.4). The pupil on the affected side is constricted. It reacts to light but does not dilate normally in response to shade or pain. In addition, denervation of the smooth muscle of the upper eyelid leads to ptosis, which can be overcome by voluntary upgaze, and enophthalmos, and of the facial sweat glands to loss of sweating on the affected side of the face. As indicated, a Horner's syndrome may appear as a result of lesions affecting the hypothalamus, brainstem or spinal cord, or as a result of damage to the emergent T1 root and cervical ganglion containing sympathetic nerve output, or to the sympathetic plexus on the carotid artery anywhere from the neck into the head.

Defects of ocular movement and diplopia

Abnormalities of eye movement may arise at one of three levels in the nervous system. Lesions of individual muscles or their nerve supply, due to damage of the IIIrd, IVth or VIth cranial nerves or their nuclei, will impair specific individual movements of the eye. This will result in a breakdown of conjugate gaze to cause double vision (diplopia). Within the brainstem, complex pathways link together centres for conjugate gaze to the individual oculomotor nuclei. For example, horizontal gaze to one side demands conjugate activation of one VIth nerve nucleus and the portion of the opposite IIIrd nerve nucleus innervating the medical rectus. These two nuclear regions are linked by fibres passing in the medial longitudinal bundle. Damage to such pathways produces disconjugate gaze known as an internuclear ophthalmoplegia. Finally, conjugate gaze to either side, or up and down, is controlled by pathways from the cerebral hemispheres arising in frontal and occipital eyefields. Damage to these pathways will cause defects of conjugate eye movement known as supranuclear gaze palsies.

Infranuclear lesions

Each eye is moved by three pairs of muscles. The precise action of these depends upon the position of the eye, but their main actions are as follows:

1. The lateral and medial recti respectively abduct and adduct the eye.
2. The superior and inferior recti respectively elevate and depress the abducted eye.
3. The superior and inferior obliques respectively depress and elevate the adducted eye.
4. The superior oblique also internally rotates, and the inferior oblique externally rotates the eye.

Weakness of an individual muscle will cause limitation of movement of one eye in a characteristic direction, and diplopia will occur due to misrepresentation of the object on the retina. The term *squint* describes a misalignment of the ocular axes, but is sufficiently great as to be obvious to the observer. When the misalignment is present at rest and equal for all directions of gaze (concomitant squint) it is not due to local weakness of the ocular muscles. Concomitant squint develops during childhood because of failure to establish binocular vision. The abnormal image from the squinting eye is suppressed, so there is no diplopia. In contrast, a misalignment of the eye that is more apparent when gazing in a particular direction indicates weakness of the muscle acting in that direction (paralytic squint), and diplopia. It should be noted that slight muscle weakness will produce diplopia before any defect of movement can be observed by the examiner.

Three rules enable the examiner to detect which of the ocular muscles is weak in a patient with diplopia:

1. The diplopia may consist of images which are side-by-side (horizontal diplopia), or one above the other (vertical diplopia) or both. Horizontal diplopia must be due to weakness of a lateral or medial rectus. Vertical diplopia, or diplopia in which the two images are at angles to one another, can be due to weakness in any of the other muscles.
2. Separation of the images is maximal when the gaze is turned in the direction of action of the weak muscle. For example, maximal separation of images on looking to the right, with horizontal diplopia, indicates weakness of the left medial or right lateral rectus.
3. When the gaze is directed to cause maximal separation of the images, the abnormal image from the lagging eye is displaced further in the direction of gaze. For example, if horizontal diplopia is maximal on looking to the right, and the image furthest to the right comes from the right eye (tested by covering each eye separately), the right lateral rectus is weak. Conversely, diplopia is minimal when the gaze is directed in such a way as to avoid the use of the weak muscle. Patients sometimes make use of this fact to prevent double vision, by adopting a convenient head posture. Thus the patient with a right lateral rectus palsy will maintain the head deviated to the right so as to be gazing slightly to the left, when the image will be single.

Although these rules sound simple, in practice it can often be difficult to analyse complex diplopia at the bedside. The use of red and green spectacles to identify the two images, and of Hess charts to plot their position, may sometimes be required to make analysis easier.

Disorders of function of individual eye muscles, and the diplopia so produced, may be due to disorder of the eye muscles themselves, or to lesions of the nerves controlling them. Lesions of the eye muscles occur in two situations. Primary ocular myopathy occurs in the group of disorders known as *chronic progressive external ophthalmoplegia*. Such patients have profound defects of all forms of eye movement, but the ocular axes remain parallel so that diplopia does not develop. In contrast, *myasthenia gravis*, which commonly affects the eyes, causes loss of conjugate gaze and inevitable diplopia. Characteristic of myasthenia is fatigue of eye muscle contraction with exercise, so that diplopia occurs towards the end of the day, or on sustained gaze in a particular direction. Ptosis is also often present in those with ocular myasthenia. Lesions of the nerves to the ocular muscles may result from disorders affecting their nuclei in the brainstem, or from damage to the nerves themselves in their course to the orbit. Such

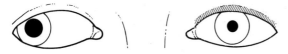

(a)   Gaze ahead : right eye turned out and down, ptosis,
        often pupillary dilatation

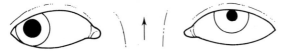

(b)   Impaired upgaze : superior rectus weak

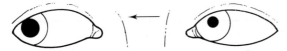

(c)   Full abduction : lateral rectus supplied by V1

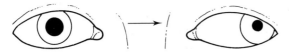

(d)   Impaired adduction : medial rectus weak

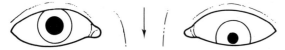

(e)   Impaired downgaze : inferior rectus weak

Fig. 3.5.   Right oculomotor palsy

lesions inevitably produce diplopia (unless the patient is blind in one eye), for conjugate gaze is destroyed.

Oculomotor (IIIrd nerve) lesions produce ptosis because the levator palpebrae is paralysed. On lifting the lid it will be apparent that the eye is deviated outwards and downwards, due to the respective actions of the intact lateral rectus and superior oblique (which are supplied by the VIth and IVth nerves) (Fig. 3.5). The pupil will usually be dilated and unresponsive to light, and accommodation is paralysed. Partial lesions of the IIIrd nerve are common, however, and in these the parasympathetic fibres to the pupil may either be spared or selectively involved.

Trochlear (IVth nerve) lesions paralyse the superior oblique muscle, producing inability to look downwards and inwards. Such patients commonly present with a complaint of diplopia when walking downstairs. The presence of

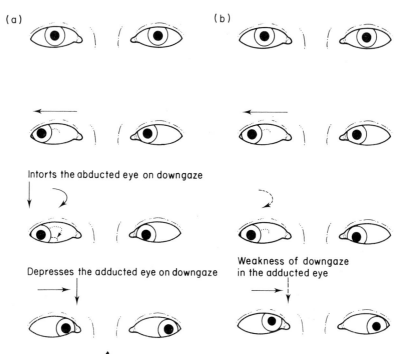

(a) (b)

Intorts the abducted eye on downgaze

Depresses the adducted eye on downgaze

Weakness of downgaze
in the adducted eye

Fig. 3.6. (a) Actions of normal superior oblique. (b) Superior oblique palsy right

intact IVth nerve function can be demonstrated by showing that the eye intorts, i.e. rolls inwards about an anterior–posterior axis, when the patient is asked to look at the root of the nose (Fig. 3.6).

Abducens (VIth) nerve lesions paralyse the external rectus, producing inability to abduct the eye (Fig. 3.7).

Internuclear lesions

The complex details of interconnection between ocular motor nuclei and pontine gaze centres (*see* below) are beyond the scope of this book. The important point is the critical role played by the medial longitudinal bundle linking ocular motor mechanisms within the brainstem. A unilateral lesion of the medial longitudinal bundle causes the characteristic features of an internuclear gaze palsy. These consist of difficulty in adducting the ipsilateral eye on horizontal gaze, with the development of coarse jerk nystagmus in the contralateral abducting eye (Fig. 3.8). The syndrome is sometimes called ataxic nystagmus of the eyes. Lesser degrees of internuclear ophthalmoplegia may be evident simply as a relative slowness of adduction compared with abduction on horizontal gaze. The adducting eye is seen to lag behind the abducting eye. Diplopia does not occur in an internuclear ophthalmoplegia, but oscillopsia, i.e. a tendency for the outside visual world to bob up and down, often occurs with

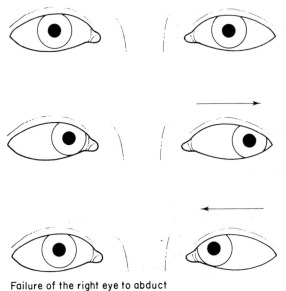

Failure of the right eye to abduct

Fig. 3.7. Right abducens palsy

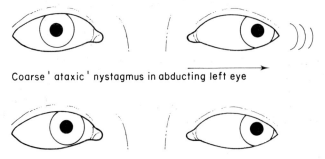

Coarse ' ataxic ' nystagmus in abducting left eye

Lag in adduction of the right eye

Fig. 3.8. Right internuclear ophthalmoplegia. Lesion of the medial longitudinal bundle

brainstem lesions. Bilateral internuclear ophthalmoplegia is almost always the result of multiple sclerosis, although vascular disease and brainstem tumours occasionally may produce unilateral internuclear lesions.

Supranuclear lesions

Four separate mechanisms exist for eliciting conjugate ocular gaze in any direction:

1. The saccadic system allows the subject voluntarily to direct gaze at will even with the eyes shut. The pathways responsible for saccadic gaze arise in the frontal lobe and pass to the pontine gaze centres.
2. The pursuit system allows the subject to follow a moving object. The pathways responsible for pursuit gaze arise in the parieto-occipital region and pass to the pontine gaze centres.
3. The optokinetic system restores gaze, despite movements of the outside world. The operation of the optokinetic system is seen in the railway train, where the eyes of the subject gazing out of the window are seen to veer slowly as the train moves, to be followed by rapid corrections back to the primary position of gaze.
4. The vestibulo-ocular reflex system corrects for movement of the head to preserve the stable visual world. Inputs from the labyrinths and from neck proprioceptors are directed to the brainstem ocular mechanisms to achieve stabilization of the visual image, despite head movement.

These systems for controlling conjugate gaze may be interrupted in many different ways. Lesions of the frontal lobes commonly disrupt voluntary saccadic gaze, while pursuit, optokinetic and vestibulo-ocular mechanisms remain intact. Diffuse cerebral disease, of whatever cause, may interfere with both saccadic and pursuit systems. Saccadic movements become slowed and hypometric, while smooth pursuit is broken up into small, jerky steps. Optokinetic nystagmus, as tested with a hand-held drum bearing vertical black and white stripes, is also disrupted in such patients. In fact, optokinetic nystagmus, tested in this way, is frequently disturbed before evidence of interruption of the pursuit system is apparent. Patients with such supranuclear gaze palsies for both saccadic and pursuit movements, often have preserved vestibulo-ocular reflex movement. This is tested by the doll's head manoeuvre, the oculocephalic reflex. The patient is asked to fixate on the examiner's face, and the head is briskly rotated from side to side or up and down. Patients unable voluntarily to direct their gaze to either side, and unable to follow a moving object in the same directions, may exhibit a full range of ocular movement to the doll's head manoeuvre. It is this preservation of vestibulo-ocular reflex eye movement in the absence of voluntary saccadic or pursuit movements that is diagnostic of a supranuclear gaze palsy. Caloric tests may also demonstrate preserved vestibulo-ocular reflex function in the brainstem (*see* p. 79).

Despite defects in gaze, the eyes remain conjugate in supranuclear palsies, so diplopia does not occur.

The centres in the cerebral hemispheres responsible for saccadic and pursuit movement control deviation of the eyes conjugately towards the opposite side of the body. Accordingly, a unilateral hemisphere lesion will cause weakness of conjugate deviation of the eyes away from the side of the lesion. As they descend towards the brainstem, these pathways cross before they reach the pons. Accordingly, damage to the region of the pontine gaze centres will cause weakness of deviation of the eyes towards the side of the lesion. The combination of damage to the pontine paramedian horizontal centre with involvement of the ipsilateral medial longitudinal bundle (internuclear ophthalmoplegia) may produce the *one-and-a-half-syndrome* (Fig. 3.9).

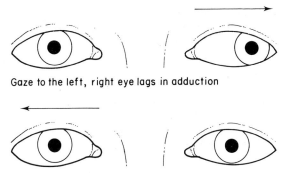

Gaze to the left, right eye lags in adduction

Gaze to the right, gaze paresis

Fig. 3.9. Right one-and-a-half syndrome. This is the combination of an internuclear ophthalmoplegia and an ipsilateral horizontal gaze paresis on the same side

The centres for conjugate vertical gaze in the brainstem lie in the midbrain. Lesions at that site cause difficulty in conjugate upgaze. The centres responsible for downgaze are less well localized, and lesions both in the midbrain and at the level of the foramen magnum can produce defects of voluntary downgaze.

Defects of vestibular function and nystagmus

The vestibular system is responsible for maintaining balance, and the direction of gaze, despite changes in head and body positions. Its components provide information on the static position of the head in space (from the otolith organs in the utricle and saccule), and on the character of dynamic changes in head position (from the semicircular canals). The information is correlated from that arising in neck proprioceptors, which provide data on the relationship of the head to the body. The integration of these various data on posture occurs in the brainstem and cerebellum. The information is used to adjust postural muscle activity to maintain balance, and eye position to maintain gaze. Damage to the vestibular system, whether it be in the labyrinth or in the brainstem/cerebellum inevitably leads to imbalance and defects of eye movement control.

Each labyrinth at rest exerts tonic influence tending to deviate the eyes to the opposite side. The effects from the two sides counterbalance each other thereby maintaining forward gaze. Sudden destruction of one labyrinth produces a forced drift of the gaze to the affected side, due to unopposed action of the normal labyrinth, followed by a rapid correction in an attempt to restore visual fixation. The jerk nystagmus provoked by such unilateral labyrinthine destruction ('canal' vestibular nystagmus) has the following characteristics: the slow phase is always directed to the abnormal ear; it is most marked when the gaze is directed away from the abnormal ear; it is predominantly horizontal or rotatory; it is independent of vision, for it persists or is enhanced when the eyes are shut in the dark or defocused using strong plus lenses (Frenzel's lenses); and it is frequently accompanied by vertigo and evidence of damage to the cochlear portion of the middle ear in the form of deafness or tinnitus. Peripheral vestibular damage causes intense vertigo, accompanied by all the other symptoms associated with 'sea-sickness' including nausea, sweating and vomiting. These symptoms are accompanied by fear. In addition, the patient is severely ataxic and often can only get around by crawling on the floor.

Compensation rapidly occurs after loss of one vestibular apparatus. The remaining intact labyrinth adapts to the new conditions so that balance is restored, and vertigo disappears over a matter of a few weeks. Indeed, even when both labyrinths are destroyed, the patient soon can walk and even dance, provided the floor is even, since visual, cutaneous and proprioceptive sensations provide the necessary alternative information.

In contrast to the dramatic and explosive symptoms caused by peripheral vestibular damage, lesions of the vestibular nerve or of its brainstem connections produce fewer symptoms. Vertigo and ataxia may be evident, but dramatic nausea and vomiting are unusual. Such brainstem damage causes 'central' vestibular nystagmus, which differs from 'canal' vestibular nystagmus in certain important characteristics: frequently it is vertical as well as horizontal; its direction changes with the direction of gaze, such that the jerk is to the right on right lateral gaze and to the left on left lateral gaze; compensation occurs but slowly; and it is improved or abolished by eye closure.

Lesions of the brainstem may cause nystagmus not only by compromising vestibular connections, but also by interfering with the mechanisms responsible for gaze. Gaze nystagmus, which is analogous to the oscillatory movement which may occur in a weak limb when the patient attempts to maintain it in a given position against gravity, occurs when the eyes are deviated in the direction of weakness of gaze. Since the pontine gaze centres are responsible for drawing the eyes towards that side, damage to this region will cause nystagmus on looking towards the lesion. In contrast, as noted above, damage to the vestibular system causes nystagmus which is maximal on looking away from the side of the lesion. As a consequence, a lesion in the cerebellopontine angle, such as an acoustic neuroma, may initially cause nystagmus on gaze away from the affected side, due to damage of vestibular fibres in the VIIIth nerve, but subsequently the nystagmus changes and becomes maximal on looking towards the side of the lesion when it has grown large enough to impinge upon the brainstem.

The otolith apparatus may be damaged alone, leaving the semicircular canals intact. In this situation, the patient complains of vertigo when the head adopts a critical posture-benign positional vertigo. Commonly this occurs at night when the patient lies on the affected ear, soon waking him. The vertigo disappears when the head posture is changed and so is transient. Benign positional nystagmus can be demonstrated in such patients, by rapidly lying them flat, turning the head with the affected ear undermost. In that position, the patient will complain of vertigo and discomfort, and jerk nystagmus will be seen. However, the symptoms and the nystagmus soon fade and disappear entirely upon repeated testing. A similar complaint rarely may occur in patients with brainstem lesions causing central positional vertigo. Again, the discomfort is evident when the head is in a critical position, but the symptoms are less marked, and no fatigue occurs.

Many of the vestibular defects described above may be deduced from careful clinical examination at the bedside. However, full assessment of vestibular function requires specialized neuro-otological investigation. This would include caloric testing in which water 7° above and below body temperature is used to irrigate the external auditory meatus. With the patient lying supine and the head flexed 30° from the horizontal, this stimulates the horizontal semi-circular canals, to produce nystagmus often with vertigo. Damage to the semi-circular canals or to vestibular nerve may abolish caloric-induced nystagmus, canal paresis. Damage to vestibular apparatus in the brainstem often produces a lesser degree of abnormality on caloric testing, in which the response to one direction is reduced to produce directional preponderance. Many other more specialized tests of vestibular function are available, but these are beyond the scope of the present book.

Muscle weakness

Weakness of muscles may be due to disease of the muscle itself (myopathy), defects in the transmission of the neuromuscular impulse at the muscle end-plate (myasthenia), damage to the motor nerve or anterior horn cell that gives rise to it (lower motor neurone lesion), or damage to the corticomotor neurone pathway (upper motor neurone lesion). The characteristic findings which allow these different lesions to be distinguished are shown in Table 3.4. The critical differences are in presence or absence of muscle wasting, changes in muscle tone and stretch reflexes, and in the distribution of weakness.

Table 3.4 Differences between upper and lower motor neurone lesions

Upper	Lower
Weak	Weak
	Wasted
	Fasciculation
Hypertonic, spastic	Hypotonic, flaccid
Clonus	
Reflexes exaggerated	Reflexes depressed or absent
Plantar responses extensor	Plantar responses flexor

Muscle wasting

The integrity of muscle fibres depends not only on their own health, but also on an intact nerve supply. Muscles waste either because they themselves are damaged (myopathy), or because of lesions of the lower motor neurones. The more proximal the damage to the lower motor neurone, the greater is the opportunity for collateral re-innervation from adjacent nerve fibres, in an attempt to overcome the consequences of denervation. Such collateral re-innervation produces abnormally large motor units, which are responsible for the involuntary twitching (fasciculation) that occurs in denervated muscles.

Muscle tone and the stretch reflex

Our understanding of the functions of the nervous system were built upon Sherrington's discovery of the stretch reflex. Muscle tone and the tendon jerks are believed to represent operation of stretch reflex mechanisms, but still there is considerable ignorance about their exact relationship.

Delivery of a tendon tap supplies the transient sudden stretch to muscle which excites primary endings wrapped around the central portion of muscle spindles. The resulting afferent volley is rapidly conducted to the spinal cord via large group 1A fibres, which synapse with anterior horn cells of both the same muscle and of synergistic muscles. The number of anterior horn cells discharged by this synchronous afferent volley depends both upon excitability of the anterior horn cell pool and the size of the afferent volley. The sensitivity of the muscle spindle endings is controlled by pre-existing tension exerted on the central portion of the spindle muscle fibres by the contractile pull of the intrafusal fibres. Contraction of the intrafusal fibres increases the tension exerted on the central receptor and, hence, increases its sensitivity to stretch. The intrafusal fibres are innervated by fusimotor nerves originating in small anterior horn cells (gamma motor neurones). Alteration of fusimotor activity therefore will change the 'bias' of muscle spindles. It follows that the amplitude of a response to a tendon tap depends on: (1) the integrity of the spinal reflex; (2) the sensitivity of the muscle spindles as determined by pre-existing activity of fusimotor neurones; and (3) the excitability of the appropriate alpha motor neurone pool.

Peripheral nerve lesions decrease the size of the tendon jerk. This is much more evident with sensory lesions than with pure motor abnormalities. Damage to sensory nerve fibres, which desynchronizes the afferent volley, soon abolishes tendon jerks. In contrast, quite extensive muscle wasting by itself may be insufficient to remove the response to a tendon tap. The tendon jerks are exaggerated (hyperreflexia) in damage to the upper motor neurone pathway, as a result of enhanced anterior horn cell excitability. The latency of the tendon jerk is more difficult to judge at the bedside, but slow muscle relaxation may be evident in patients with myxoedema and certain other metabolic disorders which delay muscle relaxation time.

Although Sherrington considered the tendon jerk to be a fractional manifestation of the stretch reflex, the basis of muscle tone as appreciated by the clinician at the bedside is unclear. Muscle tone is defined as the resistance to passive movement imposed by the examiner. Such resistance must comprise both passive elements of viscosity and elasticity arising in muscle, tendons and joints, as well as the active response of the muscle itself. Probably, muscle tone involves the combined effect of activation of both primary and secondary muscle spindle endings, both of which cause reflex muscle contraction.

Decreased muscle tone and depression of tendon jerks occur physiologically during sleep, including REM sleep, and in anaesthesia or deep coma. In all these situations, fusimotor activity and anterior horn cell excitability are likely to be decreased. Muscle tone also is diminished in cerebellar disease, perhaps as a result of decreased fusimotor spindle drive.

Increased muscle tone is characteristic of lesions of the descending motor pathways from the brain to the spinal cord. Spasticity is a resistance to attempted stretch of the muscle that increases with the applied force, until there is a sudden give at a certain tension, the 'clasp knife' or 'lengthening' reaction. Rigidity is a resistance to passive movement that continues unaltered throughout the range of movement, and so has a plastic or lead-pipe quality. Both types of hypertonia are due to excessive alpha-motor neurone discharge in response to muscle stretch. In spasticity, the tendon jerks are also exaggerated (hyper-reflexia), but in rigidity the tendon jerks are usually of normal amplitude and threshold.

The distribution of spasticity and rigidity differs. The spastic posture of the patient after a stroke, with flexed arm and extended leg, indicates that tone is increased mainly in the adductors of the shoulders, the flexors of the elbow, the flexors of the wrist and fingers, the extensors of the hip and knee, and the plantar flexors and invertors of the foot. By contrast, the posture of generalized flexion in Parkinson's disease illustrates that rigidity is maximal in all flexor muscles in the body, although it is appreciated in extensors as well.

The complete picture of damage to upper motor neurone pathways includes not only spasticity and hyper-reflexia, but also absence of the abdominal reflexes and an extensor plantar response. However, different corticoneurone pathways may be involved in the expression of these various manifestations of an upper motor neurone lesion. A lesion restricted to the 'pyramidal' pathway in the medulla, thereby sparing all other corticomotoneurone systems, only causes loss of abdominal reflexes and an extensor plantar response. Spasticity and hyper-reflexia appear when the alternative non-pyramidal cortico-motoneurone pathways are interrupted. Such damage liberates overactive segmental stretch reflex mechanisms to produce the increased muscle tone and exaggerated tendon jerks.

Distribution of muscle weakness

Careful analysis of the distribution of muscle weakness in a patient discovered to have motor signs may be invaluable. It is much easier to examine the motor than the sensory system, and deductions based upon motor deficit may dictate the pattern of subsequent sensory examination.

The distribution of weakness resulting from an upper motor neurone lesion can be recalled. The hemiplegic man has the arm flexed across the chest and the leg extended with the toes scraping the ground. Accordingly, upper motor neurone weakness selectively involves shoulder abduction, elbow flexion, wrist and finger flexion, and the small muscles of the hand, and in the leg, hip flexion, knee flexion, dorsiflexion and inversion of the foot.

Damage to the motor roots or anterior horn cells also causes distinctive patterns of weakness, depending upon the level involved (Fig. 3.10). Likewise, lesions of peripheral nerve containing motor fibres also produce a distinctive pattern of weakness. Careful attention to detail allows the examiner to distinguish weakness due to an upper motor neurone lesion from that due to root or peripheral nerve damage. The following examples will illustrate the point.

Weakness of shoulder abduction may be due to an upper motor neurone

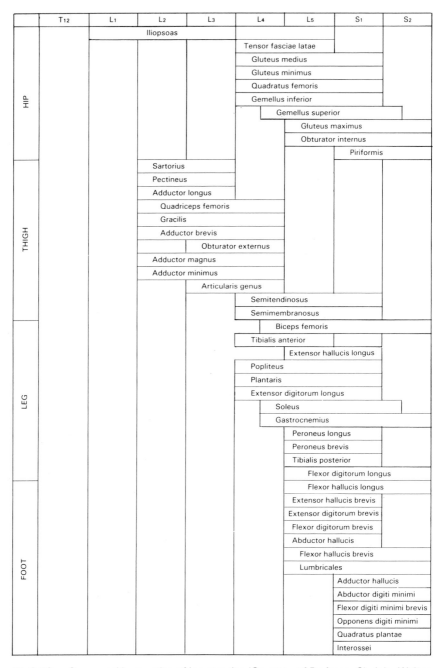

Fig 3.10a   Segmental innervation of leg muscles (Courtesy of Professor Sir John Walton and Oxford University Press *Brain's Diseases of the Nervous System* 8th edition)

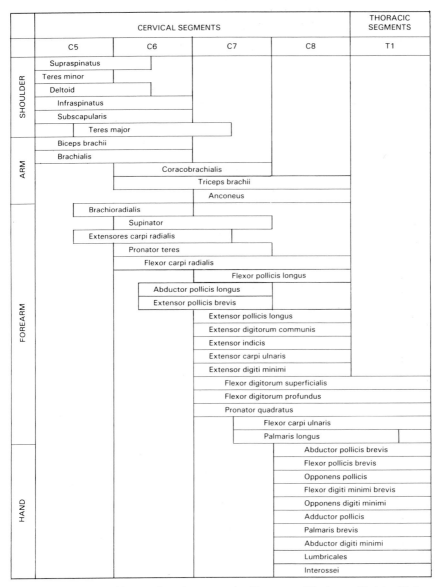

Fig 3.10b Segmental innervation of arm muscles (Courtesy of Professor Sir John Walton and Oxford University Press *Brain's Diseases of the Nervous System* 8th edition)

lesion, a C5 root lesion, or damage to the circumflex nerve. In an upper motor neurone lesion, elbow extension and wrist and finger extension will also be weak; in a C5 root lesion, the biceps will be weak and the biceps jerk will be lost; in a circumflex nerve lesion weakness will be restricted to shoulder abduction and the biceps jerk will be normal.

Elbow extension may be weak because of an upper motor neurone lesion, or damage to the radial nerve. In an upper motor neurone lesion, shoulder abduction will also be weak.

Weakness of one hand may be due to an upper motor neurone lesion, to damage to the T1 motor root or anterior horn cells, or to an ulnar nerve lesion. If an upper motor neurone lesion is responsible, there also will be weakness of wrist and finger extension, and elbow extension, and of shoulder abduction. If the ulnar nerve is involved, the thenar eminence is not wasted and the abductor pollicis brevis is strong because these are innervated by the median nerve. If the ulnar nerve is involved at the wrist, only the hand muscles will be weak. If the ulnar nerve is involved at the elbow, there will also be weakness of the long flexors (flexor digitorum profundus) of the ulnar two digits, which flex the top joints of the fingers.

Weakness of hip flexion may be due to an upper motor neurone lesion, damage to the L2/3 motor roots, or a femoral nerve lesion. If an upper motor neurone lesion is responsible, then knee flexion and dorsiflexion and eversion of the foot will be weak. If the L1/2 roots are involved, then hip adduction will also be weak, but knee flexion and dorsiflexion of the foot will be normal.

A foot drop may be due to a lesion of the upper motor neurone, of the L4/5 root, or the lateral popliteal nerve. If an upper motor neurone lesion is responsible, the hip flexion and knee flexion will also be weak. If the L4/5 roots are involved, then hip extension and knee flexion will be weak. If a lateral popliteal nerve lesion is responsible, then hip movements and knee flexion will be normal.

In addition to the very distinctive patterns of weakness due to upper motor neurone lesions, root lesions, and peripheral nerve lesions, diffuse generalized peripheral neuropathies and primary muscle disease (myopathy) also produce characteristic patterns of muscle weakness. A generalized peripheral neuropathy usually affects the longest nerve fibres first, so that the distal parts of the limbs are most affected, and the legs before the arms. Accordingly, weakness around the feet in dorsiflexion and plantar flexion with wasting of the lower limb is the commonest earliest sign of a peripheral neuropathy, to be followed by wasting and weakness of the small muscles of the hand.

In contrast, primary muscle disease selectively involves the more proximal muscles to cause weakness and wasting round the hip and shoulder girdle.

In both peripheral neuropathy and primary muscle disease, flexors and extensors are involved more or less equally. Upper motor neurone lesions, root lesions, and peripheral nerve lesions usually preferentially affect flexors or extensors with relative sparing of antagonists.

Bulbar and pseudobulbar palsy

Bilateral lower motor neurone lesions affecting the nerves supplying bulbar muscles of jaw, face, palate, pharynx and larynx cause a bulbar palsy. Speech and swallowing are impaired. In particular, speech develops a nasal quality due to escape of air through the nose. The paralysed soft palate no longer can occlude the nasopharynx. Swallowing of liquids is particularly impaired, with a tendency to regurgitate fluids back through the nose, and to cough on fluids which pass into the trachea. Paralysis of affected muscles will be evident, and the tongue will be wasted.

Pseudobulbar palsy results from bilateral damage to corticomotoneurone pathways innervating bulbar musculature. In other words, pseudobulbar palsy is the result of an upper motor neurone lesion of corticobulbar systems. A unilateral upper motor neurone corticobulbar lesion produces only transient weakness of many of the muscles supplied by the cranial nerves. Thus, after a stroke, there is no loss of power in the upper part of the face, and weakness of the muscles of the jaw, palate, neck and tongue is transient.

Bilateral damage to corticobulbar tracts causes persistent weakness and spasticity of the muscles supplied by the bulbar nuclei. As a result, there is slurring of speech, known as a spastic dysarthria, and difficulty in swallowing (dysphagia). The jaw jerk is abnormally brisk, and movements of the tongue are reduced in velocity and amplitude as a result of spasticity. In addition, patients with a pseudobulbar palsy exhibit emotional incontinence. This describes a loss of voluntary control of emotional expression such that the patient may laugh or cry without apparent provocation.

The differential diagnosis of bulbar and pseudobulbar palsies is shown in Table 3.5.

Table 3.5   Differentiation between bulbar and pseudobulbar palsies

Bulbar	Pseudobulbar
Weakness of muscles (LMN) from motor brainstem nuclei V–XII	Bilateral corticobulbar (UMN) lesions
Tongue: atrophic, fasciculating	Tongue: small, spastic, difficulty with rapid movements, protrusion
Speech: monotonous, hoarse, nasal	Speech: spastic slurring dysarthria
	Exaggerated reflexes: jaw jerk, snout, pout
Gag may be depressed	Brisk gag reflex
Lips, facial muscles may be weak. Saliva may pool and dribble	Stiff, spastic facial muscles
Spill-over of fluids, occasional nasal regurgitation	Trouble chewing, food may stay in mouth or spill out
Weak cough	May choke
	Emotional incontinence
	Often bilateral corticospinal tract signs in limbs

LMN, lower motor neurone; UMN, upper motor neurone.

Note motor neurone disease which is the commonest cause of a bilateral wasted tongue may also show UMN signs.

Sensory defects

The assessment of sensory function starts with the history, because symptoms may precede any demonstrable abnormality of simple sensation as tested by

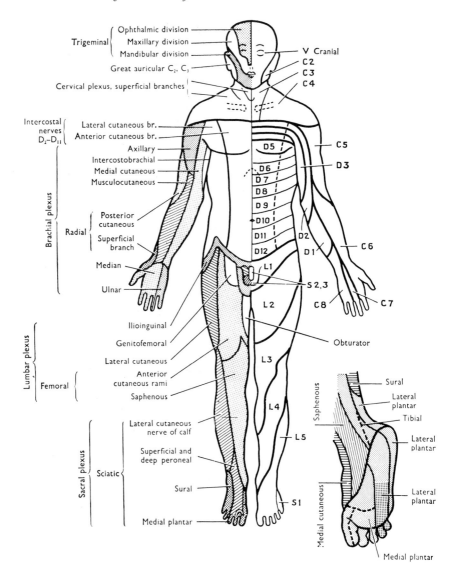

ANTERIOR ASPECT

Fig. 3.11. Cutaneous areas of distribution of spinal segments and the peripheral nerves
(a) Anterior aspect;

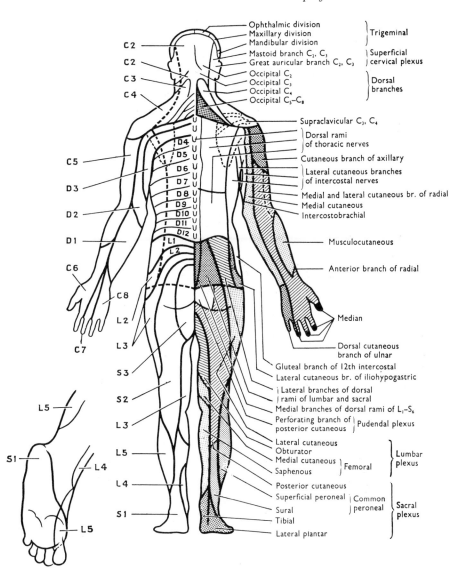

The sensory system

POSTERIOR ASPECT

(b) Posterior aspect. (Courtesy of Professor Sir John Walton and Oxford University Press: *Brain's Diseases of the Nervous System*, 9th edition. [1985])

standard clinical techniques. The patient's symptoms will suggest which area of the body, or which type of sensory function, needs the most detailed attention. The examination of the motor system will also direct attention to the appropriate sensory testing.

Sensory symptoms are of two types.

Defects of sensation

If there is impairment of all forms of cutaneous sensation the patient may complain of numbness or of freezing feelings. Many liken it to the sensation which follows dental treatment under local anaesthesia injection. If there is more specific sensory loss, it may only come to attention indirectly. Thus, inability to perceive pain usually is detected because unexpected injuries occur, such as burns of the fingers on cooking utensils or by cigarettes. Loss of temperature appreciation may be recognized by inability to perceive the heat of bath water.

Abnormal sensations

These may be qualitative changes in an existing sensation (dysaesthesiae), or spontaneous sensations (paraesthesiae). Paraesthesiae may take the form of burning, coldness, wetness or itching (all of which suggest a lesion of pain pathways), or they may consist of feelings of pins and needles, vibration, electric shock, or tightness as if wrapped with bandages (all of which suggest a lesion of the posterior column sensory pathways).

The anatomical arrangement of sensory pathways is such that the signs on physical examination usually allow one to distinguish between lesions at the following sites: a peripheral nerve or a trunk of a nerve plexus, a spinal root, the spinal cord, the brainstem, the thalamus, and the cerebral cortex. The distribution of the resulting sensory signs is illustrated in Figs 3.11–3.14.

A lesion of the peripheral nerve or of one trunk of a plexus usually causes both sensory and motor loss in its area of distribution, although one may strikingly precede the other. The sensory loss involves all sensory function, and its site roughly corresponds with the anatomical distribution of the nerve (Fig. 3.11). There is, however, considerable overlap in the area of supply of individual peripheral nerves, so that the extent of sensory loss after damage to a given nerve varies considerably from one subject to another. Partial lesions of peripheral nerves tend to affect the appreciation of touch more than that of pain.

Peripheral neuropathies tend to affect the longest fibres first, so symmetrical sensory loss starts in the legs before the arms, and begins in the feet and then the hands. The result is the classical 'glove-and-stocking' pattern of sensory disturbance (Fig. 3.12).

Lesions of a posterior spinal root cause sensory loss without motor deficit, although the appropriate tendon jerk is depressed or absent. The sensory loss will correspond roughly with the anatomical area of root supply (the dermatome) (*see* Fig. 3.11). However, there is considerable overlap of dermatomes, so that the extent of sensory deficit after individual root damage is much less than that predicted from its known distribution. Indeed, loss of a single posterior root may produce no sensory deficit that can be detected.

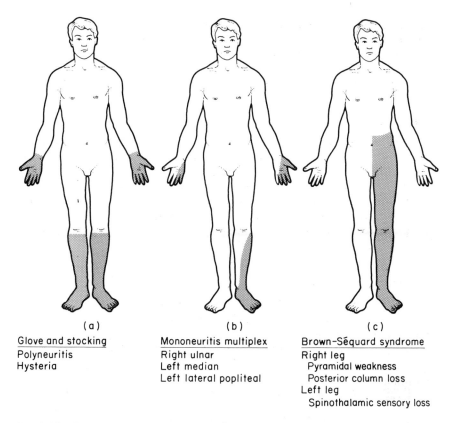

(a)	(b)	(c)
Glove and stocking	Mononeuritis multiplex	Brown-Séquard syndrome
Polyneuritis	Right ulnar	Right leg
Hysteria	Left median	Pyramidal weakness
	Left lateral popliteal	Posterior column loss
		Left leg
		Spinothalamic sensory loss

Fig. 3.12.   Patterns of sensory loss

Root damage commonly impairs appreciation of pain more than that of touch.

Complete lesions of the spinal cord cause loss of all forms of sensation, and of motor activity, in those areas supplied by the cord below the lesion (Fig. 3.13). Also, there will be a fairly well defined 'upper level' for the loss of both sensory and motor function. Partial lesions may cause a sensory loss unaccompanied by motor loss, and also may cause selective loss of one or more types of sensation. Such dissociated sensory loss occurs because the different sensory pathways follow different anatomical roots in the spinal cord.

The lateral spinothalamic tract contains the second sensory neurone conveying the sensations of pain, temperature, tickle and itch, and to some extent those responsible for appreciation of touch, from the contralateral side of the body. The posterior columns contain the central processes of the first sensory neurones conveying the sensations of joint position, vibration, and to some extent those of touch for the ipsilateral half of the body. The dorsal columns also carry the sensory fibres responsible for judgement of location of the site of the stimulus, its weight, texture, and the capacity to distinguish between two separated points.

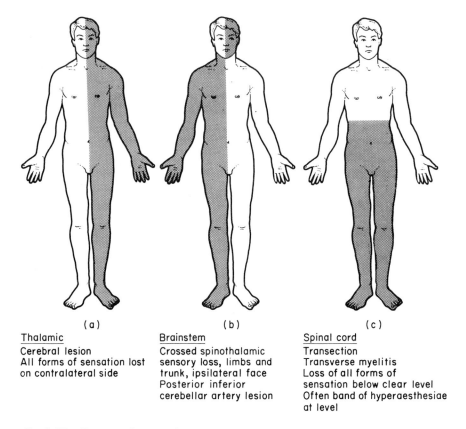

| (a) | (b) | (c) |

Thalamic

Cerebral lesion
All forms of sensation lost
on contralateral side

Brainstem

Crossed spinothalamic
sensory loss, limbs and
trunk, ipsilateral face
Posterior inferior
cerebellar artery lesion

Spinal cord

Transection
Transverse myelitis
Loss of all forms of
sensation below clear level
Often band of hyperaesthesiae
at level

Fig. 3.13.   Patterns of sensory loss

Lesions which cause dissociated sensory loss include damage to one half of the spinal cord (Brown-Séquard syndrome), damage to the anterior half of the cord, and expanding intramedullary lesions. Each of these disorders will produce a particular pattern of dissociated sensory loss, in combination with distinctive motor signs below the lesion. In the Brown-Séquard syndrome there is ipsilateral loss of vibration and position sense, and impairment of tactile discrimination, with contralateral loss of pain and temperature sensation (*see* Fig. 3.12). Voluntary motor activity is lost on the side of the lesion. With damage to the anterior half of the spinal cord, there is bilateral loss of pain and temperature sensation and of voluntary motor activity, but preservation of touch, vibration and position sense. An intramedullary lesion which interrupts the decussating fibres from the dorsal grey column to the lateral spinothalamic tract often causes preferential loss of pain and temperature appreciation in a segmental distribution corresponding to the site of cord involvement.

The anatomical level of sensory loss which accompanies spinal cord lesions is affected by a number of factors, and may be misleading. For example, in spinal cord lesions, the upper level of loss of pain and temperature is often two or three segments below the site of the lesion. This is because the fibres conveying pain and temperature cross the cord obliquely, and may ascend for a few segments before decussation. A lesion compressing the spinal cord from the outside tends to affect the most superficial fibres first. In the lateral spinothalamic tract, these are from the legs. Accordingly, extramedullary cord compression initially produces sensory disturbance in the legs which then ascends as the lesion progresses. In contrast, intramedullary lesions of the cervical cord produce loss of pain and temperature sensation in the arms, before the legs or sacral regions show any sensory deficit (suspended sensory loss) (Fig. 3.14).

Within the brainstem, the arrangement of sensory tracts changes. The first neurones of the posterior column synapse in the gracile and cuneate nuclei, and then cross to enter the medial lemniscus, now lying in close relation to the lateral lemniscus carrying fibres from the spinothalamic pathway. In addition, sensory fibres from the fifth nerve join the lemniscal system so that a unilateral lesion in the pons tends to cause loss of all varieties of sensation from the opposite half of the body. However, a lesion in the medulla may cause crossed sensory loss. This consists of contralateral loss of all sensation and ipsilateral loss of pain and temperature over the face. Such a pattern arises because fibres of the fifth nerve subserving pain and temperature descend in the spinal tract of the fifth nerve into the medulla, before synapsing in the nucleus of that tract and then ascending in the trigeminal lemniscus.

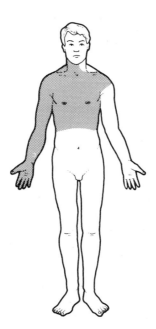

Fig. 3.14. Intramedullary spinal cord lesions. Spinothalamic sensory loss in the right arm and 'cuirasse' distribution over the chest. Lost arm reflexes. Pyramidal signs and posterior column sensory loss in the legs, i.e. dissociated sensory loss

The second sensory neurones from the opposite half of the body all terminate in the thalamus, from which the third sensory neurone fibres pass to the cortex on the same side. Thalamic lesions thus cause loss of all types of sensation on the opposite half of the body (*see* Fig. 3.13). In addition, for reasons that are not understood, thalamic damage may cause an abnormally heightened affective response to sensory stimuli. Mild sensations may become painful (hyperpathia). Thus, the single pinprick produces a perverted sensation of pain, which is poorly localized, protracted, and intensely disagreeable. In addition, thalamic lesions, may produce spontaneous thalamic or central pains.

Lesions of the cerebral cortex characteristically affect the ability to integrate sensory information, and to make judgements based upon crude sensory appreciation from the opposite half of the body. Cortical damage does not impair the ability to be able to appreciate simple touch, pain, temperature, or vibration. However, the patient cannot utilize such information to make sensory judgements. Thus, appreciation of joint position and two point discrimination is impaired. The ability to identify familiar objects placed in the hand (stereognosis), and the ability to judge the comparative size and weight of different objects placed in the hand, are compromised by cortical lesions. Another useful test of cortical sensory function is the ability to perceive two simultaneous sensory stimuli applied with equal intensity to corresponding sites on opposite sides of the body. A unilateral cortical lesion may lead to failure to perceive the contralateral stimulus, even though it is easily detected when administered by itself. Such sensory neglect, when severe, may extend to an apparent unawareness of the contralateral limb or even one whole half of the body, a form of agnosia.

Coma

Impairment of cerebral function causes depression or clouding of consciousness leading to coma. Many terms are used to describe various levels of depression of consciousness. Comatose patients are unconscious and unable to respond to verbal command, although they may show motor responses to painful stimuli. Stuporose patients are unconscious, but can be roused by verbal command or painful stimuli for short periods to produce a verbal response. When stimulation ceases, they lapse back into coma. Confused patients are alert, but disoriented for time, place and even person. Delirious patients are confused, but also restless and overactive. Another way to describe delirium is a toxic confusional state.

These various grades of depression of consciousness are difficult to define accurately in practice. A valuable method of recording prognostic data is the international Coma Scale (Table 3.6), which has proved to be easy to administer by doctors and nurses. The scale describes the best verbal, motor, and eye response to stimulation, either by verbal command or pain. Each of the three categories of response is graded on a scale ranging from normal (the patient is oriented, obeys verbal command, and shows spontaneous eye opening) to deep coma (the patient exhibits no verbal response to stimulation, no motor response to pain, and never spontaneously opens the eyes). In addition, it is crucial to record the pupillary responses to light, the reflex eye movements in both vertical

Table 3.6 Coma scale

Assessment of conscious level	
Eye opening	
spontaneous	4
to speech	3
to pain	2
none	1
Best motor response	
obeying	6
localizing	5
weak flexion	4
abnormal flexion	3
abnormal extension	2
none	1
Best verbal response	
orientated	5
confused	4
inappropriate	3
incomprehensible	2
none	1

After Teasdale and Jennett (1974)

and horizontal plane to oculocephalic (doll's head manoeuvre) and/or caloric stimulation, the blood pressure, respiration, pulse and temperature in every unconscious patient.

Other terms are used to describe the level of consciousness and physical state of patients surviving coma. A persistent vegetative state refers to a patient who shows no signs of any function of the cerebral cortex. Such patients survive coma, but do not speak or exhibit any purposeful response to the outside world. They may show periods of wakefulness, groan or grunt, and exhibit stereotyped primitive movements in response to external stimuli, but they have no intelligent communication. This state also has been called the apallic syndrome. The 'locked-in' syndrome refers to patients who have sustained extensive damage to the pons to cause complete loss of speech and quadriplegia. However, because the midbrain is intact such patients are alert and have a normal EEG. Their only means of communication is by eye movements. The pontine damage paralyses horizontal gaze, but eye-lid movement and vertical gaze is preserved. These patients can see, hear, and think normally. Akinetic mutism refers to patients who recover from serious brain insult to a level between the persistent vegetative state and conscious communication. They are speechless and immobile, except for primitive reflex movements that can be provoked, e.g. feeding. They appear to have a sleep–waking cycle, and when the eyes are open they will follow objects as if taking an interest in their surroundings. However, they never exhibit any indication of intelligent communication.

Causes of coma

Consciousness depends on stimulation of the cerebral cortex by the ascending reticular activating systems arising in the upper brainstem. A unilateral lesion of the cerebral cortex will not cause coma, unless there is space-occupation to distort the opposite hemisphere and the brainstem. Diffuse bilateral cortical damage does produce coma. Relatively small lesions affecting the upper brainstem, thereby damaging the ascending activating systems, also cause coma. However, lesions of the pons and medulla will not cause coma unless they occupy space to cause distortion of the upper brainstem.

Unconsciousness, therefore, is caused either by diffuse brain disease or by a focal upper brainstem lesion. Diffuse brain disease may be the result of some generalized extrinsic condition, whose primary cause lies outside the brain, or to diffuse intrinsic disease of the brain itself. Extrinsic conditions will include metabolic disturbances such as diabetic coma, renal or hepatic failure, and self-poisoning with alcohol or drugs. Intrinsic causes would include the diffuse cerebral effects of meningitis, encephalitis, traumatic concussion and subarachnoid haemorrhage.

Focal brain lesions causing coma most commonly are abscesses, traumatic extradural or subdural haematomas, primary intracerebral haemorrhage or post-infarct swelling, or tumours.

Pathophysiology of coma

Diffuse brain disease usually causes coma by interfering with cerebral metabolism. The energy requirements of the brain are normally supplied by the oxidation of glucose. Each 100 g of human brain utilizes 5 mg of glucose/min, and the brain as a whole consumes 15–20 per cent of the total oxygen consumption of the body at rest, which amounts to 3.3 ml O_2/100 g brain/h. The carbohydrate reserves of the brain are only about 2 g, and there are almost no reserves of oxygen. The brain is therefore critically dependent on its blood supply for its large requirements of both glucose and oxygen. The resting cerebral blood flow is about 50 ml/100 g of brain/min which amounts to nearly one-fifth of the cardiac output.

When the brain is deprived of its supply of oxygen or glucose, function declines almost immediately and consciousness rapidly is lost. Cortical neurones are highly vulnerable to lack of oxygen or glucose, and loss of consciousness probably results from widespread depression of cortical function.

Focal brain lesions cause coma in one of two ways. Focal damage to the upper brainstem destroys the ascending activating systems responsible for consciousness. Focal space-occupying lesions supratentorially, or in the posterior fossa, cause coma by impairing brainstem function as a result of pressure and distortion. Small lesions of the cerebral hemispheres usually do not produce coma, but as a tumour grows or a blood clot or abscess expands inside the skull, they begin to displace intracranial contents. Because the skull and spinal canal have very rigid walls, a mass lesion can only be accommodated by displacement of other intracranial materials. A little blood can be displaced from collapsible veins (but not from the major sinuses which are well protected by tough dural and bony walls), and the total CSF pool can be reduced. However, once these compensatory mechanisms have taken place, further growth of a mass must cause a rise of pressure within the skull and displacement of brain away from the lesion. The latter may lead to blockage of the major drainage routes of CSF, which may cause further increases in intracranial pressure.

The tentorium cerebelli and the falx cerebri act as relatively immobile partitions within the skull. An enlarging mass lesion thus causes severe distortion of the displaced brain in the neighbourhood of the dural folds. A supratentorial mass lesion pushes the brain towards the opposite side, and some of it is squeezed under the falx. The midbrain and diencephalon are squeezed through the tentorial notch into the infratentorial compartment. The upper brainstem thus is distorted by stretch and by compression against the unyielding edge of the tentorium. In addition, the inferomedial portion of the temporal lobe, the uncus, may be squeezed through the tentorial notch to compress and distort the midbrain together with the adjacent IIIrd cranial nerve. As this process of transtentorial herniation occurs, not only is the brainstem distorted and stretched, but the blood vessels supplying it, which are relatively tethered, are also torn and stretched. As a result, haemorrhage occurs in the upper brainstem as transtentorial herniation occurs and consciousness is lost.

Infratentorial posterior fossa mass lesions also cause shifts of intracranial content. They force the brainstem upwards through the tentorial notch, causing midbrain distortion, and force the medulla and cerebellar tonsils down through the foramen magnum, leading to medullary herniation. The shift of the intracranial contents through the tentorial notch or through the foramen magnum generally is referred to as 'coning'.

It is obvious that both supratentorial and infratentorial large mass lesions may result in compression, distortion and ischaemia of the brainstem as a result of coning. However, in addition to the mass itself, other important factors also may contribute to impairment of brain function in these circumstances. The volume and pressure of blood in capillaries is controlled, in part, by the tone of the cerebral arterioles and these will dilate in response to a rise in local $P\text{CO}_2$, or a fall of $P\text{O}_2$. Consequently, hypoventilation can result in a further increase in intracranial pressure. The rise in $P\text{CO}_2$ and fall in $P\text{O}_2$ that follows respiratory failure leads to cerebral arteriolar dilatation, and an increased volume of blood in the skull, which must cause further coning. A period of respiratory depression can thus be disastrous for a patient with an intracranial mass lesion. Indeed, when an intracranial mass produces coma by brainstem compression, matters are delicately poised. Once the compression begins to cause impairment of function in the respiratory centre, a 'vicious cycle' may be initiated, which can rapidly result in death. Fortunately, the development of a pressure cone is accompanied by a sequence of physical signs resulting from progressive impairment of brain function. These should give sufficient warning of the impending disaster, provided the patient is examined frequently. As will be described later, the process of coning causes an orderly sequence of loss of neuronal function which can point clearly to what is happening.

Patients at risk of coning, or in the process of coning due to large intracranial mass lesions may be treated as an emergency by shrinking intracranial contents. Assisted ventilation will reduce cerebral blood volume to give more space, and cerebral oedema around infarcts, haemorrhages, or tumours may be reduced by the use of intravenous mannitol. Mannitol, a hyperosmolar agent, withdraws oedema fluid out of the brain, and causes a brisk diuresis. Intravenous infusion of 100–200 ml of 20 per cent mannitol will rapidly reduce intracranial pressure and may stop or reverse the process of coning long enough to allow further investigation and definitive treatment to be undertaken. Steroids also reduce cerebral oedema, but their effect is slower in onset. Dexamethasone 5–10 mg intravenously followed by 4 mg 6 hourly may help to control cerebral oedema.

Examination of the unconscious patient

Because the patient cannot cooperate, a different system of examination must be employed to assess coma. A suitable sequence should include the following investigations.

Respiration and circulation: the first and most urgent need is to make sure that respiration and circulation are adequate to sustain life. If either are compromised, emergency action should be taken to ensure an airway with assisted ventilation, and an adequate cardiac output. Once emergency resuscitation has been completed, further examination can continue.

Blood pressure, pulse and temperature are recorded, and the character of respiration noted.

Damage to respiratory neurones produces a variety of abnormalities of respiration. Cheyne-Stokes breathing refers to periodic cycles of hyperventilation alternating with apnoea, the complete cycle lasting about a minute. The patient ceases respiration, then begins to breathe again, the rate and depth increasing to a peak, and then dying away again. The commonest cause is circulatory failure. A similar pattern, with a shorter cycle length of about half a minute, occurs in some patients with midbrain and internal capsular lesions. Central neurogenic hyperventilation is associated with destruction of the reticular formation of the pons and the midbrain. It causes respiratory alkalosis. Apneustic breathing describes a prolonged pause after each inspiration before the next expiration occurs. It results from damage to the caudal respiratory neurones in the pons. Ataxic breathing is completely irregular in amplitude and frequency. It indicates damage to the respiratory neurones in the medulla. Gasping respiration is characterized by an abrupt inspiration followed by expiration, then a long pause before the next breath. It occurs shortly before death.

Progressive transtentorial herniation of the brainstem thus may produce an orderly sequence of changes in respiration. As coning occurs, central neurogenic hyperventilation may give way to apneustic breathing, followed by ataxic breathing, gasping respiration and then death.

Assess level of consciousness: take note of the patient's spontaneous verbal, motor and ocular responses, and observe how they react to external circumstances and your commands. The aim will be to place the patient in the appropriate category on the Coma Scale in due course. Suitable graded stimuli are spoken commands, shouted commands, pinprick, pressing on the supraorbital notch or sternum, which causes severe pain. While watching the response of the patient to stimuli, always look for asymmetric motor reactions, or apparent neglect of such stimuli on one half of the body.

Examine the head: the skull. Palpate the skull for signs of fracture and for bruising. Note any bruising or discharge of CSF from ears, nose or mouth. This would suggest a fracture at the base of the skull.

The neck: flex the neck on the head and note any resistance to movement suggesting irritation of the meninges by infection or by blood. Obviously this test should not be carried out if there is a suspicion that cervical vertebrae may have been fractured.

The eyes: the visual fields may be examined in such patients either by advancing a bright light in each quadrant, or by making a threatening movement of the hand towards the eye. Patients whose level of consciousness allows reaction to such stimuli, will turn the head and eyes away, or blink.

Examine the optic fundi with the ophthalmoscope.

Note the size of the pupils and their response to light. The midbrain contains the IIIrd nerve, parasympathetic and pretectile nuclei, so that midbrain lesions produce obvious pupillary abnormalities. The pupils, therefore, are invaluable in indicating the presence of a focal brain lesion as responsible for coma. A unilateral supratentorial mass lesion causing transtentorial coning, leads to a IIIrd nerve palsy as the process evolves. The pupil on the side of the lesion dilates, becomes unreactive to light and accommodation, ptosis develops and the eye turns down and out. Bilateral supratentorial mass lesions, or diffuse brain swelling, which produces a central transtentorial herniation, tend to affect pupillary pathways in the diencephalon and brainstem in an orderly sequence. At first, damage to the sympathetic fibres causes the pupils to become small but reactive. Then, as the process evolves, the pupils begin to dilate and eventually become completely dilated and unreactive to light. Primary pontine lesions spare the parasympathetic pupillary systems, causing disruption only of sympathetic mechanisms. As a result, the pupils are constricted and may become very small ('pinpoint' pupils). Lesions of the lateral part of the medulla affect the descending sympathetic fibres to produce a unilateral Horner's syndrome.

Some specific poisons also affect the pupillary responses, e.g. atropine causes dilatation, opiates cause constriction, and glutethimide dilates the pupils.

The pupillary responses are, perhaps, the single most important guide to the cause of coma. It can be stated that an unconscious patient showing no focal motor deficit, who has equal, normal-sized, and reactive pupils is in coma because of diffuse brain disease. The absence of a history or signs of cerebral trauma, and normal CSF examination in such patients will exclude intrinsic causes of diffuse brain disease. In those circumstances a confident diagnosis of extrinsic diffuse brain disease or 'metabolic' coma can be made.

One other pupillary sign is worth noting. In patients whose brainstem is intact, the pupils dilate in response to painful stimuli. Thus, pinching the side of the neck will elicit the ciliospinal reflex, which stimulates both ascending and descending pathways of the brainstem.

Examine eye movements. Provided the patient is capable of some response to command, the range of eye movements can be assessed simply. However, many stuporose and/or comatose patients will not obey verbal command, so eye movements must be tested in other ways. Two techniques can be used. Eye movement may be provoked by the oculocephalic reflexes elicited by the doll's head manoeuvre. Brisk rotation of the head from side to side, or flexion and extension of the neck, will provoke conjugate eye movements in the opposite direction to the head movement. This gives the impression that the patient's gaze is focused on an object straight in front of him. Such oculocephalic

responses are attributed to the effect of vestibular input combined with proprioceptive impulses from the neck. This information eventually ascends via the
medial longitudinal bundle in the brainstem to the ocular motor nuclei. Preservation of horizontal and vertical eye movement in response to the doll's head
manoeuvre implies that the brainstem is intact. Loss of reflex conjugate upgaze
indicates damage to the midbrain. Loss of reflex conjugate horizontal gaze
indicates damage to the pons. Disconjugate eye movements may be provoked
by the doll's head manoeuvre, or may occur spontaneously in the comatose
patient. Failure of lateral deviation of one eye when gaze is reflexly provoked in
that direction indicates a VIth nerve palsy. Failure of adduction of the eye with
normal abduction suggests an internuclear ophthalmoplegia. If the doll's head
manoeuvre is insufficient to provoke eye movement, then caloric responses may
be employed to elicit vestibulo-ocular reflexes, which again depend upon an
intact brainstem. Ice-cold water is syringed into each ear in turn, making
certain that the ear-drum is normal before doing so. If brainstem function is
intact, there will either be nystagmus in the direction away from the irrigated
ear, or a conjugate deviation of the eyes to the irrigated side. Again, those with
specific ocular motor nerve palsies may show a disconjugate response to caloric
stimulation. In addition to examination of voluntary or reflex eye movements,
spontaneous eye movements should be carefully recorded in the unconscious
patient. Tonic deviation of the eyes conjugately to one side suggests a focal
lesion, either of the cerebral hemisphere or of the brainstem. With a hemisphere
lesion, the opposite limbs will be paralysed and the eyes will look away from
them towards the side of the lesion. In a brainstem pontine lesion, the opposite
limbs will be paralysed, but the eyes will look towards them, i.e. away from the
side of the lesion. Other abnormalities of spontaneous eye movement are
described in coma.

The face: look for signs of unilateral facial paralysis (drooping of one side of
the mouth which is puffed out with each breath). Test the corneal reflexes with a
wisp of cotton-wool, and the facial response to pinprick or supraorbital
pressure. Both of these stimuli should cause screwing up of the same side of the
face.

The ears: examine the ear-drums with an auroscope, looking for evidence of
middle ear infection, such as an opaque, bulging drum, or a ruptured drum
with purulent discharge.

The mouth: smell the breath for alcohol, ketones, or other distinctive odours.
Look for lacerations of the tongue which suggest an epileptic fit in the recent
past. Check the presence of a 'gag' reflex.

Examine the limbs: establish whether all four limbs move, either
spontaneously or in response to painful stimuli. Squeezing the Achilles tendon
or a finger nail, or rubbing the sternum are useful means of provoking reflex
movement. Such stimuli should always be applied at various sites to allow for
local anaesthesia. Failure to move an arm or leg on one side in response to
stimuli on each side in turn, indicates a hemiplegia. Absence of any limb
movement in response to all strong stimuli occurs with bilateral severe damage
to the brainstem, as in the 'locked-in' syndrome, but also occurs in very deep
coma without any focal brain damage.

Provided the limbs are not paralysed, stimuli may provoke appropriate or inappropriate reflex responses. When there is no motor defect, painful stimuli will cause withdrawal of the limb, attempts to remove the source of pain with the opposite limb, screwing up of the face, and even verbal responses. The earliest motor sign of focal cerebral damage is the appearance of stereotyped limb movements in response to painful stimuli. Destructive lesions involving the internal capsule cause decorticate rigidity. A painful stimulus provokes flexion and adduction of the arm with extension of the leg on the affected side. Damage to the upper brainstem causes decerebrate rigidity in response to a painful stimulus. The neck retracts, and the teeth clench. The affected arm extends, adducts, and the forearm pronates. The affected leg extends and the foot plantar flexes. Spontaneous spasms of decerebrate rigidity may occur with severe brainstem lesions, often accompanied by shivering, hypertension and hyperpyrexia.

Muscle tone can be assessed in the unconscious patient by passive manipulation of the limbs, or by noting the response to dropping the limb to the bed. Lift the arms and legs, individually or together, and note the speed with which they fall to the bed when dropped. Hemiplegic limbs, which are flaccid in the acute stage, fall harder and faster than normal limbs.

Examine the tendon jerks and plantar responses. However, remember that it may take some days for hyper-reflexia and Babinski's sign to appear after an acute lesion of corticomotor neurone pathways. In the stage of shock following an acute hemiplegia, the limbs are flaccid, the tendon jerks are normal or absent, and the plantar may be unresponsive.

General examination: examine the heart, lungs and abdomen.

Always test the urine for protein, glucose and ketones, and examine it with a microscope for pus cells and casts.

If the course of coma is not apparent at this stage, *always measure the blood glucose* concentration and administer glucose intravenously. Most casualty departments have an absolute rule that a blood glucose must be done on all unconscious patients. In addition, give thiamine and other vitamin B components in the form of intramuscular high potency parentrovite. Many unconscious patients admitted to some casualty departments are victims of chronic alcohol abuse, and may have Wernicke's encephalopathy.

The differential diagnosis of coma

The important features distinguishing diffuse brain disease and focal brain lesions causing coma are shown in Table 3.7. The important features distinguishing a supratentorial focal brain lesion from an infratentorial focal lesion causing coma are shown in Table 3.8.

The initial clinical assessment and examination may have revealed the obvious cause of coma. If not, blood glucose is measured, and glucose and thiamine administered.

Now is the time to obtain as much information as possible on the background of the patient. Witnesses to the circumstances in which the individual was found must be questioned. These will include policemen, ambulance attendants, relatives and friends. The patient's clothing must be searched, for evidence such as a diabetic or steroid card, or an empty bottle for sleeping tablets. If known,

Table 3.7   Differentiation of diffuse and focal brain lesions leading to coma

Diffuse
  Absence of focal or lateralizing signs: motor or sensory
  May be bilateral changes in tone, reflexes and extensor plantar responses
  Brainstem functions often preserved initially, especially ocular movements and
    pupillary responses
  Often self-poisoning, metabolic causes, infection, bleeding or epilepsy, so CT brain
    scan often negative
Focal
  Focal or lateralizing signs usually present to suggest hemisphere or brainstem damage.
    Include flaccid weakness and loss of response to pain on one side
  Reflex asymmetry, including plantar response
  Tonic deviation of eyes to one side
  Derangements in ocular motility and pupillary responses
  Often supratentorial mass (abscess, tumour, haematoma) or infratentorial mass
    (haematoma, tumour), so CT brain scan positive

Table 3.8   Differentiation of supratentorial focal from infratentorial lesion in patients
with a depressed conscious level

Supratentorial
  Focal mass has to expand to compress the other hemisphere and cause brainstem
    compression to produce coma
  May be clear unilateral focal signs
  Often brainstem reflexes initially preserved: pupillary responses, ocular movements,
    gag, corneal, etc
  Eyes may be tonically deviated to side of lesion (away from hemiplegia)
  May be focal epileptic seizures
  Sometimes decorticate rigidity
  Late: unilateral oculomotor palsy with uncal cone
Infratentorial
  Small lesions damaging the reticular formation may cause early coma with often signs
    of midbrain or even foramen magnum coning
  Brainstem reflexes impaired: abnormal pupils (e.g. bilateral pinpoint), impaired ocular
    motility, lost corneal, gag, etc
  Impaired doll's head and cold caloric reflexes
  Eyes may be tonically deviated away from the side of a pontine lesion (towards
    hemiplegia)
  Hyperventilation, irregular breathing patterns: apnoea
  Decerebrate rigidity

the patient's general practitioner can be approached for further information
and other relatives contacted. Any containers brought by relatives or witnesses
should be kept for analysis in patients suspected of self-poisoning.

If the cause of coma is still not apparent, then a series of investigations should
now be set in train (*see* later), and the patient kept under close observation.
Subsequent events may clarify the situation, so it is particularly important to
repeat parts of the initial examination at intervals to assess progress.

The most sensitive index of change is the state of consciousness, but heart
rate, blood pressure, temperature, limb movements, pupillary size and reaction
to light, should all be regularly observed and recorded.

Investigations in coma

In those in whom the cause of coma is not evident, the direction of investigation is determined by whether examination suggests that it is due to diffuse brain disease, or a focal brain lesion. If a focal lesion is suspected, examination of the CSF may be dangerous. Reducing CSF pressure by lumbar puncture may precipitate further coning and death. Accordingly, when focal brain lesions are suspected to be the cause, investigations should be directed towards the head in the form of skull X-rays, EEG, radioactive brain scan or CT scan. The most important of these is a CT brain scan. When a mass lesion has been excluded by these techniques, then the CSF should be examined for the presence of blood or pus.

If diffuse brain disease is suspected to be the cause of coma, and there are no signs of a focal mass lesion, then lumbar puncture is mandatory to exclude meningitis, encephalitis or subarachnoid haemorrhage. This is particularly so in any drowsy or unconscious patient with meningism.

If diffuse brain disease is suspected, and there is no meningism and the CSF is normal, then the following metabolic and other investigations should be undertaken: full blood count, erythrocyte sedimentation rate, blood glucose, urea and electrolytes, liver function tests, blood alcohol and ammonia levels, and a screen for drug levels that might be responsible for self-poisoning. If the patient has a temperature, or there is some other clue to infection, blood cultures should be set up. A urine sample should be sent for routine analysis, also for estimation of drug levels, osmolality and even porphyrins. The EEG is a valuable test in suspected 'metabolic' coma. The finding of a focal abnormality may provide the diagnosis towards a focal brain lesion as the cause. Generalized abnormalities may be found in any metabolic disorder, or in meningitis and encephalitis. Epileptic discharges may be detected. Certain rare encephalitic diseases may show diagnostic changes of periodic widespread discharges.

While awaiting the results of these various investigations, the patient should be continually monitored, as described above. Adequate airway and ventilation should be maintained. This may require an oropharyngeal airway, an endotracheal tube, or even assisted respiration. Fluid and caloric supplements should be given with continued added vitamins. Initially this may require intravenous infusion, but a nasogastric tube may be used subsequently. The bladder should be catheterized and regular fluid balance charts instituted. The patient should be regularly turned every 2 h to prevent bedsores.

Cerebral death

Rapid and efficient resuscitation is now widely available and saves lives. However, it also reclaims some individuals whose brain is so severely damaged that they will never recover an intelligent existence. For all intents and purposes, their brain is dead, but the heart continues to beat. Eventually, even the heart will cease beating. Such patients may be said to have suffered cerebral death.

The importance of defining cerebral death is twofold. First, once it can be established with certainty that cerebral death has occurred, the patient's relatives may be informed that there is no point in continuing resuscitation and life-support. After discussion, it may be deemed appropriate to cease artificial ventilation. Second, once the diagnosis of cerebral death has been established beyond doubt, the possibility of using that patient's organs for transplantation arises.

The criteria for cerebral death must be fool-proof. If there is any doubt, the diagnosis should not be made. Irreversible brainstem damage from a known cause is synonymous with cerebral death.

To diagnose cerebral death the *cause* of the brain damage must be known. Often this is obvious as after major trauma or a subarachnoid haemorrhage. Such a cause must be *irreversible*: this will exclude patients who are hypothermic, have received recent doses of neuromuscular blocking drugs, depressant drugs or who have a possible metabolic or endocrine defect causing coma.

The affected patient will be on a ventilator as spontaneous breathing has failed and will not be 'fighting' the machine. There must be no signs of any residual brainstem function.

1. The pupils are fixed, dilated and unreactive.
2. There are absent corneal reflexes.
3. There are absent oculocephalic (doll's head) and oculovestibular (cold caloric) reflexes.
4. There is an absent 'gag' reflex or no response to a suction catheter in the trachea.
5. No purposeful movements should be elicited, nor facial grimaces to painful stimuli applied to the limbs, trunk or face.
6. The patient's medullary respiratory centre will not respond to a rise in arterial carbon dioxide ($P_a CO_2$) of greater than 6.65 kPa (50 mmHg) if the patient is disconnected from the ventilator, i.e. to an adequate chemical stimulus for that centre.

Such tests should be repeated after an interval to ensure that they remain absent.

4

Diseases of muscle and the neuromuscular junction

There has been a surge of interest in diseases of muscle over the past 25 years. In part this stemmed from the introduction of cortisone as a therapeutic agent and its benefit in some muscle disorders. Henceforward, the realization that many muscle diseases were treatable accelerated the need for accurate diagnosis and led to parallel developments in neurophysiology and muscle pathology. Subsequently there has been increasing interest in the genetics of familial muscle disease and the identification of carriers of recessively inherited conditions.

Diagnosis and investigation

Patients with muscle disorders nearly always complain of weakness. Limb weakness is most common, proximal and girdle musculature being selectively or preferentially affected. This results in complaints of difficulty in lifting the arms above the head to brush hair or hang out washing, and problems rising from a low chair or climbing stairs. Involvement of the muscles innervated by the cranial nerves produces drooping of the eyelids, double vision, difficulty with chewing and swallowing and alteration of the voice. Weakness of facial muscles impedes sucking, kissing or blowing up ballons. The head may flop due to neck weakness. It is always important to find out how long symptoms have been present, their rate of progression, and whether there is fluctuation or fatiguability. Many muscle disorders are insidious and the patient may not consult a doctor until the disease has been present for some years. Enquiries should always be made about muscle pain, and also sensory disturbance, as the differentiation from primary neuropathic disorders may be difficult.

On examination it is important to assess the individual muscles throughout the body. Although patients may complain of weakness in only one part, it is frequently found that the loss of strength is more extensive. Particular attention should be paid to the presence or absence of fasciculation, to wasting, to the distribution of muscle weakness and its degree. Muscles should be palpated for tenderness and the state of the tendon reflexes carefully elicited. It is also important to exclude any sensory change which never occurs in primary muscle disorders.

The investigation of muscle disorders does not usually have to be too extensive. Some myopathies are associated with systemic illness so that a blood count, erythrocyte sedimentation rate (ESR) and chest X-ray should be carried out. It is also important to perform a biochemical screen with particular reference to serum potassium and calcium levels as electrolyte alterations may produce muscle weakness. Thyroid function tests may show thyrotoxicosis. An ECG may indicate cardiac muscle involvement.

There are three investigations which are specific for muscle disorders: the serum creatine kinase level, electromyography (EMG), and muscle biopsy. The level to which the creatine kinase is elevated in the blood will depend on the rate of muscle breakdown and the mass of muscle involved by the disease process. Extremely high levels are seen in the more active forms of muscular dystrophy and polymyositis, but by contrast, some of the metabolic myopathies and the congenital non-progressive myopathies give normal levels. Electromyographic testing of muscles can give important information. Typically in muscular dystrophy there is a so-called myopathic pattern in which the action potentials are reduced in amplitude as well as being of short duration and polyphasic. In polymyositis fibrillation may be seen, although this is more commonly an indication of muscle denervation. Nerve conduction rates are always normal in primary muscle disease. Specific electrophysiological tests of myoneural function may be used in the diagnosis of myasthenia gravis (*see* below). Muscle biopsy may be needed to clinch the diagnosis in some disorders. It is important to select a muscle which is clinically affected. In acute disorders a more severely affected muscle is likely to show the pathological process clearly, while in chronic myopathies a less involved muscle is to be preferred. Open muscle biopsy has the advantage of producing a large specimen which can be used for a number of different investigations. Needle biopsy produces a relatively small number of muscle cells, but it is easily repeated and can be helpful where the muscle involvement is patchy. The information obtainable from routine paraffin sections of muscle is limited, and it is important that tissue is taken for histochemical study and possible biochemistry and electron microscopy.

Muscular dystrophy

The muscular dystrophies have now been recognized for about 100 years. They are inherited disorders which are characterized by progressive muscle weakness. The cause is not known and, as yet, there is no effective treatment. Such features as the pattern of muscle involvement, age of onset and mode of inheritance have led to the classification of these conditions.

Pseudohypertrophic muscular dystrophy

The commonest form of muscular dystrophy is the pseudohypertrophic or Duchenne type. The inheritance is by an X-linked recessive gene so that boys are affected through their carrier mothers. Accurate diagnosis is essential for future genetic counselling.

Although the disorder is present before birth, early development is usually normal although there may be some delay in walking. Symptoms commonly develop between the ages of 3 and 6. A previously mobile boy becomes less so

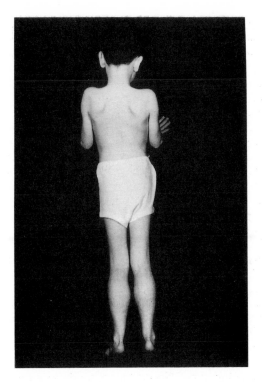

Fig. 4.1. Prominent calves, wasted thighs and thinning of scapulohumeral muscles in Duchenne dystrophy

and is noticed to regress to using his hands to climb up stairs. At this stage he may have difficulty standing from a low chair or the squatting position and his gait becomes waddling. Weakness of hip and knee extension causes the characteristic sight of a child who pushes himself off the floor with his hands and climbs up his legs.

Examination shows weakness of the pelvic girdle and thigh muscles and commonly of the shoulder girdle and proximal upper limb muscles as well. Early wasting may be apparent, but by contrast the calves are well formed and may even give the appearance of hypertrophy, having a rather solid and wooden feel (Fig. 4.1). The tendon reflexes are depressed. The serum creatine kinase level is always greatly elevated and the electromyogram shows a typical myopathic pattern. The ECG is commonly abnormal. Muscle biopsy may be required if there is no family history of the disorder as it is important to make sure that the child is not suffering from polymyositis. Pathologically there is marked variation in muscle fibre size, splitting of fibres and both fibrous and fatty infiltration. Some cellular infiltration may be seen but not to the extent that is apparent in polymyositis (Fig. 4.2).

The disease is inexorably progressive. There is a gradual spread of both muscle wasting and weakness, although the cranial nerves tend to be spared

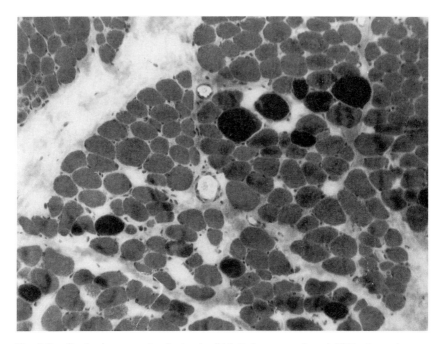

Fig. 4.2. Duchenne muscular dystrophy (H & E, frozen section × 120): shows large 'waxy' strongly eosinophilic (black) fibres together with great variation in fibre size. The large areas without muscle fibres are of fat replacement and fibrosis due to progressive fibre loss

until a late stage. The boy is usually confined to a wheelchair by his early teens and will seldom survive beyond the age of 20. Treatment is largely supportive and consists mainly of physiotheraphy to maintain as much muscle strength as possible and prevent joint contractures. With the lack of mobility obesity commonly becomes a problem.

In recent years, particular attention has been paid to the identification of carriers. Occasionally women who have one or more boys with muscular dystrophy will show minor muscle weakness on careful examination. The serum creatine kinase level may be slightly raised, and in some carriers minor EMG abnormalities have been found. About 60 per cent of carriers can be identified by using these tests. A milder form of X-linked muscular dystrophy was first described by Becker in Germany and has been increasingly recognized in this country. The onset is usually later in the first decade, and progress is less rapid so that survival into middle age with relatively little disability is quite common (Fig. 4.3). An autosomal recessive form of pseudohypertrophic muscular dystrophy affecting both boys and girls is rare.

Facio-scapulo-humeral muscular dystrophy

Facio-scapulo-humeral muscular dystrophy is a much more benign condition than the pseudohypertrophic type. It differs in its later onset, slower progression

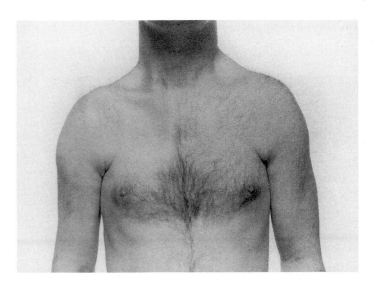

Fig. 4.3. Asymmetric wasting of pectoral muscles in man of 40 with Becker dystrophy

and dominant inheritance. Although symptoms may start in childhood, presentation is more commonly seen in the second and third decades. Insidiously developing muscle weakness principally affects the shoulder and pelvic girdles as well as the upper arms and thighs. The patients complain of difficulty lifting their arms above their heads and lessening ability to climb stairs or hills. Examination always shows bilateral facial weakness involving eye closure and mouth movements, although this may not have been noticed by the patient. Muscles of the shoulder girdle and upper arms are always wasted, and there is usually a characteristic elevation of the scapulae due to the unopposed action of the relatively preserved trapezius muscles. The pectoral muscles are particularly picked out, but the clavicular head may be spared, and this selectivity of muscle involvement is particularly characteristic of this form of muscular dystrophy. All these muscles show weakness which is usually quite severe, and movements of the hip and knee are similarly affected. Distal muscles in the limbs tend to be strong although there may be selective involvement of the anterior tibial muscles which can be unilateral.

The diagnosis can usually be made from clinical examination and the family history, although the picture can sometimes be mimicked by other forms of inherited myopathy. The creatine kinase level is usually normal or only slightly elevated but the EMG always shows multiple myopathic potentials. Muscle biopsy is only needed in doubtful cases. Although the muscle involvement is progressive, it can be very slow with little alteration over a period of years. Most patients will be significantly disabled 20 to 30 years after onset and may be confined to a wheelchair. Life expectancy is usually shortened, but it is not uncommon to see relatives of patients who are only so slightly affected that they do not realize they have the condition.

Limb girdle muscular dystrophy

Limb girdle dystrophy is less common than the previous two conditions. It is usually inherited in an autosomal recessive fashion with both sexes being affected. As its name implies there is selective involvement of the girdle and proximal limb muscles, the face being normal and the distal muscles relatively spared, at least in the early stages. Onset is usually in the second decade, and at diagnosis there is usually quite marked wasting and weakness of the affected musculature, the well preserved forearms and lower legs standing out in contrast. The tendon reflexes are usually depressed and later become absent. The creatine kinase level is usually normal or slightly elevated and typical myopathic potentials are seen on electromyography. The condition may be closely mimicked by the chronic forms of spinal muscular atrophy which develop in childhood or early adult life, and muscle biopsy may be required if the EMG findings are not characteristic, for an accurate prognosis and for genetic counselling.

Ocular myopathy

Ocular myopathy is the name given to a rather heterogeneous group of conditions in which the main features are progressive bilateral ptosis accompanied by symmetrical limitation of eye movements without pupillary involvement. Both sporadic and familial cases occur and onset varies from childhood to middle age. Because both eyes are symmetrically affected diplopia is seldom noticed, and patients seek medical aid when the drooping lids interfere with their vision. Progress is usually very slow, and perusal of old photographs may show the ptosis has been developing for several years before advice is sought. Although ocular myopathy may be an isolated condition it is often accompanied by weakness elsewhere in the body. The term oculopharyngeal myopathy is used when there is concomitant weakness of bulbar muscles causing difficulty with swallowing and speech, and oculoskeletal myopathy when the proximal limb muscles are involved. Other reported associations of progressive external ophthalmoplegia include cardiomyopathy with or without heart block, and both central and peripheral nervous system syndromes. Indeed, in some cases, it is not certain whether the ptosis and impairment of eye movements are due to primary muscle disease or are secondary to some cranial nerve or nucleus degeneration. The diagnosis is made on the clinical picture, the creatine kinase level usually being normal and the electromyogram unhelpful. Muscle biopsy findings in reported cases have been variable, and most frequently show an abnormality of the mitochondria on electron microscopy, but such findings are of more scientific than practical value. As mentioned above, the disorder tends to be slowly progressive, and the most useful procedure that can be carried out for the patient is a small operation to hitch up the eyelids and improve the vision.

Metabolic, endocrine and toxic myopathies

Metabolic myopathies

The term metabolic myopathy is used when muscle weakness with or without pain and stiffness occurs in association with changes in body chemistry. There are two main groups: first, those patients in which the muscle disease is primary, and second, cases in which muscle weakness results from biochemical alterations secondary to systemic diseases.

The *periodic paralyses* are rare conditions which are familial and usually inherited via a dominant gene. Onset is usually in the first or second decade and the patient is subject to attacks of paralysis of varying severity which affect the limbs but usually spare the respiratory and cranial muscles. In the commonest form there is hypokalaemia at the time of muscle weakness which usually develops during the night or in the early part of the morning. It is often precipitated by a heavy carbohydrate intake or rest after unaccustomed exercise. The weakness or paralysis often persists for several hours. In a severely affected person attacks of variable severity may occur nearly every day, but they often lessen in later life. In between attacks there is no abnormality, but in occasional patients a permanent myopathy may ensue. The exact cause of the condition is unknown. Biopsy often shows multiple vacuoles in the muscle fibres, and it is most likely that there is some abnormality of the muscle surface membrane which allows abnormal shifts of electrolytes and water. Treatment of the acute attack is by potassium chloride which can usually be given orally, but may have to be given by careful intravenous infusion if there is vomiting. The severity and frequency of attacks can be lessened by taking a low salt diet with oral potassium supplements.

In some patients with periodic paralysis the attacks of weakness are accompanied by a raised blood potassium level. Again the onset of such episodes is usually in childhood and they may be quite brief or last for several days. Such attacks may be precipitated by cold, fasting or pregnancy. In some families there is an association with paramyotonia and a permanent myopathy is quite common in adult life. In an attack the ECG may show the peaked T waves of hyperkalaemia, and the best treatment is intravenous glucose and insulin to reduce the potassium level. Rarer still is the normokalaemic variety of periodic paralysis when the weakness is improved by large doses of sodium.

An association between hypokalaemic periodic paralysis and thyrotoxicosis has been recognized, nearly always in persons of oriental origin. Males are much more commonly affected than females, and the paralytic episodes only appear when the thyroid gland is overactive. Treatment of the thyrotoxicosis abolishes the episodes of muscle weakness.

Muscle weakness may also be secondary to alterations in blood potassium levels caused by systemic diseases. Loss of strength is only usually apparent when the serum potassium exceeds 7 mmol/l or is reduced below 2 mmol/l, and it affects all body musculature, although it is usually most apparent in the limbs. Symptoms are usually persistent although there may be some fluctuation. The tendon reflexes are usually preserved and the serum creatine kinase level normal as are electromyographic studies. Causes of hypokalaemia include use of diuretics, hyperaldosteronism, various renal disorders and severe intestinal potassium loss. Hyperkalaemia is commonly secondary to renal or adrenal insufficiency, but may be iatrogenic. The muscle weakness improves if the serum potassium level is corrected by treatment of the underlying disorder.

Calcium excess or deficiency in the bloodstream can produce muscle weakness very similar to that seen with changes in potassium. Dietary deficiency, intestinal malabsorption or renal disease produce a low serum calcium level with secondary hyperparathyroidism. Patients complain of weakness, fatiguability and muscle pain which particularly affects the proximal limb muscles. Muscular atrophy develops after a time, the gait becomes slow and waddling, and muscle tenderness is a common feature. In primary hyperparathyroidism the serum calcium level is persistently raised and there may be accompanying proximal limb muscle weakness. Excess osteoblastic activity results in a raised serum alkaline phosphatase, but electromyographic studies are seldom helpful and muscle biopsy merely reveals non-specific fibre atrophy. Treatment of the underlying condition to bring the serum calcium level back to normal results in return of muscle strength.

Glycogen storage diseases

Excess glycogen in various body tissues is the hallmark of a number of rare disorders which are all inherited through an autosomal recessive gene. They result from deficiency of one or other enzyme which is essential for the breakdown (or occasionally build up) of glycogen to produce glucose. The majority of affected patients present in infancy with failure to thrive, floppiness and hepatosplenomegaly. In such cases early death is frequent. In a number of different glycogen storage disorders, onset may be in later childhood or even adult life, and the principal symptoms are of muscular origin. The following enzyme disorders have been reported to produce myopathy: acid maltase deficiency, debranching and branching enzyme deficiency, myophosphorylase and phosphofructokinase deficiencies. Myophosphorylase deficiency specifically affects muscle and causes pain, weakness and stiffness in muscles which are exercised. The discomfort usually subsides with rest but may persist for several days. In some patients a persistent myopathy with severe muscle weakness may ensue. Suspicion of the diagnosis may be strengthened if the forearm muscles are exercised ischaemically, distal to an arterial tourniquet, and the muscles fatigue rapidly and there is no rise of lactic acid in venous blood from the affected area. Muscle biopsy is essential for diagnosis as histochemical staining will demonstrate the excess glycogen, and the exact enzyme deficiency is revealed by biochemical analysis. Frequent small meals with a high carbohydrate content may help symptoms, but there is no completely effective treatment.

Disorders of lipid metabolism

In systemic carnitine deficiency there is a failure of body synthesis of this chemical, causing hepatic dysfunction and encephalopathy. In the milder and principally myopathic form there is progressive muscle weakness developing in childhood or later. Muscle biopsy shows lipid excess and biochemically there is a deficiency of muscle carnitine. Oral prednisolone is reported to help the muscle symptoms in some cases. A related condition is carnitine palmityltransferase deficiency which is inherited via an autosomal recessive gene. Onset of symptoms is usually in the first or second decade and consists of muscle aching and fatigue with exercise, along with recurrent attacks of myoglobinuria. Strength is usually normal between the attacks when the creatine kinase level is moderately raised. Muscle biopsy may show excess lipid and the enzyme deficiency requires biochemical analysis for identification.

Another rare disorder of muscle metabolism may come to light when patients are given a general anaesthetic. In the malignant hyperpyrexia syndrome there is a rapid rise in body temperature associated with muscle rigidity, hyper-kalaemia and metabolic acidosis. The serum creatine kinase level rises rapidly and there is both myoglobinaemia and myoglobinuria. The exact abnormality has not yet been identified, but cases have been described following the use of halothane, ether, cyclopropane and succinylcholine. Investigation of patients who have been affected in this way by anaesthetics has not been very helpful, but about three-quarters of the cases have a slightly raised creatine kinase level and there are often mild and non-specific changes on muscle biopsy. The condition seems to be inherited through an autosomal dominant gene with variable penetrance.

Endocrine myopathies

Disturbance of muscle function is common in various endocrine disorders. Muscle weakness is present when looked for in the majority of patients with thyrotoxicosis. Occasionally it is the presenting symptom and the loss of strength is predominantly proximal in the limbs with maintained reflexes. The serum creatine kinase level is usually normal, although the EMG may show short duration polyphasic potentials. Muscle biopsy changes are mild and non-specific. Treatment of the thyrotoxicosis results in a return of muscle strength.

A condition peculiar to thyroid disease is exophthalmic ophthalmoplegia. Many patients with thyrotoxicosis show rather prominent eyes with lid lag. In only about 4 per cent is there variable paralysis of ocular movements which fails to improve (and may indeed worsen), as the thyrotoxicosis comes under control. The eyes may be painful and there is frequently chemosis and oedema of the eyelids. Secondary corneal ulceration, papilloedema and even blindness may follow. The cause is thought to be a delayed hypersensitivity response and histologically the orbital tissues are swollen with a mixed cellular exudate. In some patients the condition is subacute and self-limiting, although full recovery is rare. Treatment is generally not very satisfactory, but immunosuppression, irradiation of the orbit and surgical decompression have all been advocated (*see* p. 163).

The association between thyrotoxicosis and hypokalaemic periodic paralysis has already been discussed, and the link with myasthenia gravis will be dealt with later in the chapter.

Hypothyroidism also affects the body musculature producing weakness, cramps and aching pain. Muscular movements tend to be sluggish and the tendon reflexes are depressed with a slow relaxation phase. The muscles may ridge on percussion, a phenomenon known as myoedema. In contrast to thyro-toxicosis, the creatine kinase level is usually raised in hypothyroid muscle disease, and the EMG reveals myopathic potentials. Thyroid treatment results in a steady return to normal.

Muscle weakness is present in about two-thirds of patients with Cushing's disease. The onset is usually insidious with a rather non-specific pattern of predominantly proximal weakness in the limbs. Hypertension, truncal obesity and skin ecchymoses are common accompanying features. Both the creatine kinase level and EMG studies tend to be normal, and muscle biopsy shows non-specific atrophy of type 2 fibres. A very similar picture is seen with prolonged steroid treatment, and has been particularly recognized in patients taking fluorinated steroids such as dexamethasone and triamcinolone. Treatment of the underlying endocrine disturbance usually results in a slow return of muscle strength. Difficulties may arise when steroid therapy is being used to treat poly-myositis or one of the collagen vascular diseases in which muscle weakness may occur. In such cases it may prove difficult to know whether a deterioration in muscle strength is due to the treatment or the underlying disorder.

In Addison's disease generalized weakness is commonly found, is related to the underlying electrolyte disturbance, and improves if this is corrected. In the early stages of acromegaly there is an increase in muscle bulk with good or even greater than normal strength, but as the disease progresses generalized muscle wasting and weakness develop.

Toxic myopathies

Certain drugs may produce muscle damage. This can be acute or subacute, affect proximal limb and trunk muscles, and be accompanied by muscle pain and tenderness. Necrosis of muscle fibres leads to elevation of the creatine kinase with or without myoglobinuria, and myopathic potentials on electro-myography. Drugs reported to produce this clinical picture include clofibrate, epsilon aminocaproic acid and vincristine, the latter substance more usually leading to peripheral neuropathy. In emetine-induced muscle necrosis, there is frequently coexistent cardiac damage. Pain and cramps in the limb muscles, with or without weakness, are a frequent complication of danazol therapy and have been reported with cimetidine and lithium.

A painful inflammatory myopathy may occur as part of the lupus syndrome produced by procainamide. D-penicillamine can produce a similar picture, although a more common complication of this drug is myasthenia gravis. Perhaps the most frequent drug-induced muscle disorder is a chronic painless proximal myopathy due to prolonged steroid treatment (*see* Endocrine myopathies). Long-term chloroquine therapy has produced a similar clinical picture. Histologically there is widespread vacuolation, principally affecting type 1 muscle fibres. Most of the drug-induced muscle syndromes described above respond to withdrawal of the offending substance.

Alcohol in excess may produce a toxic effect upon muscle. Most commonly there is an acute myopathy which follows binge drinking and it is characterized by severe muscle pain and weakness with myoglobinuria. The acute muscular degeneration also results in very high creatine kinase levels in the blood. Recovery is the rule but persisting muscle weakness may develop with repeated attacks. A subacute myopathy is less common, and chronic muscle weakness in an alcoholic is likely to be due to the more frequently associated peripheral neuropathy.

Inflammatory myopathies

The inflammatory myopathies are a heterogeneous group of conditions of which the best known is idiopathic polymyositis. Indeed, polymyositis itself

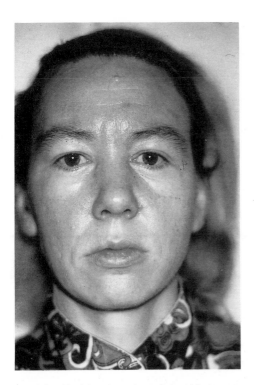

Fig. 4.4. Facial oedema in patient with dermatomyositis

comes in various guises and is frequently associated with other diseases. The incidence is about 5 per million population and males outnumber females. Although it may occur at any age, there is quite a high incidence in childhood and again in middle years. The combination of inflammation and muscle fibre damage produces weakness which principally affects the girdle and proximal limb muscles. There is frequently weakness of the flexor muscles of the neck producing difficulty in raising the head from the bed and the bulbar muscles may be involved with dysphonia, dysarthria and difficulty in swallowing. The disease may be acute with muscle pain and tenderness, subacute, or chronic and mimicking muscular dystrophy or others forms of long-standing myopathy. There is frequently an associated rash and in such cases the term dermatomyositis is used. The skin involvement may take various forms, commonly an erythema of the face, upper chest and forearms. When seen a violaceous coloration of the eyelids is characteristic. Sometimes there is a scaly erythema of extensor surfaces, with the elbows, backs of hands and knees being particularly affected. The bases of the finger nails frequently show hyperaemia and the skin may be oedematous and shiny or occasionally sclerotic (Fig. 4.4.). Arthralgia is a feature in nearly half the cases. Cardiac muscle is sometimes involved as judged by ECG changes, but clinical heart disease is rare. In the childhood form, there may be an associated vasculitis producing damage to the gastro-intestinal tract. Because of the varying forms of polymyositis and its different associations, there have been many attempts to classify the different forms of disease. A commonly used classification is:

1. Polymyositis on its own.
2. Dermatomyositis or polymyositis associated with a connective tissue disorder such as systemic lupus erythematosus, rheumatoid arthritis, progressive systemic sclerosis or Sjögren's syndrome.
3. Polymyositis or dermatomyositis associated with malignant disease.

Most childhood cases are of type 1, whereas after the age of 50 the association with neoplasm elsewhere in the body (particularly bronchial carcinoma) rises.

On investigation the serum creatine kinase level is usually raised and may reach extremely high levels in acute forms of the disease. Myopathic short duration potentials are virtually always seen on electromyography, and in about 75 per cent of cases there is fibrillation in the relaxed muscle (more commonly seen with denervation). About half the patients show bursts of fibre activity on muscle percussion, a feature known as pseudomyotonia. Muscle biopsy is usually needed to establish the diagnosis with certainty. The pathological findings consist of muscle fibre necrosis associated with both interstitial and perivascular infiltration with lymphocytes and macrophages (Fig. 4.5). Small basophilic regenerating fibres are commonly seen. Unfortunately, the muscle

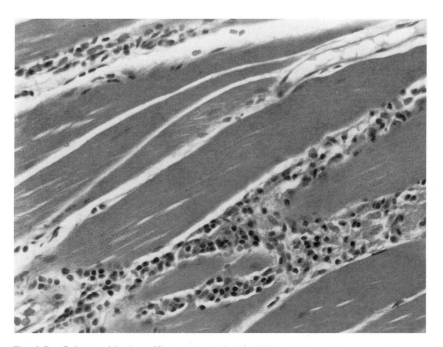

Fig. 4.5. Polymyositis: (paraffin section, H & E × 300): portion of three necrotic fibres with many large nuclei of macrophages and slightly more numerous round dark nuclei of lymphocytes. The intervening fibres are microscopically normal

involvement is sometimes patchy so that the characteristic changes may not be seen in a single biopsy specimen.

The disease is usually progressive without treatment, but can pursue a relapsing and remitting course. Contractures may develop if physiotherapy is not given, and in occasional cases there is calcification in the muscles. The mainstay of treatment is steroids. Initially, prednisolone should be given in high dosage, an adult requiring between 60 and 120 mg daily. Such a dose may be required for several weeks before the disease appears to be coming under control with improvement of the weakness and a drop in the creatine kinase level. At this stage the daily steroid dose can be gradually reduced, and a maintenance dose of between 5 and 15 mg daily continued. Treatment is often necessary for many years, although occasionally the disease seems to burn itself out. When effective control is not maintained by prednisolone, the addition of another immunosuppressive drug such as azathioprine may be needed. Improvement in muscle strength, and the rash if present, nearly always takes place. The long-term prognosis in uncomplicated polymyositis is good. The outlook is more doubtful where there is an associated collagen disease or underlying malignancy. The prognosis for life then depends on the stage of that disorder, and the overall mortality rate in polymyositis is around 25 per cent.

The cause of polymyositis is uncertain. It is generally thought to be an auto-immune disorder, but it has little in keeping with experimental myositis that can be produced in animals. There are reports of it being precipitated by drugs and virus infections, but more frequently it arises out of the blue.

Viral myositis

Coxsackie, ECHO and influenza viruses have been implicated in producing an inflammatory disorder of muscle. The onset is usually acute with pain in the muscles but little in the way of weakness, and the best known is Bornholm disease or epidemic pleurodynia caused by coxsackie B infection. The serum creatine kinase level is usually elevated and recovery is quite rapid. There are a few reports in the literature of chronic myositis which appears to be of viral origin.

Granulomatous myositis

In sarcoidosis, muscle biopsy may reveal the presence of multiple granulomas. Indeed, such changes are said to occur in about 30 per cent of patients with sarcoid, although few of them show clinical signs of a myopathy. Muscle granulomas may also be seen in Wegener's disease, and an idiopathic granulomatous myopathy has also been described.

Tropical myositis

This condition is common in tropical countries. Multiple abscesses develop anywhere in the skeletal musculature. There is local pain and swelling due to the formation of pus. Staphylococcal infection is nearly always present, and treatment consists of antibiotics with incision of the abscesses as necessary.

Congenital myopathies

The term 'congenital myopathy' is used to describe a number of pathologically different muscle conditions which bear clinical similarities. In many patients the condition is inherited, although frequent sporadic cases have been reported. Usually the disease is present at birth producing a rather floppy baby whose motor movements are reduced and whose motor development is delayed. Muscle weakness persists into childhood and adult life, but is seldom progressive. In these patients the creatine kinase level is usually normal as is the EMG, although sometimes mild myopathic changes may be recognized.

In *central core disease* there is usually some infantile hypotonia and walking is delayed to the age of 3 or 4 years. On histochemical staining of a muscle biopsy there is a central pale core in most of the type 1 muscle fibres caused by the absence of mitochondria and oxidative enzymes. The cores extend throughout the length of the affected muscle fibres. By contrast in mini-core or multi-core disease both type 1 and type 2 fibres contain several small cores with reduced staining which only extend over a few sarcomere lengths. Non-progressive weakness from birth is the usual picture. There may be some wasting of the limb muscles with impairment of tendon reflexes, and both the face and neck flexion may be weak. The disease is usually inherited through a recessive gene.

Nemaline myopathy is characterized histologically by the presence of rod bodies which occur in pallisades which are best seen with a trichrome stain. They principally occur in type 1 fibres. Infantile hypotonia is followed by delayed motor development, there tends to be universal muscle involvement and the limbs look slender. Facial weakness and nasal speech are quite common and associated abnormalities include a high arched palate, scoliosis and pes cavus. The disease sometimes progresses and respiratory failure has been reported in a number of patients. Inheritance is autosomal dominant.

Centronuclear myopathy was originally called myotubular myopathy because the muscle fibres bear a resemblance to the myotubes of fetal muscle. Type 1 fibres predominate, there is quite large variation in fibre size and the string of centrally placed nuclei (as opposed to the usual sub-sarcolemmal position) is characteristic. In the autosomal recessive form developmental delay is followed by ptosis, restriction of ocular movements and facial weakness. The more severe X-linked form of the disease usually leads to early death.

Other rare forms of congenital myopathy include fingerprint inclusion myopathy, reducing body myopathy, and congenital fibre type disproportion in which hypotonic children with a non-progressive myopathy have very small type 1 muscle fibres. In some genetic myopathies the muscle fibres look normal or only show non-specific changes.

The mitochondrial myopathies are a group of disparate conditions in which electron microscopy reveals the mitochondria to be enlarged and often of unusual configuration (megaconial) or excessive (pleoconial). It is not always clear whether the mitochondrial abnormality is primary, or secondary to some other metabolic disturbance. Children are usually affected from birth. One of the more common clinical presentations is the Kearns-Sayre syndrome in which ptosis and ophthalmoplegia are accompanied by skeletal muscle weakness. Associations include pigmentary degeneration of the retina, nerve deafness, dementia, ataxia, raised CSF protein and cardiomyopathy. In other patients with mitochondrial abnormality, there may be progressive muscular weakness and fatigue with onset in the first decade and slow progression. Rarely, there may be hypermetabolism with normal thyroid function, or hypotonia with salt craving and periodic muscular weakness, or a myopathy associated with lactic acidosis. A predominantly distal myopathy with hyperglycaemia has been described, and some patients have a pattern of muscle weakness which is similar to facio-scapulo-humeral dystrophy.

Benign congenital hypotonia

In the assessment of a newborn baby muscle tone, posture and motor activity are all important. A floppy baby is one that fails to take up a normal curled position and has flaccid limbs. There is decreased resistance to passive movements and general loss of wakeful activity. Most commonly this clinical picture results from cerebral depression, and in such babies there is usually loss of Moro, rooting and sucking reflexes. In about one-quarter of such babies the floppiness and loss of movement result from a peripheral lesion. This may be due to infantile spinal muscular atrophy or some form of congenital myopathy. In some babies, however, the floppiness and weakness gradually resolve as the child grows, and the term benign congenital hypotonia has been used to describe such infants. In general they retain active limb movements and the tendon reflexes can be elicited. The creatine kinase level, EMG studies and muscle biopsy are all normal. Although motor development is delayed there is improvement leading to normal or near normal muscle strength over a period of months or years.

Myotonic syndromes

Myotonia consists of persistent muscle contraction after relaxation of voluntary effort or electrical stimulation. It causes muscular stiffness which eases with exercise and is most commonly seen in a number of inherited disorders. It is easily detected by electromyography which shows a characteristic after discharge of electrical potentials which has been likened to the noise of a dive bomber.

Myotonia congenita or Thomsen's disease is usually present at birth but may not be recognized until early or late childhood. Patients complain of stiffness and immobility particularly when they have been resting for a while, and it tends to be worse in cold weather. Difficulties may be experienced in starting to walk, run or climb stairs. After a short while, normal mobility is regained, and many patients can be quite athletic. Involvement of the upper limbs frequently causes difficulties in relaxing grip, especially when turning a door handle. The jaw muscles may feel stiff on starting to eat and myotonia of the tongue produces intermittent dysarthria. Occasionally, there are difficulties in swallowing and movements of the eyes. There is no muscle wasting, and often the body musculature is so well developed that it almost looks hypertrophic (Fig. 4.6). On initial muscle testing the strength may appear a little reduced, but with repeated

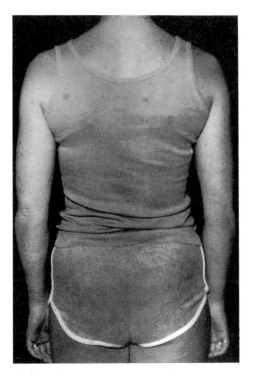

Fig. 4.6. Congenital myotonia with well developed body musculature in girl of 18

effort it becomes normal. The myotonia is usually widespread and can be demonstrated in various ways. Percussion of a limb muscle produces a characteristic dimple which may take several seconds to disappear. If the patient squeezes the examiner's fingers the grip only relaxes in a stiff and awkward manner. Percussion of the tongue produces a localized area of narrowing which again takes several seconds to disappear (Fig. 4.7). The condition is autosomal dominant, and symptoms usually become less troublesome by middle age.

A rather different form of myotonia with autosomal recessive inheritance was described by Becker. Onset is usually later than in the congenital variety, and again generalized muscle hypertrophy may be seen. The symptoms are basically similar, but examination often reveals some muscle weakness of neck flexors, grip and ankle and toe movements. Paramyotonia is similar to but less common than myotonia congenita. The symptoms from the myotonia only appear when the patient is cold, and they are interspersed with attacks of generalized body weakness. In many families these episodes of weakness are accompanied by hyperkalaemia as in periodic paralysis, but sometimes the serum potassium is low or normal. Indeed there seems to be a relationship between the two conditions, some families showing paramyotonia with only occasional attacks of weakness, and others have periodic paralysis with or without myotonia.

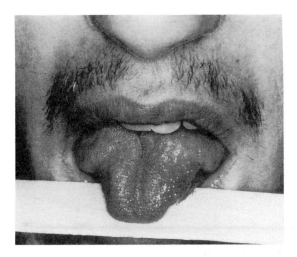

Fig. 4.7. Percussion myotonia of tongue in myotonic dystrophy

Myotonic muscular dystrophy

Dystrophia myotonica is a fascinating condition in which muscle dystrophy is combined with myotonia and various other non-neurological features. It is the commonest form of muscular dystrophy seen in adult life. Presentation is very variable, and often patients have had symptoms for several years before they seek medical aid or the diagnosis is recognized. A common complaint is weakness of the legs with difficulty in walking. Weakness and loss of use in the hands is also a frequent early feature. Occasionally, patients will complain of difficulty in grip relaxation but this symptom usually has to be uncovered by direct questioning. A few patients will present with dysphagia.

The diagnosis can virtually always be made from clinical examination. There is bilateral ptosis with a myopathic facies causing weakness of eye closure and inability to purse the lips (Fig. 4.8). The masseter and temporalis muscles often show thinning giving the patient a rather wasted appearance. The sternomastoid muscles are usually wasted and neck flexion is weak. The limbs tend to be generally thin and there is usually weakness particularly of the distal muscles. Sometimes the quadriceps muscles can be quite weak. The tendon reflexes are depressed. Myotonia of grip is nearly always demonstrable, and percussion myotonia of the limb muscles or tongue is often seen. What is often characteristic of a patient with myotonic dystrophy is the mental attitude. Many patients have low or subnormal intelligence. They tend to be apathetic with lack of insight, and are often rather suspicious in their attitude. Non-neurological features include frontal balding in males, and cataracts which take the form of scintillating whitish subcapsular particles at the back of the lens which may require a slit lamp to be seen. The testicles are often atrophic. Clinical involvement of the heart is uncommon, but conduction defects on ECG are relatively frequent. Diabetes mellitus occurs in about 5 per cent of patients with

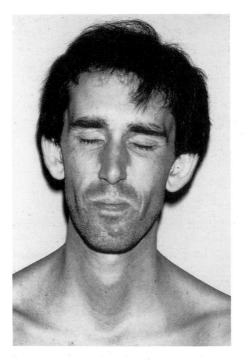

Fig. 4.8. Dystrophia myotonica: facial appearance and inability to close eyes tightly

myotonic dystrophy and other endocrine abnormalities have been described. X-ray of the skull frequently shows a small pituitary fossa and there may be hyperostosis of the skull vault. EEG abnormalities have also been described.

Myotonic muscular dystrophy is a dominantly inherited condition. Its severity varies, and in some families the disease shows anticipation with earlier onset in succeeding generations. The disease may also become more severe so that a grandparent merely has cataracts while the grandchild develops a severe and progressive form of the disease in childhood. The majority of patients develop symptoms between the second and fourth decades. When muscle weakness is mild there may be difficulty in the differential diagnosis from straightforward myotonia, especially if there is no clear family history. The presence of cataracts on slit lamp examination confirms the dystrophic nature of the disease, and these are seen in 90 per cent of cases. Occasionally, affected mothers will have children who are affected from birth. In the early stages myotonia is not present and the picture is one of a floppy and immobile infant. The mother may be only mildly affected but examination of her will make the diagnosis in the child.

Dystrophia myotonica is a progressive disorder, but as mentioned above it is very variable. Severely affected patients with early onset may be confined to a wheelchair in their 20s. Others, in whom symptoms develop later, may remain mobile and fairly active into old age, but this is uncommon. The muscle dystrophy cannot be effectively treated. The cataracts can be treated surgically. Myotonia can be lessened by the use of various drugs, the most commonly used ones being procainamide, quinidine and phenytoin. Patients with congenital myotonia often find one or other of these drugs helpful, although fairly large doses may have to be used. Against this has to be balanced the possible long-term side-effects, particularly of procainamide, and some patients are mildly affected and prefer to do without therapy. By the time patients with myotonic muscular dystrophy come to diagnosis the main feature is often weakness and the myotonia causes relatively little disability. In such cases trials of procainamide usually prove to be unhelpful.

Myasthenia gravis

Myasthenia is a not uncommon condition with a prevalence of about five per 100 000. Females outnumber males by two to one. Onset of symptoms is usually insidious but sometimes subacute and occasionally acute. The characteristic features are muscle weakness with fatiguability, so that symptoms commonly develop in the afternoon or evening in muscles which are being used repetitively. Paradoxically a few patients will complain that their symptoms are worse first thing in the morning. Almost any skeletal muscle in the body may be affected, but there is a predilection for the eye muscles. Variable drooping of the eyelids accompanied by double vision is the commonest mode of presentation. Other early features include fatigue on chewing with difficulty in swallowing and slurring of speech. The head may flop due to weakness of neck muscles, and the trunk, girdle and proximal limb muscles can also be affected. Commonly the disease starts in the external ocular muscles and spreads to involve other parts of the body, but quite often it remains limited to the eyes, and occasionally it can be generalized from the start. Complete or partial remission of symptoms may take place with recurrence months or even years later. The signs on examination will vary according to the severity and spread of the disease, and also the time of day at which the patient is seen. Common features include unilateral or bilateral ptosis, loss of ocular movements with sparing of the pupils, and weakness of face, jaw and neck musculature (Fig. 4.9). Attempts at smiling may produce a snarl-like appearance, and occasionally the tongue shows a triple furrow. Limb and trunk muscles are variably affected. Fatiguability of a particular muscle or muscle groups may be demonstrated by asking a patient to carry out a particular action for 2 or 3 min.

The clinically suspected diagnosis can usually be confirmed by an edrophonium test: 10 mg of this drug are given intravenously and a positive result occurs when then there is improvement in some or all of the affected muscles for about 5 min. An alternative is 1.5 mg of intramuscular neostigmine preceded by atropine to prevent gastrointestinal side-effects. The duration of improvement is usually 2 or 3 h. Electromyographic studies have been used extensively in the past to further the diagnosis of myasthenia. There are two forms of test. In the first a peripheral nerve is repetitively stimulated between 10 and 20 times a second, and the amplitude of the evoked muscle action potential recorded. In the normal person this amplitude stays constant during the stimulation, but in patients with myasthenia there is a progressive decrement. In

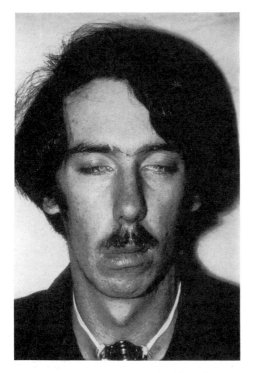

Fig. 4.9.   Bilateral ptosis and facial weakness in myasthenia gravis

the other form of test, electrical recordings are made from single muscle fibres, and the failure of some nerve impulses to evoke a muscle fibre action potential produces a characteristic picture, the jitter phenomenon. Unfortunately, neither of the above tests is absolutely reliable, and to some extent they have fallen out of favour. If the response to edrophonium is uncertain, a trial of an oral anticholinesterase drug can be instituted.

For a long time it was suspected that myasthenia gravis was an autoimmune condition. This supposition was eventually confirmed by the finding that 90 per cent of patients have antibodies in their bloodstream to the acetylcholine receptors on the muscle fibre membrane. Indeed the presence of these anti-bodies is now the most certain test to confirm the diagnosis. Pathologically the myoneural end-plates show complex abnormalities on electron microscopy. There are frequently discreet small groups of lymphocytes in the muscle tissue. The circulating antibodies in the blood can be linked to changes in the thymus which are present in about 75 per cent of patients. The thymus gland which is normally involuted in adult life shows hyperplasia with active germinal centres. In addition, a frank thymoma (usually benign) is present in between 10 and 15 per cent of cases. There is a slight association with certain HLA haplo-types, although familial myasthenia is not common. Nearly 10 per cent of patients with myasthenia have associated thyroid disease of one sort or another, and there are also associations with rheumatoid arthritis, pernicious anaemia, diabetes, etc. Neonatal myasthenia occurs in a small proportion (one in eight) of babies born to myasthenic mothers. It is presumably due to passage of the acetylcholine receptor antibodies across the placental membrane, and resolves spontaneously, although treatment may be required for a few days. Myasthenia at birth is otherwise rare and it is not often seen in childhood being most common in the third and fourth decades, although it can occur at any age.

The treatment of myasthenia is sometimes easy but can be very difficult. Initially the patient is put on a long-acting anticholinesterase drug such as pyridostigmine in a dose of 60 mg three or four times a day which can be increased to twice or three times that level. If symptom control is satisfactory no further action is required initially. Failure to achieve symptomatic relief, and worsening and spread of the disease point to the need for additional therapy, and the choice lies between immunosuppression and thymectomy. Operative removal of the thymus gland undoubtedly results in improvement of muscle weakness in many cases, although the response can be delayed for months or even years. About 60 per cent of patients benefit, and it is usually the younger patients with more generalized disease which has been present for less than 12 months who show the best results. Alternatively the disease may respond to steroids. At one time ACTH was given in high dosage resulting in an initial deterioration in muscle strength followed by a rebound improvement as the drug was discontinued. Nowadays it seems safer and better to start with a very low dose of prednisolone and only increase by small increments every few days. By this method adequate control of symptoms can often be achieved. Alternate day steroid treatment has proved very effective: patients can often be controlled on doses of prednisolone 40–60 mg on alternate days with minimal side-effects. Occasionally, added immunosuppression with azathioprine or cyclophosphamide is needed. In the past few years plasmapheresis has come into its own as a temporary treatment in severe cases of myasthenia. It is possible to reduce the antibody level in the bloodstream by exchanging between 15 and 20 litres of plasma over a period of a week or 10 days with concomitant improvement in clinical state. Relapse usually follows after a few weeks so that plasma exchange is only a holding operation while more definitive treatment takes effect. In some patients the myasthenia seems to burn itself out after a period of years so that little or no treatment is required.

Myasthenic syndrome

Various other neurological conditions are associated with fatiguability. It is well recognized in multiple sclerosis and is a common feature in polymyositis and in some forms of neuropathy. The name myasthenic syndrome is given to a condition which shares some features with true myasthenia gravis but differs in others. Muscle fatiguability is common but sometimes there is an improvement in muscle strength after initial exertion. In contrast to myasthenia gravis the eye muscles are virtually always spared, the bulbar muscles may be affected, but the main impact of the disease is on the girdle and proximal limb musculature. Whereas in myasthenia gravis the tendon reflexes are normal, in the myasthenic syndrome they are depressed. The first cases of this syndrome to be recognized were nearly all associated with a small cell lung carcinoma. Sometimes the tumour only appears months or years after the muscle weakness. In about 40 per cent of patients no occult malignancy is found on investigation or follow-up.

The diagnosis can be suspected clinically in patients who have a myopathy in which fatigue is a prominent feature. Repetitive nerve stimulation produces an increment in the evoked muscle action potential, in contrast to the decrements seen in myasthenia gravis. It seems that the mechanism of the disorder is a failure of release of normal quanta of acetylcholine molecules from the terminal nerve endings in the muscles. Quite why this should occur is uncertain but it may be an autoimmune disturbance. In the past, guanidine, which stimulates the release of acetylcholine, has been widely used in treatment. Unfortunately, it is difficult to get the drug in absolutely pure form and common side-effects are rashes, gastrointestinal disturbance and blood dyscrasias. Some patients respond to steroid therapy.

Carcinomatous neuromyopathy

It has long been recognized that occasional patients with malignant disease may develop neurological disorders, and the association is now widely recognized. The paraneoplastic syndromes, as they are called, do not result from a direct effect of tumour tissue on the nervous system, and the exact mechanism of their development is ill understood. The central nervous system may be affected, but involvement of the peripheral nervous system or muscle is much more common (*see* p. 137). The neurological symptoms may precede the recognition of the underlying tumour, or may develop when the malignancy is already being treated. Such syndromes have been recognized in about 5 per cent of patients with small cell carcinoma of the lung, and a less frequent association is present with carcinoma of the breast, stomach, ovary, kidney and prostate.

Paraneoplastic peripheral neuropathy is usually acute or subacute with both motor and sensory involvement. Much less commonly it may be purely motor and there are occasional recorded cases of sensory neuropathy producing incoordination and ataxia from proprioceptive loss. The myasthenic syndrome is associated with carcinoma in about 50 per cent of cases, and has been described earlier in this chapter. Many patients with advanced carcinoma show severe generalized muscle wasting amounting to cachexia. Despite their appearance these muscles often retain good strength and the tendon reflexes are intact. In other patients, selective proximal muscular weakness may develop with depression of the tendon reflexes. The creatine kinase level and EMG studies are often normal, and muscle biopsy only shows minor and non-specific changes. This picture is most frequently seen in men over the age of 50, and underlying malignant disease should always be suspected in such patients. It is usually a subacute illness, but an acute necrotizing myopathy has been described. Polymyositis and particularly dermatomyositis are well recognized as complications of malignant disease. Again the association is most commonly seen in the middle-aged and elderly.

Carcinoma, particularly of the lung, may produce endocrine abnormalities. These include Cushing's syndrome, hypercalcaemia and inappropriate secretion of antidiuretic hormone resulting in hyponatraemia. These metabolic and endocrine disturbances may have a secondary effect on muscle producing generalized weakness.

The mainstay of management of the paraneoplastic syndromes is treatment of the underlying malignant disease. Successful eradication of the tumour sometimes produces marked clinical improvement, although this is not always the case. Recurrence of tumour tissue is likely to result in deterioration in the neurological symptoms and signs. Steroids should always be used in polymyositis and dermatomyositis, although the response tends to be less gratifying than that seen in pure polymyositis or collagen disorders. Some cases of paraneoplastic peripheral neuropathy will also respond to steroid therapy, although the improvement may be temporary.

5

Peripheral neuropathy

Neuropathy describes pathological damage to the peripheral nerve which may involve motor fibres travelling from their anterior horn cell in the spinal cord to the muscle, sensory fibres ascending from the periphery to the neurones in the posterior root ganglia, and autonomic fibres concerned with the control of the pupils, bowel, bladder, circulation, sweating and sexual function.

Neuritis, strictly an inflammation of nerves, is often used synonymously with the term neuropathy. The term 'neuropathy' may be classified in a number of ways relating to the cause, fibre size, temporal profile, pathogenesis, pattern and distribution. Most forms of neuropathy are a symmetrical polyneuropathy or peripheral neuropathy involving the most distal parts of the nerve in an even fashion, so symptoms start in the extremities. A mononeuropathy describes a single nerve lesion: if many unrelated nerves are involved in a patchy fashion, the term 'mononeuritis multiplex' may be used, e.g. lesions of the right radial, lateral popliteal and left ulnar nerves. Mononeuritis multiplex is particularly likely to arise in conditions where vascular lesions affecting the vasa nervorum occur, e.g. polyarteritis nodosa, diabetes mellitus, sarcoidosis, but it may also occur in leprosy.

The causes of polyneuropathy are numerous (Table 5.1). The most common found in the UK are due to diabetes, other metabolic upsets (uraemia), to B12 deficiency, drugs (e.g. isoniazid, nitrofurantoin), alcohol, or to an occult carcinoma, lymphoma or dysproteinaemia. About 50 per cent of patients presenting to hospital with a peripheral neuropathy show no obvious cause. In some of these follow-up may give an answer.

Pathogenesis

Many neuropathies show a mixture of damage to the insulating myelin sheath, segmental demyelination, and damage to the parent neurone, or its axonal process, axonal degeneration. In some neuropathies the major damage is demyelination, e.g. lymphomas, protein disorders; in others the damage is axonal, e.g. connective tissue disorders, toxic or metabolic upsets. Such damage can be differentiated by electrophysiological studies or by histological examination.

Table 5.1 Causes of polyneuropathy

Inherited
  Peroneal muscular atrophy or Hereditary sensori-motor neuropathy
  Other hypertrophic forms: Déjérine–Sottas
  Amyloidosis (some forms)
Metabolic
  Diabetes mellitus
  Uraemia
  Porphyria
  Hepatic
  Myxoedema
Nutritional
  B12 deficiency
  B1 deficiency
  Multiple deficiency states: malnutrition, malabsorption
  Vitamin E lack
Toxic
  Drugs: isoniazid, nitrofurantoin, perhexilene, dapsone, vinca alkaloids, disulfiram
  Alcohol
  Toxins: lead, gold, acrylamide, organophosphates
Infective
  Leprosy
  Diphtheria
  Glandular fever
Postinfective
  Guillain-Barré syndrome
  Chronic and relapsing demyelinating neuropathies
Inflammatory
  Polyarteritis nodosa
  Rheumatoid arthritis
  Systemic lupus erythematosus
  Sarcoidosis
Neoplastic
  Carcinoma
  Lymphoma
  Dysproteinaemia
  Leukaemia

Symptoms and signs

These are similar in most neuropathies although the tempo and extent may be determined by the cause. Motor symptoms involve weakness starting in the extremities, with difficulty walking so the feet 'slap' as a foot drop develops. Patients may trip, particularly on uneven surfaces and find running difficult. As weakness ascends, difficulties appear on steps or in getting out of a low chair or the bath, later in standing up. In the hands, the ability to use the fingers in fine manipulative tasks is impaired, later the grip is affected. There may be problems in carrying, lifting or even raising a hand to the face. The legs are affected more severely than the arms in most nutritional, metabolic and toxic neuropathies, although in porphyria and lead poisoning the arms can be more affected. The weakness is of lower motor neurone (LMN) type with reduced tone, wasting, fasciculation and depressed or absent reflexes.

Sensory symptoms often start in the feet, then spread to the hands, with pins and needles, tingling, numbness, pains or less commonly bizarre sensations, e.g. liquid trickling, ants under the skin; later there may be loss of sensation with sometimes postural loss causing unsteadiness and impaired balance, sensory ataxia. Severe postural loss in the fingers may cause pseudo-athetoid movements (like piano playing) if the arms are held outstretched with the eyes closed. There is usually sensory loss in a glove-and-stocking distribution which may ascend (*see* Fig. 3.12) and this may involve all modalities. Pain may be a striking feature of some peripheral neuropathies, particularly those caused by diabetes, alcoholism, thiamine deficiency (B1), uraemia, myeloma, carcinoma and amyloidosis. Such affected patients complain bitterly about 'burning pains' commonly in the feet aggravated by any contact with a 'supersensitive' hyper-aesthetic quality. Neuropathies involving small and unmyelinated fibres are more likely to cause pain and autonomic disturbance.

In autonomic disturbances there may be complaints of dizzy, faint feelings aggravated by standing erect and produced by postural hypotension, urinary incontinence and constipation arising from sphincter control problems, impotence in the male, impaired or absent sweating, dry eyes, blurred vision with abnormal or absent pupillary reactions. To elicit signs of autonomic involvement the blood pressure and pulse should be taken standing and lying, and the pupillary reactions recorded.

Peripheral nerves may be easily palpable at certain accessible sites – the ulnar nerve at the elbow, the lateral popliteal nerve at the head of the fibula. At such sites a diseased nerve may be obviously thickened or distorted by a local swelling or neuroma. In certain chronic neuropathies, particularly congenital disorders, there may be associated skeletal abnormalities with sometimes pes cavus, a talipes equinus, tight heel cords from contractures of the tendo Achilles, and even trophic skin changes. Neuropathic joints (Charcot's arthropathy) arise from painless disorganization of weight-bearing joints.

Investigations (Table 5.2)

These are designed to show the cause, confirm the diagnosis and indicate the pathogenesis. The electrophysiological measurement of motor and sensory conduction velocities, of amplitudes of action potentials and needle sampling of muscles (to show denervation) will confirm the presence of a neuropathy and indicate the pathogenesis. Blood samples should be taken for elucidation of the common metabolic disturbances – B12 deficiency, serum proteins and electro-phoresis – and the detection of connective tissue disorders. It is also wise to perform a few screening tests for an occult carcinoma (e.g. chest X-ray) or lymphoma. Specific inquiries should be made about the intake of any drugs, alcohol excess, or exposure to toxic chemicals. If these measures fail to give the answer, further investigation for rare metabolic causes may be indicated (e.g. phytanic acid for Refsum's disease). Examination of family members may give unsuspected evidence of a hereditary neuropathy. In a few highly selected patients a nerve biopsy or muscle biopsy may be undertaken. Nerve biopsy means sampling a portion of a peripheral nerve which will leave some damage, so a predominantly sensory nerve is chosen, either the sural or radial cutaneous

Table 5.2 Investigations of a polyneuropathy

Blood
    Full blood count and ESR
    Urea, liver function
    Fasting and 2 h post glucose load sugar levels
    Serum B12 level
    Serum proteins and electrophoresis
    Autoantibodies, DNA binding, antinuclear factor
    Others as indicated, e.g. vitamin E, plasma lead, lipid profile
Urine
    Glycosuria, protein, porphyrins
Cerebrospinal fluid
Chest X-ray
Electrodiagnostic studies (EMG and nerve conduction studies)
Examination of family members
Nerve or muscle biopsy

Not all these studies may be necessary

branch. Biopsy may give a specific answer to the cause, although more often only indicates the pathogenesis. A vasculitis, infiltrating granuloma, or certain rare conditions such as amyloidosis or metachromatic leucodystrophy, may be diagnosed by biopsy.

Guillain-Barré syndrome, acute polyradiculoneuropathy

This is the most common cause of an acute polyneuropathy which usually presents as a rapidly progressive motor paralysis (ascending) spreading from the limbs sometimes to involve the trunk and respiratory muscles. It may also spread to involve the facial and bulbar muscles. Paralysis of the respiratory and/or bulbar muscles, if not recognized and treated, will kill the patient. It is essential to make the diagnosis and where appropriate treat the patient by intubation with a cuffed endotracheal tube and mechanical ventilation. If such severely affected patients can be nursed through the acute stage of the illness they have an excellent chance of a full recovery. The course of this illness well illustrates the pattern of an acute neuropathy.

About two-thirds of affected patients give a history of a preceding acute infection, usually of the upper respiratory tract or a gastrointestinal upset, occurring in the previous 10–21 days, leading to the term postinfective polyneuritis. The condition has also followed surgery and glandular fever. It is thought that the infection sets up a disordered immune response leading to acute segmental demyelination of the motor roots with infiltration by inflammatory cells. Later, the peripheral nerves may be involved. With severe damage, axonal degeneration may also occur. The damage leads to increasing weakness usually affecting the legs more than the arms, but often all four limbs. The weakness often affects proximal muscles earlier than distal. It commonly progresses over a period of days, to a maximum (often up to 21 days) and then starts to improve. In about one-half of cases there will be bilateral facial weakness.

Facial weakness is a warning that respiratory involvement may occur. In one-third, bulbar weakness with difficulties in swallowing develops. About one-third have respiratory muscle weakness requiring artificial ventilation. Associated with the weakness are depressed or absent reflexes. As a bedside rule do not diagnose acute polyneuritis if the ankle jerks are still present.

Sensory symptoms are common at the onset, although the sensory signs may be very mild and are usually far less than the motor ones. About 15 per cent of cases show severe position sense loss. Back pain, sometimes severe, may be a presenting symptom, and complaints of muscular aching in the limbs are common. In the early stages the Guillain-Barré syndrome may be misdiagnosed as hysteria, particularly if the signs are mild.

Autonomic disturbances arise in about 25 per cent with the development of urinary retention, which may require catheterization, and constipation. More important circulatory upsets may occur with disordered or paroxysmal disturbances of heart rate and rhythm. There may be postural hypotension. A small number of patients have been found with unusual abnormal signs which include papilloedema (perhaps related to a high CSF protein) and even extensor plantar responses.

In general, the neurological deficit progressively worsens in the first 7–21 days, then stabilizes before beginning to improve. Recovery occurs over months. Complete recovery occurs in those with less severe damage and in the young. Very severely affected individuals, especially those who are elderly, may be left with some residual deficit.

Assessment of respiratory function is vitally important. A simple bedside test of respiratory function is to ask the patient to take a deep breath and then count aloud for as long as possible. The best measure is that of vital capacity, and a falling value (less than 50 per cent predicted normal) is the warning. Any adult with a capacity of 1.0 litre or less requires urgent admission to an intensive care unit with facilities for artificial ventilation, and the ability to measure blood gases. Hypoxia may precede hypercarbia and a PO_2 of less than 8.0 kPa (60 mmHg) is significant. The PCO_2 which is normally 5–6 kPa (37–45 mmHg) may rise to above 6.6 kPa (50 mmHg). A rising PCO_2 or hypoxia may cause agitation, restlessness and confusion. Remember that hypoxia and hypercarbia indicate that respiratory failure has occurred. Impending respiratory failure in those with muscle weakness is indicated by increasing distress, a rising respiratory rate and tachycardia. Be particularly careful not to sedate such patients as this may depress the brainstem respiratory centre. If in doubt measure the blood gases and vital capacity in such patients.

Bulbar function can be assessed at the bedside by watching a patient drink a small sip of water. If there is significant weakness, there will be spill over into the trachea causing choking and coughing. Severe soft palate weakness may allow nasal regurgitation of fluids. With bulbar paralysis it is necessary to insert a cuffed endotracheal tube to close off the airway from the entry of oral secretions and food. In most patients a nasotracheal tube is better tolerated but, if this is likely to remain in place for more than a few days, it is better to perform an elective tracheostomy with insertion of a cuffed tube directly into the trachea. All such endotracheal tubes will prevent the patient from speaking, until they are removed.

Patients will show an elevated CSF protein, often very high 1.5 g/litre, usually with no cellular increase, the 'albumino-cytologique dissociation', although about 10 per cent have a transient lymphocytosis. Nerve conduction studies will show abnormalities: slowing, block, diminished or absent action potentials, or even signs of denervation. F wave latencies, looking at proximal conduction, are commonly prolonged or absent in the early stages before peripheral abnormalities can be detected. The electrophysiological studies lag behind the clinical picture and in the first few days conduction may appear near normal, but within a week or two is prolonged. There may be a mild rise in the creatine kinase. Sometimes there may be inappropriate secretion of antidiuretic hormone causing a low sodium level.

Treatment

There has been debate about the most appropriate treatment: initially steroids were suggested but a trial has suggested they are ineffective. More recently, plasma exchange has been found to shorten the duration and severity of the illness if used early (within 2 weeks of onset). Where there is good agreement is that all patients require close observation in the initial phase with all facilities available for ventilatory support, and the care of the totally paralysed patient. Severely affected patients require regular turning, intensive physiotherapy, nasogastric feeding, and often a catheter and aperients. Subcutaneous heparin may reduce the risks of thrombotic complications and so pulmonary emboli. The mortality of the condition (less than 2 per cent) is linked with respiratory failure, infective complications, pulmonary emboli and circulatory collapse, the latter linked with autonomic involvement. In some 85–90 per cent the condition 'burns out' with good recovery over a few months. Patients requiring ventilation have a mean stay in hospital of 2 months. About 8–10 per cent of patients are left with residual weakness: some 5 per cent have recurrence.

A variant of acute inflammatory polyneuropathy has been described by Miller Fisher and is characterized by the development of an ophthalmoplegia with impaired ocular movements, often pupillary abnormalities, ataxia, and areflexia. Such affected patients will again usually recovery spontaneously.

Chronic inflammatory demyelinating neuropathies

These may be a variant of the Guillain-Barré syndrome producing a very similar clinical picture, but either following a progressive course (50 per cent), a relapsing and remitting course (30 per cent) or, in the remainder, a monophasic illness, the zenith being reached after some 6 months. All ages may be affected with a male predominance and peak incidence in the over 50s.

Symmetrical weakness and sensory symptoms appear but often distal and proximal muscles may be equally involved with signs of a sensorimotor neuropathy. In a few patients the distribution may be that of a mononeuritis multiplex. Peripheral nerves may sometimes appear thickened. These inflammatory demyelinating neuropathies need to be differentiated from the heredofamilial group (hypertrophic peroneal muscular atrophy type I) and from the demyelinating neuropathies associated with paraproteinaemias.

Electrical tests will confirm slowing from demyelination with dispersion of the compound muscle action potentials, and often focal conduction block. In over 90 per cent the CSF protein is raised.

Many patients respond to steroids in high dosage, initially prednisolone 100 mg/day, which is then reduced. Immunosuppression and plasmapheresis have also been used.

Other causes of acute neuropathy

These include those associated with uraemia, a carcinoma (most often an oat-cell carcinoma of the lung, but also from breast and gastrointestinal tract), lymphoma or leukaemia, and porphyria.

Many neuropathies show a much slower evolution and these are well illustrated by the most common cause of peripheral nerve damage in the UK – diabetes mellitus.

Diabetic neuropathies

These may present in a number of different forms. The most common is a distal symmetrical sensory-motor neuropathy. There may also be a mononeuropathy multiplex: this includes diabetic amyotrophy. Less often there may be an autonomic neuropathy or a cranial neuropathy.

The neuropathy usually arises from axonal degeneration but a number of studies on mononeuropathies and cranial nerve lesions have suggested that the pathogenesis in these arises from thrombosis of the feeding vasa nervorum leading to patchy areas of infarction in the affected nerves. However, in some studies significant segmental demyelination has also been found. Small myelinated and unmyelinated fibres may be affected in keeping with severe pain and autonomic disturbances. Various suggestions about a metabolic disturbance have also been put forward.

Distal symmetrical sensorimotor neuropathy

The incidence of this increases with the duration of diabetes but also depends on the criteria used for diagnosis. A large number (over 60 per cent) of long-standing diabetics may show absent ankle jerks and loss of vibration sense in the toes. In more florid cases there is the gradual development of sensory loss in the toes and feet, often in a short-sock distribution, with later sensory loss in the fingers. This may be associated with distal weakness so that patients may show a slight foot drop and difficulty standing on tiptoe on one foot. Pain in the feet is common; in some this is intense and pricking, stabbing, burning or tingling may be described. Such pains are often worst at rest in bed. There may be associated hyperaesthesiae of the affected areas. A few patients complain of abnormally cold feet. Severe sensory loss may lead to the presence of neuropathic joints. In the diabetic foot, particular problems may arise from the combination of neuropathic sensory loss (with the absence of pain), ischaemia from bad circulation and secondary infection leading to painless perforating ulcers and even gangrene.

Diabetic amyotrophy

This is usually an acute femoral neuropathy or disturbance of the lumbar plexus presenting with severe pain in the thigh, often awakening the patient at night. It usually starts on one side but occasionally occurs sequentially in both. There is associated weakness and wasting of the quadriceps muscles, but also weakness commonly in the hip flexors, with a depressed or absent knee jerk, and sensory loss in the thigh. In some patients there may be associated signs of a more distal neuropathy with absent ankle jerks and vibratory loss in the feet.

Autonomic neuropathy

Diabetes is the commonest cause of an autonomic neuropathy. Here patients may develop postural hypotension with complaints of weakness, dizziness or faint feelings often precipitated by a change in position. There may be bladder disturbance with hesitancy, straining, a sense of poor emptying which may lead to retention with overflow from a large flaccid insensitive bladder. Bowel upsets include nocturnal diarrhoea and, conversely, constipation. If there is pupillary involvement there may be light-near dissociation, like an Argyll Robertson pupil. Sweating disturbances include impaired sweating and the reverse, excessive facial sweating triggered by eating, gustatory sweating. In the male, erectile failure may lead to impotence.

Investigation of such changes involves measuring the blood pressure, standing and lying; a postural drop of more than 30 mmHg is significant. Inability to show variation in the R-R interval on the ECG during the Valsalva manoeuvre, on deep breathing or on standing up, indicates a failure of these circulatory reflexes. Urodynamic studies may confirm a large atonic bladder.

Cranial neuropathies

Most commonly these affect the oculomotor and abducens nerves producing the acute onset of double vision often associated with pain. The oculomotor nerve is the most frequent palsy and is usually associated with pupillary sparing, although this is not inevitable. The facial nerve may also be affected with an acute lower motor neurone palsy (Bell's). Most of these nerve lesions recover completely within 3–4 months.

Patients with diabetes mellitus and perhaps a subclinical neuropathy are more prone to develop *entrapment syndromes*, e.g. carpal tunnel.

Investigations

In all forms of diabetic neuropathy the CSF protein may show a mild elevation, 0.5–2.0 g/litre. The level of glycosylated haemoglobin, HbA_1, is often elevated. Nerve conduction studies usually show motor slowing, denervation in affected muscles, and absent or reduced amplitudes of sensory action potentials.

Treatment

This is always by scrupulous control of the diabetes which commonly involves treatment with soluble insulin. Regular analgesics together with drugs such as clonazepam or carbamazepine may be used to try to control severe pain. An antidepressant, e.g. amitriptyline, at bedtime may also be helpful. In many patients the pain eases in time and there may be slow recovery although lost reflexes and distal sensory loss may persist.

Toxic neuropathies

Certain drugs or exposure or ingestion of various neurotoxic chemicals or poisons may provoke a neuropathy. In most instances this is an axonal degeneration with little slowing of conduction, but often there are signs of denervation on muscle sampling. In most instances recognition and removal of the cause allows the slow recovery by nerve regeneration, although this may be incomplete. Many drugs have been incriminated. The most common include isoniazid (used in the treatment of tuberculosis), particularly where high doses (20 mg/kg) are used. This can be prevented by the concurrent administration of pyridoxine. Others are nitrofurantoin (more common if there is uraemia), disulfiram (used in alcoholism), gold (used in rheumatoid arthritis), vinca alkaloids (used in lymphomas and leukaemias), and metronidazole (used in anaerobic infections).

Toxic chemicals include acrylamide (used as a grouting agent), arsenic (found in insecticides and weed-killers), carbon disulphide (used in the viscose-rayon industry), lead, which may produce a predominantly motor neuropathy with bilateral wrist drop and foot drop (lead is found in paints, storage batteries and used in smelting), and organophosphates (which are mostly found in insecticides but also in lubricating oils).

Alcoholic neuropathy

This is intermingled with the nutritional neuropathies produced by thiamine and other vitamin B deficiencies. In malnutrition, starvation or severe forms of malabsorption, multiple vitamin deficits may produce a polyneuropathy. Thiamine deficiency may also produce a cardiomyopathy with tachycardia, exertional dyspnoea and peripheral oedema, and an encephalopathy (Wernicke's) with nystagmus, ocular palsies, ataxia and mental confusion with amnesia. In patients with Wernicke's syndrome, some 80 per cent will show signs of a peripheral neuropathy (*see* p. 407).

Alcoholic neuropathy is characterized by severe pain in the feet often associated with burning, tingling, stabbing and a degree of hyperaesthesiae. Weakness is common with foot drop and lost ankle jerks, and often lost knee jerks. The limb musculature is often poor and there may be other stigmata of chronic alcoholism, e.g. hepatic enlargement, spider naevi, tremulousness.

A strong index of suspicion may be necessary but discussion with relatives may give support to the diagnosis of alcohol excess. Many patients show a macrocytosis in their blood film with abnormal liver function tests, particularly the gamma glutamyl transpeptidase (γ-GT). An abnormal red cell transketolase may support the presence of thiamine deficiency. Conduction studies will commonly show axonal degeneration, mild conduction slowing and absent or diminished sensory action potentials.

Treatment involves abstinence and large doses of thiamine with a good diet. Recovery may occur but is slow and often incomplete.

Uraemia

With the advent of dialysis many patients with chronic renal failure and uraemia survive for long periods. A neuropathy may develop and the onset may either be slow or rapid. Commonly there are complaints of painful tingling sensations in the feet, sometimes burning, constricting bands or even restlessness. There is usually a mild distal weakness with absent ankle jerks, later a more general loss of reflexes, and lost vibration sense in the feet. Spread into the hands is common.

There is usually axonal degeneration. The CSF protein may be raised. Dialysis will usually halt the progression or allow improvement but a successful renal transplant is followed by recovery.

Porphyria

This is a dominantly inherited metabolic disorder with the increased production and excretion of porphobilinogen. Acute intermittent porphyria presents in attacks often with abdominal pain and sometimes with confusion and a psychosis, and even epileptic seizures. These may be linked with an acute poly-neuropathy mimicking a Guillain-Barré syndrome. The weakness may appear more proximal and affect the arms more than the legs. Limb and back pains may occur. The weakness may spread into the face, trunk and respiratory muscles so patients may need artificial ventilation. Autonomic involvement with a tachycardia, postural hypotension and even hypertension may sometimes be seen.

The neuropathy may be precipitated by ingestion of certain drugs – barbitu-rates, sulphonamides, and alcohol. The detection of porphobilinogen in the urine confirms the diagnosis. The CSF protein is normal or only slightly raised. Conduction studies suggest axonal degeneration.

There is a mortality and morbidity but careful nursing and full support, as for a Guillain-Barré patient, will usually be followed by recovery over many weeks. Patients must be advised on safe drugs for further use, and relatives should be screened for the disorder.

Vitamin B12 deficiency

The spinal cord, peripheral nerves, brain and optic nerves may all be damaged in pernicious anaemia. *Subacute combined degeneration* (SACD) describes the pathological process in the spinal cord where the posterior and lateral columns are involved. Thus patients with SACD may have signs of cord damage in addition to those of a peripheral neuropathy.

B12 deficiency may also arise from dietary deficiencies in vegans, after gastrectomy, in certain types of malabsorption, and in parasitic infestations of the gut.

Commonly there are complaints of peripheral tingling or sensory upset in the extremities, which spread proximally and there may be a glove-and-stocking sensory loss. These may be accompanied by weakness. As the cord becomes involved, an ataxic paraparesis may appear with lost ankle jerks and extensor plantar responses. There are usually signs of posterior column sensory loss.

Conduction studies confirm the peripheral nerve involvement with mild slowing of conduction. There is often a macrocytic anaemia (not always) with megaloblastic changes in the bone marrow. The serum B12 level is low and a Schilling test may confirm a failure of B12 absorption.

Massive doses of B12 by injection, hydroxocobalamin 1000 μg daily for 10 days and then monthly indefinitely, will prevent deterioration and usually improve any peripheral neuropathic features. More severe cord damage may not recover.

Vitamin E deficiency

This has been recognized as an uncommon cause of a predominant sensory neuropathy which may be associated with cerebellar ataxia. It may be associated with abetalipoproteinaemia and also rarely arises in patients with intestinal malabsorption.

Infective causes

Leprosy

World-wide one of the most common causes of peripheral neuropathy is *leprosy* (Hansen's disease). This is due to infection with *Mycobacterium leprae* usually from skin contact, but also possibly by nasal discharge and even flies. It is most often found in patients from India or Africa. In most affected patients it will produce a mononeuritis multiplex with invasion of multiple nerves causing a thickening with granuloma formation (tuberculoid infection) and later failure of function in that nerve. In time, severe sensory loss from such nerve damage may lead to disfiguring loss of tissue, digits and gross distortion of facial features. Patients may present with patchy sensory loss which may appear in hypopigmented skin lesions, weakness and wasting in the territory of affected nerves. The nerves may be palpably thickened. Leprosy may also present with widespread dermatological lesions (lepromatous infection) and here a symmetrical polyneuropathy may appear.

Diagnosis is by biopsy of a nerve granuloma or skin lesion. Treatment is now highly effective in early cases before severe damage occurs. Drugs commonly used include dapsone, rifampicin and ethionamide (the last two being anti-tuberculous drugs).

Diphtheria

This has largely been eliminated by immunization. However, patients may be affected by the diphtheria toxin produced by *Corynebacterium diphtheriae* which will lead to cranial nerve damage with pharyngeal and laryngeal palsies, and to involvement of the ocular muscles causing diplopia and blurred vision (the latter from the loss of the pupillary reactions in focusing). Such features arise some one to two weeks after the throat or nasal infection.

A peripheral neuropathy may also appear 5–8 weeks after the infection with marked distal sensory symptoms and signs, and later weakness. Treatment is similar to that for a Gullain-Barré syndrome.

A number of viral infections may be associated with a peripheral neuropathy. These include *glandular fever* (infectious mononucleosis) and infective hepatitis.

Malignancy

A carcinoma, lymphoma, leukaemia or dysproteinaemia may produce a peripheral neuropathy. In some instances there may be actual infiltration of the affected peripheral nerve by malignant cells which may 'cuff' the nerve. This may cause a single or multiple nerve lesion and involve cranial nerves. The leukaemias, lymphomas and myeloma perhaps are most often incriminated. The other pattern of peripheral nerve damage seems to be as a remote 'toxic' effect of the tumour. This is supported by the observation that removal of such a tumour may allow regression of the neuropathic symptoms. The carcinomas most commonly involved arise from the bronchus, breast, gastrointestinal tract, but also the uterus, cervix, kidney, thyroid and prostate. Such a peripheral neuropathy is also found in some 8–10 per cent of patients with a lymphoma. Various clinical patterns are recognized (*see* p. 124):

1. A sensorimotor neuropathy, usually subacute with an onset in the extremities, starting in the legs. The neuropathy may be the presenting symptom of the carcinoma.
2. A predominantly sensory neuropathy affecting the posterior root ganglia and large fibres. This produces tingling with pains and aching in the limbs, most often the feet, accompanied by a sensory ataxia with loss of joint position sense. It should be recalled that some forms of chemotherapy for these malignant conditions may also produce a peripheral neuropathy, e.g. vinca alkaloids, cisplatin.

Disorders of protein metabolism

About 15 per cent of patients with multiple myeloma may have a peripheral neuropathy usually a subacute sensorimotor pattern, or mononeuropathy. In a few patients it may be associated with amyloid deposits around peripheral nerves.

Macroglobulinaemia, cryoglobulinaemia and paraproteinaemias may also be associated with a peripheral neuropathy, again usually of sensorimotor pattern. Those associated with paraproteins IgG and IgM may be linked with a relapsing and remitting course arising predominantly from a demyelinating process.

Various forms of treatment have been used including steroids, immuno-suppressant drugs and even plasma exchange.

Connective tissue disorders

Peripheral neuropathy occurs relatively commonly in these conditions. The pathogenesis is varied, but in many instances reflects a vasculitis involving the vasa nervorum with patchy infarction of a number of nerves, a mononeuritis multiplex. However, local entrapment by swollen diseased joints, deposition of amyloid, or even toxic neuropathies from the drugs used, may also need consideration, particularly in rheumatoid arthritis.

Rheumatoid arthritis

About 10 per cent of patients develop a neuropathy. Affected patients usually have clear signs of inflammatory joint disease and sometimes skin lesions indicative of an active vasculitis. Various patterns of peripheral nerve involvement are recognized. These include:

1. A digital neuropathy affecting the sensory digital nerves producing sensory symptoms. This occurs in about 20 per cent.
2. A distal sensory neuropathy largely involving the legs again with sensory symptoms and signs, occurring in about 30 per cent.
3. Local entrapment lesions, particularly the carpal tunnel.
4. A distal sensorimotor neuropathy which appears to be progressive and have a bad prognostic outlook. It commonly starts in the legs and may be associated with features of an active vasculitis. It affects about 10 per cent.
5. A mononeuritis multiplex. Patchy involvement of a number of peripheral nerves.

Rheumatoid arthritis may also cause *atlanto-axial subluxation* producing symptoms and signs of a high cervical cord lesion. These may include extensive sensory symptoms with discriminative loss in the fingers, accompanied by pyramidal signs in all four limbs with exaggerated reflexes and extensor plantar responses.

Systemic lupus erythematosus (SLE)

About 10 per cent of patients with SLE will show features of a peripheral neuropathy. It is usually associated with systemic upset, fever, malaise, a skin rash and lesions, arthritis and joint pains. The pattern is one of a distal sensorimotor neuropathy or a mononeuritis multiplex.

Polyarteritis nodosa (PAN)

Some 75 per cent of patients with PAN show signs of peripheral nerve damage. This may be the presenting symptom. Most often there is a mononeuritis multiplex or a distal symmetrical sensorimotor neuropathy. The presentation of these vascular nerve lesions may be acute and painful with the later appearance of numbness and weakness in the territory of the affected nerves. Many patients also show features of renal damage, a high ESR and eosinophilia.

Investigations

The diagnosis of the different connective tissue disorders rests on the clinical picture, laboratory tests and often the histology obtained from a biopsy. There appears to be some overlap in the tests designed to demonstrate an immunological disturbance, e.g. many patients with SLE show a positive test for rheumatoid factor and even a false positive Wassermann's reaction.

In many of these patients the blood count may show a normochromic normocytic anaemia and the erythrocyte sedimentation rate (ESR) is commonly raised (it may act in part as an index of the disease activity). The white count may be low in SLE and raised in PAN where some 30 per cent may show an eosinophilia. Antinuclear factor (ANF) and DNA binding are commonly positive and raised in SLE, although ANF may be positive in PAN and rheumatoid arthritis. Rheumatoid factor is strongly positive in rheumatoid arthritis (also positive in about 30 per cent of PAN patients) and the IgG and IgM levels in the rheumatoid factor in rheumatoid arthritis may be good markers of the disease activity.

Most of these conditions show hyperglobulinaemia, the IgG and IgM fractions being those chiefly affected.

Conduction studies and needle sampling of muscles will confirm the presence of peripheral nerve lesions or denervation. Biopsy of skin, muscle or peripheral nerve (usually the sural) may establish the diagnosis of an active vasculitis particularly if the tissue included contains an affected segment of small artery.

Treatment

This involves the use of appropriate anti-inflammatory analgesics, often the non-steroidal anti-inflammatory drugs (NSAIDs), for relief of pain, and often the use of steroids, and immunosuppressants (azathioprine) to try to control the inflammatory disturbances.

Hereditary neuropathies

The most common of these is *peroneal muscular atrophy* (PMA), or Charcot-Marie-Tooth disease. This classicially presents in adolescence and, with time, the distal wasting of the leg muscles leads to the description of an inverted champagne bottle. Motor symptoms usually predominate but associated with the condition are a number of other features. These include thickened, hypertrophic nerves, skeletal deformities with pes cavus (high arched feet) in two-thirds, clawed toes, contractures of the tendo Achilles (tight heel cords) and scoliosis, the latter in some 15 per cent.

Patients show wasting and weakness of the extremities, the feet being affected first, but commonly there is also involvement of the small hand muscles resulting in clawing. The reflexes are lost and there is usually loss of vibration in the toes at an early stage, with more prominent sensory loss (impaired pain and position sense) occurring later.

Conduction studies have differentiated two groups:

I. These show a marked slowing of conduction indicating significant demyelination.
II. These show a predominant axonal degeneration with little or no slowing of conduction.

The inheritance most often is dominant, but autosomal recessive types and mutations may be found. A number of variants have also been described: these include the Roussy-Levy syndrome where the features of PMA may be combined with prominent tremor and ataxia.

PMA is very slowly progressive and treatment is purely symptomatic. Insert splints and various aids may help selected patients.

There are also a number of rare inherited neuropathies where a metabolic fault has been incriminated. These usually are inherited as an autosomal recessive. They include:

Refsum's disease where phytanic acid accumulates in the central and peripheral nervous system.

Metachromatic leucodystrophy where there is an accumulation of galactosyl sulphatide in the central and peripheral nervous system.

Tangier disease where there is a deficiency of high density lipoprotein.

Amyloidosis where there is deposition of amyloid. This has a dominant inheritance. Amyloid involvement of peripheral nerves may also occur in rheumatoid arthritis and myeloma where it is not inherited.

Bassen–Kornzweig disease where there is hypocholesterolaemia with absence of low density lipoproteins (abetalipoproteinaemia) and vitamin E deficiency.

Fabry's disease where there is alpha-galactosidase A deficiency.

Ataxia telangiectasia where there is defective DNA repair.

Many of these rare disorders have other neurological features, e.g. cerebellar disturbance.

There is also a group of rare inherited sensory neuropathies where loss of pain sensation may lead to considerable damage from neuropathic joints (insensitive to pain) and painless trophic ulcers. Many of these appear to have a dominant inheritance.

The unknown cause group

In a large number of patients presenting with a peripheral neuropathy of subacute or chronic pattern, no cause may be found. Some of the more common causes will already have been excluded by their general practitioner. In this undetermined group the usual blood tests and other investigations (*see* Table 5.2) will have been undertaken, and there is no evidence of an hereditary cause. In a few, biopsy of the sural nerve or a muscle may sometimes give the answer, although more often such biopsy only confirms the presence of a neuropathy. If there is no clear answer, then follow-up in a proportion may establish a diagnosis. A few will show protein abnormalities, and others the presence of an occult carcinoma.

In the unknown group treatment is often given by 'flooding' the patient with B vitamins, adding active physiotherapy, and providing aids such as insert splints for foot drop, outside irons with springs for the more severe ankle weakness, and the use of elbow crutches and walking frames. The more severely disabled may require a wheelchair and a home assessment visit for the provision of appropriate aids.

6

Nerve and root lesions

Pathogenesis of pressure palsies

Compression of peripheral nerves may occur acutely or as a more chronic process. This may cause damage varying in severity. Mild compression is easily recognized and has been personally experienced by most people either when they sit with their legs crossed compressing the lateral popliteal nerve on the head of the fibula, or by leaning heavily on the elbow compressing the ulnar nerve on the bone of the medial epicondyle. With any duration of compression the blood supply to the nerve is compromised, tingling develops and later numbness and weakness appear in the territory of the affected nerve. With relief from the compression, there is usually rapid and complete recovery.

Moderate compression will produce damage to the insulating myelin sheath (segmental demyelination) producing a local conduction block or slowing with preservation of the continuity of the axon. This is called a *neurapraxia*. Usually the large fast conducting myelinated fibres are involved but small and unmyelinated fibres may be spared so there is often preservation of some sensation. Repair is by remyelination and is usually complete with full recovery within a number of weeks or even months.

More severe compression will damage the myelin sheath and the axon leading to axonal (Wallerian) degeneration distal to the site of injury. There will be a conduction block in the distal part of the affected nerve and the muscles supplied by the nerve become inexcitable, later showing signs of denervation with the development of wasting and fasciculation. The nerve trunk remains in continuity. Small and unmyelinated nerve fibres are commonly involved. This type of damage is termed an axonotmesis. Repair is by regeneration over many months at 1–2 mm/day and may be incomplete.

If the nerve is severed or torn apart, causing the connective tissue framework to separate and disrupting the continuity of axons and myelin sheaths, the ends of the nerve are free; this is termed a neurotmesis. In this situation unless the two ends are sutured together or lie in close proximity, repair by regeneration is likely to be poor.

Nerve conduction studies will usually give appropriate information about the pathogenesis of such lesions and may demarcate the site of damage if there is a local conduction block. It should be remembered that the electrical signs of denervation caused by axonal degeneration, may take 5–7 days to appear in affected muscles after a severe injury. Electrodiagnostic tests performed too early, within 2–3 days of injury, may prove misleading.

Many compressive nerve lesions are a mixture of axonal degeneration and demyelination.

Acute compression may arise in unconscious patients from direct pressure of the weight of an inert limb particularly against a sharp edge or unyielding surface. Patients with a depressed conscious level from sedative drugs, excess alcohol or a general anaesthetic are particularly at risk. The 'Saturday night paralysis' of the drunk is the classic example. Here the radial nerve in the upper arm is compressed against the humerus as the arm hangs over a chair back. Such damage may be of varying severity so that such pressure palsies may take weeks or even months to repair.

Chronic compression or entrapment is likely to arise at certain sites where peripheral nerves travel in fibro-osseous tunnels or over bony surfaces so the nerve may be constricted, stretched or deformed. The damage may be persistent or intermittent and the term entrapment is often used in lesions where surgical release of the compression may afford relief. In chronic entrapment the affected nerve may appear thickened at the site and this may be palpable. It should be emphasized that nerves already 'sick' or damaged from some other neuropathic process are more liable to compression, i.e. two faults summate. Thus patients with a diabetic neuropathy are particularly prone to develop a carpal tunnel syndrome. Occasional neoplastic or granulomatous infiltration of nerves may produce local compressive lesions, e.g. leprosy, lymphoma.

Acute traction or stretch injuries can sometimes produce severe nerve damage as when the brachial plexus is injured by a motor cyclist landing at speed on his shoulder. In such injuries the nerve roots may actually be torn out of the spinal cord with complete loss of continuity. Such severe injuries will produce signs of denervation in the affected arm muscles and there may be no recovery.

Carpal tunnel syndrome (CTS)

In its distal part the median nerve may be compressed in the fibro-osseous carpal tunnel at the wrist. The median nerve arises from the C6, 7, 8 and T1 roots. The tunnel is narrower in women where there is a greater incidence of CTS, and this may be further compromised by rheumatoid arthritis, myxoedema, acromegaly, past wrist injuries and even deposition of amyloid. Nearly one-half of the patients with a CTS have an underlying cause: the most common is diabetes mellitus. People who repeatedly work the hands and wrists in certain occupations may develop thickening of the adjacent tendons and this may in part explain why CTS symptoms may be provoked by increased manual work, e.g. house painting, washing, hop-picking. CTS may also appear during pregnancy.

The classical early symptoms are painful paraesthesiae in the fingers and thumb (strictly sparing the little finger) which is worse after use of the hand and on waking. Such symptoms may also awaken the patient from sleep. Relief is found by most patients in hanging the hand down, shaking it about or changing position. Unpleasant aching may spread into the forearm and even the upper

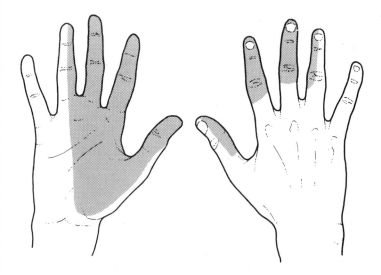

Fig. 6.1. Area of sensory loss in right median nerve lesion

arm, raising the question of a more proximal cervical root lesion. Often the patient describes the pain and sensory symptoms in all their fingers. Initially there are no signs but inflation of a tourniquet (blood pressure cuff) around the upper arm will often provoke similar sensory symptoms within minutes. Forced flexion of the wrist (Phalen's test) may also be used to provoke similar sensory symptoms.

In time the thenar pad muscles may waste and become weak, particularly abductor pollicis brevis, and some sensory signs may appear in the tips of the thumb, index, mid and ring fingers (Fig. 6.1). EMG studies will confirm the diagnosis with absent or diminished sensory action potentials and delay in the distal motor sensory latencies in the median nerve across the wrist. In the more severely affected there may be denervation in abductor pollicis brevis.

Treatment will depend on the severity of the lesion and whether there are any added factors, e.g. diabetes, pregnancy. In mildly affected patients a degree of rest and the use of a wrist splint at night may afford relief. In a few patients local injection of steroids under the carpal ligament may also be of benefit together with a reduction in the amount of manual work performed. In more marked cases, surgical decompression will be necessary. This will usually relieve pain and sensory upset, although severe muscle wasting (in the thenar pad) may not recover, particularly in the elderly. Occasionally surgery may not produce relief of symptoms raising the possibilities of incorrect diagnosis or inadequate decompression. Further conduction studies may be useful in such instances.

Ulnar nerve lesions

The ulnar nerve arises from the roots of C8 and T1. The most common ulnar nerve lesion is compression of the nerve by the fibrous arch of flexor carpi ulnaris (the cubital tunnel) which arises as two heads from the medial epicondyle and the olecranon. Other ulnar nerve lesions at the elbow may reflect long-standing damage to the joint, often from an old fracture, causing deformity and angulation. This may result in a wide carrying angle with stretching and angulation of the nerve in its bony groove at the elbow where it may be palpably thickened. Recurrent dislocation of the nerve from its groove is another mechanism and external pressure may arise either from repeated trauma, or often from patients confined to bed supporting their weight on their elbows. Ulnar lesions may also arise after an anaesthetic where presumably the nerve has been acutely compressed at the elbow while the patient was unconscious.

Patients may complain of tingling or numbness involving the little finger, part of the ring finger and sometimes the ulnar side of the hand, distal to the wrist. Weakness may appear in the ulnar innervated small hand muscles causing difficulties in the use of the hand for fine manipulative tasks. In time there may be wasting of the first dorsal interspace muscles, later the dorsal interossei and hypothenar pad. This will be associated with weakness of varying degree. With severe muscle wasting the hand is deformed, 'clawing' with flexion of the little and ring fingers, associated with the inability fully to extend the tips, as the lumbricals of these two fingers are involved. The other fingers will appear slightly abducted from weakness of the interossei. Often the ulnar innervated long finger flexors, flexor digitorum profundus to the ring and little fingers, may be affected. Weakness usually involves the thumb adductors, the interossei – with difficulty abducting and adducting the outstretched fingers – and the hypothenar pad muscles. The area of sensory loss is shown in Fig. 6.2.

At the elbow the ulnar nerve may be thickened or unduly sensitive. There may be obvious deformity of the elbow with restricted joint movements. If the

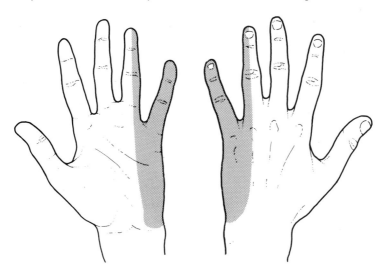

Fig. 6.2.   Area of sensory loss in left ulnar nerve lesion

forearm flexors are involved, the muscles of the medial side of the forearm will be wasted.

EMG studies will usually show an absent or diminished ulnar sensory action potential and ascending nerve action potential. There may be electrical signs of denervation in the first dorsal interosseous and abductor digiti minimi. Commonly there is slowing of motor conduction across the elbow. In milder cases there may be a significant decrement in the amplitude of the evoked muscle action potential from stimulation of the ulnar nerve above and below the elbow and at the wrist.

Treatment of ulnar nerve lesions is less satisfactory. If there has been acute compression or repeated external pressure, then a period of rest and careful attention to avoiding any local pressure on the nerve at the elbow may be worth a trial. In more severe lesions, exploration of the nerve at the elbow may allow decompression if such a lesion is exposed. If this is not found, the nerve may undergo anterior transposition, resiting it more anteriorly across the elbow. However, such measures seldom reverse any major wasting or weakness in the small hand muscles although pain, paraesthesiae and discomfort may be eased. In milder lesions, recovery may take place but some of these lesions treated conservatively may do as well. Surgical treatment may sometimes prevent further progression of ulnar nerve damage.

Ulnar nerve lesions at the wrist

These are far less common, but occasionally the deep palmar branch of the ulnar nerve may be compressed in Guyon's canal which runs between the pisiform and the hook of hamate. The nerve may be compressed here by a ganglion, a neuroma or more frequently by repeated external pressure often with an occupational relation, e.g. the twist-grip of a motor cycle throttle, the 'proud' edged handle of a butcher's cleaver.

The deep palmar branch is motor and will cause wasting and weakness of the interossei, particularly the first, and adductor pollicis, but sensation will be spared. The hypothenar muscles are usually spared although the third and fourth lumbricals may be affected.

Electrically the ulnar sensory action potential (SAP) is present but there is a prolonged distal motor latency to the first dorsal interosseous with a normal latency to abductor digiti minimi, and normal motor conduction in the ulnar nerve in the forearm.

If there is no history of repeated trauma, surgical exploration of the nerve may be necessary.

Sciatic nerve

The sciatic nerve is the largest peripheral nerve and arises from the roots of L4, 5 and S1 and 2. It leaves the pelvis through the greater sciatic foramen and runs posteriorly down the thigh where just above the knee it divides into the medial and lateral popliteal divisions. It lies close to the back of the hip joint and can be damaged if that joint suffers extensive trauma or following hip surgery. In its upper part, the sciatic nerve is covered by gluteus maximus, but the nerve may

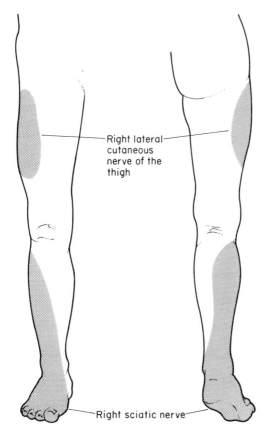

Fig. 6.3. Areas of sensory loss in lesions of right lateral cutaneous nerve of the thigh, and right sciatic nerve

be directly damaged by a buttock injection misplaced too medially. The sciatic nerve may also be damaged by direct pressure in the unconscious patient.

A high lesion of the sciatic nerve will affect the hamstrings and all the leg muscles below the knee; calf and anterior tibial as well as the small foot muscles. This will produce a 'flail' foot with distal wasting and weakness. There will be sensory loss involving the foot and posterolateral aspect of the lower leg (Fig. 6.3). Electrically there will be denervation of the affected muscles with impaired conduction in the medial and lateral popliteal nerves and absent sural and lateral popliteal nerve action potentials.

Lateral popliteal nerve

The lateral popliteal or common peroneal nerve is the most commonly affected peripheral nerve in the leg, perhaps because of its vulnerable site at the head of the fibula, where it lies on a hard bony surface with only a surface covering of skin. External compression from a single prolonged exposure, e.g. leaning on a sharp surface, continued squatting, or repeated trauma, e.g. sitting cross-legged, wearing high stiff boots, may produce a lesion. It may also be compressed by a ganglion (which may arise from the superior tibiofibular joint) or even from the tendinous edge of peroneus longus.

The presentation may be with a painless foot drop which may become more noticeable if the patient is tired or has walked any distance. This may cause the patient to trip. There is weakness of tibialis anterior and often the evertors with a preserved ankle jerk. The sensory loss is variable (Fig. 6.4): if the deep peroneal branch is affected there may only be numbness on the dorsum of the web between first and second toes.

Electrically, denervation may be found in tibialis anterior and extensor digitorum brevis. There may be a local conduction block or slowing in the

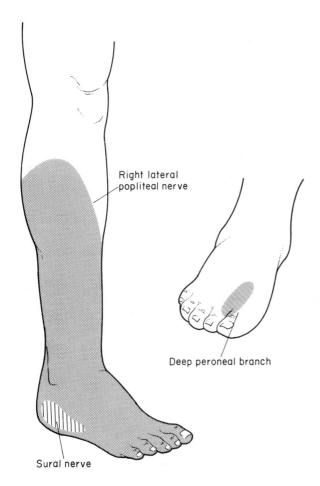

Right lateral popliteal nerve

Deep peroneal branch

Sural nerve

Fig. 6.4. Areas of sensory loss in lesions of the right sural, lateral popliteal and deep peroneal branch nerves

region of the head of the fibula. Usually the lateral popliteal nerve action potential is lost. The sural nerve action potential is preserved and medial popliteal conduction should be unaffected which will help to localize the lesion.

Physiotherapy, an insert splint or foot drop appliance, may be useful while waiting for recovery if an external compressive lesion, or acute trauma has been incriminated. In a few instances the lateral popliteal nerve may have to be surgically explored to exclude a ganglion or compressive lesion.

Tarsal tunnel

Rarely the posterior tibial nerve may be compressed in the tarsal tunnel in the sole of the foot. This usually will provoke tingling, pain and sometimes 'burning' in the sole of the foot and toes which may be worse at night and aggravated by inversion of the ankle. Note the similarities to a carpal tunnel syndrome. In severe cases there is weakness of abductor hallucis and sensory loss distally over the sole and toes. Electrically, there may be a prolonged distal motor latency to abductor hallucis and in younger patients the medial plantar sensory action potential will be absent. Decompression may be effective treatment.

Femoral nerve

This arises from the L2, 3 and 4 roots passing through the psoas muscle and under the inguinal ligament lateral to the femoral artery, to supply the anterior thigh muscles. It may be compressed by an abscess, a haematoma (often from over-anticoagulation) in the psoas, or damaged acutely by fractures of the pelvis, knife wounds to the groin or from thrombotic lesions of the vasa nervorum, e.g. diabetes mellitus.

A femoral nerve lesion will produce weakness of the knee extensors, the quadriceps group, with muscle wasting, a depressed or absent knee jerk, and sensory loss in the anterior thigh and medial part of the knee. There may be mild weakness in the hip flexors. Patients will experience difficulty walking, particularly going up stairs, and the leg may seem to buckle. Electrically, it is possible to show denervation in the quadriceps and a prolonged distal motor latency when the nerve is stimulated in the groin.

Lateral cutaneous nerve of the thigh (meralgia paraesthetica)

This sensory nerve arises from L2 and 3 and leaves the abdomen under the inguinal ligament adjacent to the anterior superior iliac spine. At this site it may be compressed or stretched within its fascial tunnel. Sometimes this is provoked by obesity or pregnancy. It may also be entrapped or compressed by a neuroma. Patients complain of tingling and numbness in a patch about the size of a hand on the anterolateral aspect of the thigh above the knee (*see* Fig. 6.3). There is no weakness or reflex changes.

In most patients explanation, reassurance and sometimes weight loss are often all that are necessary. In a few patients where pain is troublesome, surgical exploration may be required.

Thoracic outlet compression

The lower trunk of the brachial plexus arises from C8 and T1. It passes across the posterior triangle of the neck behind the subclavian artery running between scalenus anterior and medius. If there is an extra cervical rib attached to the transverse process of C7 or a fibrous band attached to an elongated transverse process, either of these may compress the lower cord of the plexus. They may also compress the subclavian artery producing vascular symptoms. Symptoms may be predominantly neurological, vascular or a combination. The condition is more common in women.

Neurological features

These include aching and pain radiating down the inner forearm to the ulnar side of the hand, associated with tingling and sometimes numbness. Sensory loss can be demonstrated on the medial side of the forearm proximal to the wrist unlike that found in an ulnar nerve lesion. There is often wasting and weakness involving all the intrinsic muscles of the hand, the thenar and hypothenar pads and the medial forearm muscles.

Vascular features

These include Raynaud's phenomenon with complaints of coldness and colour changes in the fingers or more severe upsets from arterial or venous obstruction. The radial pulse may disappear in certain arm positions on the affected side and a bruit may by audible in the supraclavicular fossa. Rarely distal emboli may affect the fingers.

Electrically, there will be denervation in the thenar pad muscles as well as in the ulnar innervated muscles. The ulnar sensory and nerve action potentials will be small and the F wave latencies prolonged. Evoked potential studies may show delay proximally. X-rays may show the cervical ribs or an elongated transverse process of C7. Arteriography may show compression of the sub-clavian vessel.

In severe symptomatic cases surgical treatment with decompression of the lower cord of the plexus is necessary.

Brachial plexus damage

This may arise in a number of ways. Occasionally there may be a direct injury from a penetrating wound but, more commonly, acute lesions arise in motor cycle accidents when the patient lands on his shoulder sustaining an acute traction injury so that the roots may be actually torn out of the cervical cord. If such severe damage occurs this may be irreversible but less severe damage may allow some recovery. Most commonly young men are affected and the upper C5 and 6 roots, or C5, 6 and 7 may be damaged, although C8 and T1 may also be involved. Unfortunately in more than half of such injuries C5 to T1 are affected.

Depending on the extent of the root damage, there will be paralysis of muscles supplied by the affected roots, loss of reflexes and sensory loss. The latter may appear less extensive because there is considerable overlap of dermatomes. If the root has been avulsed, the affected muscles waste leaving a 'flail' limb with often unpleasant pains with a causalgic quality. The presence of a Horner's syndrome may indicate T1 damage. Plain X-rays may show the presence of any fractures, or a fracture-dislocation of the cervical spine or clavicle. Electrical studies will confirm denervation in affected muscles. If the nerve root has been avulsed proximal to the dorsal root ganglion, the sensory action potential may be preserved. Somatosensory evoked potentials may confirm the presence of proximal damage. Myelography may demonstrate multiple traumatic meningoceles at the sites of the avulsed roots.

The outlook is often poor: about one-half of patients with extensive plexus injuries show no recovery, the remainder show varying degrees of improvement, often in more proximal muscles. A variety of measures and appliances may be used to help those with disability. Some patients with a complete lesion may undergo amputation of the affected useless limb. Most recently, attempts at surgery to repair selected plexus lesions have been made.

The *brachial plexus* may also be damaged by *neoplastic infiltration*, often spread from carcinoma of the breast or bronchus, or from malignant lymphomas. Commonly this leads to a painful progressive loss of function with weakness, wasting, tingling and sensory loss, the distribution depending on the pattern of involvement. A Horner's syndrome may arise if T1 is affected. The reflexes are commonly depressed or absent. Quite frequently the arm distally may become swollen and there may be palpable thickening or even a mass in the supra-clavicular fossa.

Conventional radiology often fails to demonstrate a lesion of the plexus, although a soft tissue apical shadow may be present on chest X-rays. (Fig. 6.5).

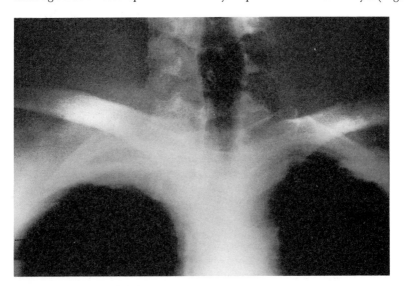

Fig. 6.5. Apical chest X-ray to show shadowing at the right apex. This patient presented with wasting of the small muscles of his right hand and had a right Horner's syndrome. The shadow was caused by a lymphoma

These may also show destruction of the first rib. CT scanning may demonstrate a mass. Electrical studies may indicate a proximal lesion which commonly has produced denervation in affected muscles.

It is always worth testing and charting individual arm muscles in such lesions to elucidate the pattern of root or plexus involvement (*see* Fig. 3.10).

A further cause of brachial plexus damage is *radiation fibrosis* following radiotherapy in patients treated for breast carcinoma. Here there may be a relatively slow painless and progressive weakness with sensory loss pointing to a proximal lesion often starting some 12 months after treatment. The total radiation dose may have exceeded 6000 cGy. Commonly, the affected limb is swollen from lymphoedema and it may be difficult to differentiate brachial plexus damage from neoplastic infiltration from that caused by radiation, although the former is painful. Treatment is symptomatic.

Neuralgic amyotrophy (brachial neuritis)

This is an uncommon condition most often found in younger patients where there is the onset of acute painful patchy damage to the brachial plexus on an inflammatory basis. It is thought either to have a link with viral infections or disordered immune responses. It may follow a clear viral infection or immunization. It is also rarely seen as a familial disorder in association with multiple pressure palsies.

The onset is with excruciating severe pain usually in the shoulder, base of the neck, or arm. Initially this is unremitting keeping the patient awake and requiring strong analgesics. The pain lasts days, up to 2–3 weeks and as it remits the patient is aware of patchy weakness of affected muscles. There is associated depression or loss of reflexes and varied sensory loss. The pattern of weakness is patchy and a whole muscle may be affected which may help to differentiate this from an acute cervical root lesion arising from a disc prolapse. In a small number both arms may be affected. In most patients over a period of months, often 6, there is recovery, but in some others the progress is slow, up to 18 months suggesting that repair here is by regeneration.

Electrical studies will confirm denervation in affected muscles, commonly with slowing in affected motor nerves and prolonged or absent F waves. The CSF may be normal, although a mild lymphocytic pleocytosis and protein rise have been found.

Treatment is symptomatic: analgesics and rest until the acute pain has settled. Physiotherapy directed towards strengthening the affected muscles is helpful.

Cervical root problems

The muscles of the arm are supplied by the C5,6,7,8 and T1 roots. These leave the spinal canal through the intervertebral foramina and may be irritated, stretched or compressed causing symptoms and signs referred to that root. It should be emphasized that the pain from such a lesion is referred into the myotome which may be different from the site of sensory symptoms (paraesthesiae, numbness) which are referred to the dermatome (*see* Fig. 3.11).

In the cervical spine there are eight exiting nerve roots from the seven vertebrae so that the root exits above the body of the vertebra concerned, i.e. the C6 root exits between C5 and 6. Below T1 the root exits below, i.e. T1 exits between T1 and 2.

The most common causes of cervical root damage are:

1. Compression by an acute soft disc prolapse.
2. Compression by a hard bony spur in degenerative spondylitis.
3. Compression by a neuroma, lymphoma, extradural tumour or metastasis.

Cervical root symptoms

Pain in the neck or arm is very common affecting over 10 per cent of the population. However, only a small number of these have pain arising from cervical root irritation. More often pain may arise from the soft tissues or joints. With cervical root disturbances the initial symptoms are usually increasing pain, often referred to the base of the neck, shoulder, scapula or upper arm. Later there may be weakness of affected muscles, depression or loss of the appropriate reflex, and sensory symptoms, tingling and numbness. Commonly affected roots compressed by spondylotic spurs or disc protrusion are C6 (C5/6 disc space), C7 (C6/7), C5 (C4/5) and C8 (C7/T1). In younger patients there may be an acute soft disc prolapse. If this extends laterally it will compress the affected root. The root is initially irritated causing referred pain, but if the compression becomes more severe, the nerve root may infarct leading to loss of pain but more severe weakness with signs of denervation in the affected muscles, reflex loss and sensory impairment. It is worth recalling the charts for the root innervation of the arm muscles (Fig. 3.10) and for the dermatome distribution (Fig. 3.11). Table 3.1 gives the reflex levels.

A central cervical disc protrusion will lead to encroachment onto the spinal cord producing a myelopathy with spastic leg weakness, sensory changes in the feet and sometimes disturbed bowel and bladder function. These will be accompanied by long tract signs, increased reflexes, clonus, extensor plantar responses and sensory loss in the feet.

Most patients with neck problems, particularly acute root irritation, show pronounced spasm of the nuchal muscles causing greatly limited neck movements. Lateral flexion is particularly affected for most rotation occurs at the atlanto-axial joint and proximally. Sometimes a 'wry neck' may develop.

In older patients degenerative changes in the spine lead to narrowing of the intervetebral space with bulging of the disc, and hypertrophy of the surrounding ligaments causing these to thicken. The bony margins of the vertebrae become raised producing hard osteophytic spurs which may compress nerve roots, the spinal cord or both. The last causes a spondylotic radiculomyelopathy. Again symptoms and signs depend on the root involved and whether there is spinal cord compression. Failure to notice spinal cord compression may lead to irreversible damage with even a tetraplegia and lost sphincter control.

Cervical spondylosis may be aggravated by trauma, particularly if this is repeated. Occasionally patients may give a highly relevant history of trauma causing acute but transient neurological symptoms, e.g. paresis in an arm or legs with sensory upset, which recover only to be followed some time later by further symptoms which may slowly progress.

Investigations

Good quality X-rays of the cervical spine with oblique views will demonstrate spondylotic degenerative changes, encroachment of the exit foramina by osteophytic spurs or any malalignment. Bony collapse from unexpected malignant infiltration will also be shown. However, it should be emphasized that as patients get older, all will show some spondylotic changes in the cervical spine so it is important to put these in the clinical context of the patient's symptoms and signs before attributing all arm or neck pain to the blanket term 'cervical spondylosis'.

The sagittal diameter of the cervical canal is an important factor in the possible development of a myelopathy. A diameter of 10 mm or less on a true lateral film suggests the cord is compromised. Myelography, using water-soluble contrast, will show most acute root or cord compressive lesions. This is now being increasingly supplemented by spinal CT scans. Electrical studies may show denervation in appropriate root territories and help to exclude peripheral nerve entrapment or a more widespread neuropathic disorder.

Treatment

In many instances treatment of an acute root lesion from a disc or spur, in which pain is the dominant feature, consists of bedrest, flat, combined with regular analgesics (strong if necessary) and muscle relaxants, e.g. diazepam. This may often allow the pain to settle within a few days. Later this may be aided by splinting the neck in a collar for 2–3 weeks. As the pain settles, heat and gentle exercises in physiotherapy may help recovery. Halter traction to the neck has its advocates: it certainly confines the patient to bed, flat, and may help relieve pain more quickly, although in a few patients there is complaint that this actually aggravates their symptoms.

In patients with progressive root signs, particularly if there are signs of any cord involvement, persistent severe pain or failure to respond to medical treatment, myelography is necessary. In those patients with a large symptomatic disc lesion surgical decompression may be used. This either may be by a foraminotomy freeing the root at the exit foramen, or may involve more extensive excision of the disc by an anterolateral approach which may be combined with a bone graft at the affected disc level, Cloward's procedure. Posterior decompressive laminectomy (deroofing the spinal canal) may also be used if there is extensive narrowing of the canal with multiple disc impressions. However, less than 5 per cent of patients with cervical root symptoms come to surgery.

Many older patients with cervical spondylosis and a mild radiculo-myelopathy may be managed conservatively using a cervical collar and physiotherapy.

Lumbar root lesions

The other mobile part of the spine, apart from the neck, is the lumbar region. Here nerve roots may be irritated, stretched or compressed provoking symptoms and signs in the territory of the affected root. *Sciatica* describes the pain referred down the course of the sciatic nerve from the back of the buttock, down the back of the leg to the foot. This pain most commonly arises from compromise of the L5 and S1 roots.

In the lumbosacral region a lateral disc prolapse may effect a nerve root, or sometimes roots. A central disc prolapse will extend into the lumbar sac compressing the cauda equina and producing symptoms and signs in both legs, and more alarming disturbances of bowel and bladder control. Such symptoms of sphincter disturbance are a medical emergency and patients should be admitted to hospital urgently with a view to myelography and surgical decompression before irreversible damage occurs.

Over 95 per cent of lumbar disc protrusions occur at the L4/5 and L5/S1 levels affecting the L5 and S1 roots, less often the L4 roots. In the lumbar region, roots can be involved at a higher level so that myelography is essential before deciding on surgery; e.g. an L4/5 disc protrusion can involve the L5 or the L4 root. Lumbar disc protrusions may follow an acute injury or strain, particularly lifting. Many patients may have a preceding history of low back pain and intermittent sciatica which in the past has responded to rest or physiotherapy. Small disc protrusions will settle with rest but a large extruded fragment is likely to give continuing trouble.

Other causes of root pain need consideration although these are less common. Diabetic infarction of nerve roots or the femoral nerve, diabetic amyotrophy or plexopathy, may present with acute pain in the thigh and be accompanied by wasting, impaired reflexes and sensory upset (*see* p. 133). Neoplastic involvement of nerve roots may arise in the spinal canal, often secondary to bony metastases with collapse of the vertebrae, most often from primary growths of bronchus, breast, prostate, kidney, gastrointestinal tract or lymphomas. The lumbosacral plexus on the side wall of the pelvis may be involved with gynaecological or colonorectal malignancy. Such tumours cause severe pain which is often not relieved by rest, unlike the pain of a disc. In time the lymphatic pathways and even the iliac veins may be obstructed leading to swelling of the affected leg.

Root symptoms

S1 root lesions will produce pain down the posterior aspect of the buttock, thigh and leg to the heel. There will also be tingling or numbness in the sole of the foot, particularly the lateral side and outer two toes. There will be weakness of plantar flexion, leading to the inability to stand on tiptoe on one leg, with also some weakness of the hamstrings and glutei. The ankle jerk will be depressed or absent. Sensory impairment is often on the sole and lateral border of the foot.

L5 root lesions produce pain in the hip down the lateral side of the leg to the ankle. There will be sensory upset on the dorsum of the foot, including the great toe, and the lateral aspect of the shin. Weakness involves the dorsiflexors of the great toe (which has an exclusive L5 innervation) and often slight weakness of the ankle dorsiflexors, evertors and hamstrings. The patient may have difficulty walking on their heels. The ankle jerk is usually preserved; rarely it may be slightly depressed. Sensory impairment is usually over the dorsum of the foot extending onto the lateral side of the lower leg.

L4 root lesions produce pain radiating into the anterior aspect of the thigh, knee, shin and medial side of the calf. There may be tingling and numbness on the medial side of the calf with sensory impairment. There is weakness of the ankle dorsiflexors (tibialis anterior) and the quadriceps. The knee jerk is usually reduced or absent.

With L4, 5 and S1 root lesions there are commonly associated root tension signs with the inability to flex the fully straightened leg to a right angle at the hip. In older patients and those with hip disease this may not be possible because of local restriction from the joint. If nerve roots are stretched by a disc protrusion, then straight leg raising is commonly limited on the affected side with pain referred in a sciatic radiation. Such pain may be aggravated by dorsiflexion of the foot. It should be noted that in patients exaggerating their symptoms with the suspicion of a functional component, straight leg raising may be grossly restricted lying on the couch, yet if the patient is then asked to sit up to demonstrate the site of their back pain, they may be able to do this with legs flexed at the hip to 90° and the knees fully extended. Spinal movements are often restricted with lumbosacral root lesions, particularly trunk flexion. There may also be sometimes a scoliosis or pelvic tilt.

Upper plexus or lumbar root lesions are uncommon but produce weakness in the hip flexors, adductors and quadriceps. Such patients have difficulty getting out of a low chair, the bath or climbing upstairs. The lumbar plexus may occasionally be damaged during surgery in the pelvis or if a massive retroperitoneal haematoma develops in a patient with a bleeding diathesis. If the upper lumbar roots are stretched (L2,3) the presence of root tension signs may be detected by a femoral stretch test. Here the patient lies prone with the knee flexed to a right angle, and the thigh is then extended at the hip. A positive test will produce pain in the front of the thigh.

All patients with lumbosacral root symptoms should be specifically questioned about their bowel and bladder function, and in the male about potency. A rectal examination, or pelvic examination where appropriate, should be undertaken to exclude any palpable local mass. At the same time this will enable sensation to be checked in the lower sacral dermatomes, the tone of the anal sphincter to be assessed, and the anal reflex elicited. The last is tested by pricking or scratching the pigmented perianal skin and eliciting a localized contraction of that muscle which can be seen. There is an old aphorism 'beware of the patient who sits on their signs' for if the buttocks and anal reflex are not tested, sacral lesions whether arising in the conus, cauda equina or more distally, may be missed.

Investigations

Blood should be taken for a full blood count, ESR, fasting blood glucose, and where appropriate estimation of the acid and alkaline phosphatases, serum proteins and electrophoresis. Plain X-rays of the spine may show degenerative changes, a narrowed disc space, or occasionally point to other pathology by the appearance of vertebral collapse, loss of pedicle or abnormal density. A chest X-ray is appropriate in adults. If there is progressive or persistent neurological deficit, continuing pain or diagnostic doubt, myelography may be undertaken to visualize the spinal cord and roots. CSF can be obtained at the same time and occasionally cytology may point to a malignant process, or other changes in the fluid may indicate alternative pathology. Spinal CT scans sometimes with intrathecal contrast, and MRI scans may sometimes prove helpful in the diagnosis of severe root pain.

Treatment

This will depend on the cause, but most acute disc lesions respond to strict bedrest for 2–3 weeks, accompanied by analgesics and muscle relaxants. Traction has its advocates. Surgery may prove necessary where medical treatment has failed, where there is progressive or persistent neurological deficit and where a large disc is demonstrated, or there is persistent unremitting root pain. This is discussed further (*see* p. 196).

7

Cranial nerve syndromes

Cranial nerve I

Anosmia

The olfactory nerves arise in the nasal mucosa at the top of the nose; from this area the olfactory tract passes along the olfactory groove of the cribriform plate to the cerebrum. In most instances the sense of smell relies on the inhalation of very small particles of the substance under test. Although many patients refer to the taste of foods, in nearly all instances this involves smell, as taste only differentiates sweet, salt, bitter and acid.

Smell may be lost (anosmia), diminished (hyposmia) or distorted (dysosmia). There also may be olfactory hallucinations, most often found as part of the aura of complex partial seizures. These are usually unpleasant, very brief, and may arise from the uncinate lobes. Olfactory hallucinations may also occur in psychiatric disorders.

Temporary anosmia is found most commonly with local nasal disease and many people will have experienced this loss with an acute 'cold'. It may be uni- or bilateral. Head injuries may cause anosmia, most often by shearing the delicate olfactory fibres. Such loss is often permanent; it is commonly associated with fractures in the floor of the anterior fossa.

Anosmia may also arise with subfrontal tumours and those on the floor of the anterior fossa. These include olfactory groove or subfrontal meningiomas, frontal gliomas, giant aneurysms, skull metastases and nasopharyngeal carcinoma. These mass lesions may present with dementia and the most important localizing sign may be anosmia. If the tumour is very large it may cause papilloedema or even optic nerve damage with optic atrophy.

Cranial nerve II

Papilloedema

By definition this is swelling with elevation of the optic disc. This may arise from:

1. Raised intracranial pressure
   Mass lesions: tumours, abscesses, haematomas
   Diffuse brain swelling
   Infections: meningitis, encephalitis
   Obstructive hydrocephalus: blocked CSF pathways, posterior fossa masses, aqueduct stenosis
   Venous thrombosis: sagittal sinus thrombosis
   Benign intracranial hypertension
2. Local optic nerve swelling: includes nerve head-papillitis
   Inflammation: acute demyelination
   Ischaemia: giant cell arteritis, vascular disease
   Neoplastic: cuffing of the optic nerves by tumour cells, e.g. leukaemia, lymphoma, carcinoma
3. Medical disorders
   Severe anaemia, e.g. pernicious anaemia
   Polycythaemia
   Carbon dioxide retention with chronic pulmonary insufficiency
   Guillain-Barré polyneuritis
   Drugs: usually causing benign intracranial hypertension e.g. tetracycline, excess vitamin A, steroid withdrawal
   Lead poisoning
   Accelerated hypertension

As the optic disc swells, the veins become engorged and venous pulsation is lost. The margins of the disc become indistinct and then radial streak haemorrhages may appear around the edge.

Papilloedema may be asymptomatic but usually there are symptoms related to the cause, particularly if there is a mass lesion. With a papillitis there will be severe loss of visual acuity, accompanied by a significant field defect, usually central. With raised intracranial pressure (ICP) impairment of acuity is a very late development: initially there may only be some enlargement of the blind spots, but later some concentric constriction of the fields with a fall in acuity. Occasionally, with a very high ICP, there may be transient visual obscurations with acute loss of vision, usually for a few seconds, provoked by bending, coughing or straining – measures that all produce a transient rise in ICP.

Papilloedema may develop very rapidly, e.g. with cerebral haemorrhage, but more commonly arises slowly over days or weeks, e.g. with a tumour. It must be emphasized that only some 50 per cent of cerebral tumours cause papilloedema. The disc swells because the rise in ICP is transmitted through the subarachnoid sheaths of the optic nerves with an added obstruction of the venous return.

Optic neuritis

This is an acute inflammation of the optic nerve. If the process involves the nerve head, the papilla, it is termed a papillitis. The nerve head is visible through an ophthalmoscope and with papillitis there is swelling of the optic disc. If the inflammation is behind the nerve head, a retrobulbar neuritis, the optic disc appears normal initially.

Symptoms and signs

Optic neuritis commonly affects younger patients aged 15–40. Most complain of acute impairment of vision with a fall in acuity which may vary from mild (6/9–6/12) to severe with almost complete visual loss (to hand movements (HM) or perception of light (PL)). The impairment of vision may progress over hours or days, usually reaching its worst within one week. There is often tenderness of the globe and pain on eye movement on the affected side. The pain usually lasts a few days. In most instances there is a central field loss (scotoma), sometimes extending to the blind spot, centrocaecal. There may be a massive field loss with only a thin peripheral rim of preserved vision in severely affected eyes.

Even if the acuity is only moderately impaired there will be reduced colour vision and an afferent pupillary defect (*see* p. 67). In most instances of acute neuritis the optic disc appears normal unless there is a papillitis. Usually there is involvement of only one optic nerve, but occasionally, there may be bilateral involvement, either simultaneously or sequentially.

Aetiology

The most usual pathogenesis is an acute demyelination of the optic nerve. In some instances this may be the initial symptom of multiple sclerosis (MS); about 25 per cent of patients with MS may present in this way. However, if patients with an optic neuritis are followed up over a number of years some 50–75 per cent develop MS.

Other far less common causes include local infection or inflammation of tissues around the optic nerves (e.g. orbital cellulitis, herpes zoster, meningitis, sphenoid sinusitis); direct viral infections (e.g. varicella-zoster, mumps, measles); infections (e.g. tuberculosis, syphilis); granulomatous inflammatory conditions (e.g. sarcoidosis); and intraocular inflammations (e.g. uveitis). In a proportion of patients no cause is found.

Prognosis and treatment

In most instances recovery of vision occurs over a number of weeks, often 6–8, and about 90 per cent of patients recover vision to an acuity of 6/9 or better. In many of these patients there is some residual impairment of colour vision, an afferent pupillary defect, and some pallor of the optic disc, i.e. evidence of a degree of atrophy with a scarred nerve head. A small number of patients may be left with severe visual loss. Visual evoked potentials will usually show a prolonged latency and this may persist.

Steroid treatment in the acute phase of the illness may shorten the course, relieving pain and allowing a more rapid recovery of acuity, but it is probable that the degree of return of vision in the long term is not influenced by whether or not steroids are used. Steroids may be given as intramuscular injections of ACTH, tablets of prednisolone or dexamethasone, or even by retro-orbital injections. The doses are those used in MS (*see* p. 349).

Ischaemic papillitis

In older patients acute swelling of the nerve head may follow occlusion of the posterior ciliary arteries and the peripapillary choroidal vessels of the optic nerve, leading to infarction of the anterior part of the optic nerve. The retina is supplied by the retinal artery. Such vascular lesions will usually cause acute severe visual loss which is painless. However, in some patients there may be complaints of pain in or around the eye or headache, particularly if there is a giant cell arteritis.

The eye shows a severe drop in acuity or even blindness, with most often an altitudinal field defect. The nerve head is swollen and there may be many small flame-shaped haemorrhages. The arteries may appear thin and tortuous. As the disc swelling subsides, optic atrophy follows.

In such patients this loss of vision is always an emergency and the ESR must be measured urgently. If this is high, giant cell arteritis (GCA) may be the cause and patients should be started immediately on steroids, prednisolone 60 mg daily. It is important to stress that an arteritis may affect the second eye in 75 per cent of patients unless they are treated promptly with steroids. However, ischaemic papillitis may also arise from atheroma (idiopathic), diabetes mellitus, or other rare forms of vasculitis.

A *central retinal artery occlusion* may also cause an acute painless loss of vision in older patients. Usually this will cause complete blindness with a lost direct pupillary response. The retina appears pale, swollen and the arteries are thinned. A cherry red spot at the fovea may be present. Often there is occlusion of a branch of the retinal artery leading to a depressed acuity with partial field loss. Again, it must be stressed that giant cell arteritis needs exclusion, although other vascular causes may be responsible. The prognosis of these vascular lesions is poor.

Optic atrophy

This indicates that the optic nerve has been damaged. The signs are those of impaired vision with reduced acuity, a field defect and pallor of the optic disc. There are many causes including:

1. Following raised intracranial pressure: consecutive optic atrophy
   a. Mass lesions
   b. Infections: meningoencephalitis, syphilis.
2. Following vascular lesions: central retinal artery occlusion, papillitis.
3. Inflammatory lesion: optic neuritis.
4. Toxic: drugs (ethambutol, chloramphenicol, isoniazid, digitalis), tobacco, alcohol.
5. Inherited: Leber's optic atrophy.
6. Trauma.
7. Vitamin deficiency, metabolic: B12 lack, diabetes mellitus.
8. Ocular causes: glaucoma, macular degenerations.
9. Optic nerve, chiasmal compression
   a. Optic nerve glioma, cuffing by neoplastic cells, optic canal meningioma

b. Chiasmal involvement by pituitary tumours, aneurysms, parapituitary tumours.

Slowly progressive visual loss always requires full investigation to exclude a *local ocular cause*, or *compression* of the *optic nerve or chiasm*.

Slowly progressive visual deterioration may also arise with toxic and deficiency causes. This is well illustrated in *tobacco-alcohol amblyopia*. This is found most commonly in older patients, often chronic alcoholics whose dietary calories largely arise from alcohol coupled with a degree of malnutrition. It is also found in heavy smokers using strong tobacco to roll their own cigarettes. There is a progressive fall in acuity accompanied by bilateral centrocaecal scotomas. These latter are often difficult to chart but are most easily found with red targets. Such field defects commonly cross the vertical meridian of the field.

Abstention from alcohol, cessation of smoking, a good diet with added thiamine injections, and hydroxocobalamin injections may prevent further deterioration and often allow a degree of recovery although this may prove incomplete.

Leber's optic atrophy

This is a rare inherited form of visual loss largely with an X-linked inheritance. Males aged 15–30 are commonly affected, and females are carriers. However, some 15 per cent of patients may be female.

It usually presents with acute loss of vision in both eyes either occurring sequentially or together over weeks, sometimes months. The acuity falls, often to 6/60, and there is a dense central scotoma. Acutely the optic disc may appear swollen: later it is pale from progressive atrophy. It may sometimes be difficult initially to differentiate this condition from an acute optic neuritis. Complete blindness is rare and some patients show a fluctuating course.

It has been suggested that the inability to detoxify cyanide may be the inherited metabolic defect. Treatment is with massive injections of hydroxocobalamin (B12) which possibly slows up or even arrests the process.

Cranial nerves III, IV and VI: ocular motor palsies

Damage to these nerves will cause weakness or paralysis of the ocular muscles they supply, producing diplopia if the two eyes are not in parallel. The frequency of some of the causes of these ocular motor palsies is:

Cranial nerve	III	IV	VI
Trauma	13	28	11
Vascular	17	15	9
Neoplasm	18	10	31
Aneurysm	18		3
Undetermined	20	34	22
Other	14	13	24

(figures as percentages)

Diplopia may also arise from weakness of the ocular muscles, e.g. dysthyroid eye disease, or from disturbance of the neuromuscular junction, e.g. myasthenia gravis. If there is a very slow onset and progression, and particularly if this occurs early in childhood, there may be suppression of the image from the weak eye, amblyopia. This is often accompanied by a visible squint, strabismus. In a divergent squint the eyes are deviated away from each other, exotropia; in a convergent squint the eyes are turned towards each other (cross-eyed), esotropia. If one eye is obviously higher (above) than the other, this is termed hypertropia, or below the other, hypotropia. A latent squint may be demonstrated by asking a patient to fix on an object and then covering each eye in turn. If the uncovered eye moves to fix on the target, a latent squint has been elicited. The cover test will also distinguish between a concomitant squint (where the affected eye will show a full range of movement when its fellow is covered) and a true paralytic squint. The testing of diplopia has been described in Chapter 3.

Oculomotor palsy

In a complete oculomotor palsy the eyelid droops to cover the eye and the globe is turned down and out due to the actions of the unparalysed lateral rectus and superior oblique muscles (*see* Fig. 3.5). The pupil may be enlarged and unreactive if the pupillomotor fibres (these lie around the periphery of the nerve) are compressed. There will be paralysis of the superior and inferior rectus, the medial rectus and inferior oblique muscles. Vascular lesions which may infarct the third nerve, e.g. in diabetes mellitus, an arteritis, may produce a complete oculomotor palsy with pupillary sparing. Compression of the nerve by a mass or aneurysm often involves the pupil.

Trochlear nerve palsy

The superior oblique depresses the adducted eye and intorts the abducted eye. This will cause diplopia on downgaze with vertical separation of the images. There may often be an associated head tilt to the opposite shoulder. Trauma is a relatively common cause.

Abducens nerve palsy

The lateral rectus abducts the eye causing diplopia with horizontal separation of images maximal on gaze to the affected side. The sixth nerve has a relatively long course on the base of the skull, through the cavernous sinus and into the orbit via the superior orbital fissure. On this course it may be involved in trauma, compression from masses and damaged as an effect of raised intracranial pressure.

Ocular motor palsies may arise centrally within the pons and midbrain from strokes, neoplasms, plaques of multiple sclerosis and even thiamine deficiency. Usually such lesions produce other signs, particularly involvement of other cranial nerves, a Horner's syndrome, cerebellar signs and sometimes long tract signs in the limbs. At the base of the brain the nerves may be damaged in

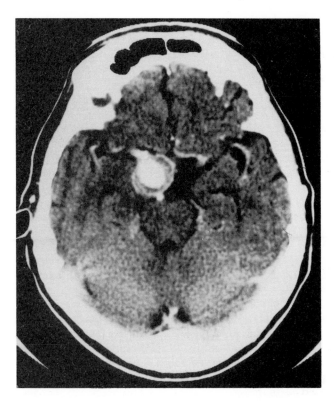

Fig. 7.1. CT brain scan with enhancement showing a large aneurysm at the termination of the internal carotid artery. The patient presented with a painful partial oculomotor palsy with pupillary involvement

meningitis or from basal neoplasms, e.g. nasopharyngeal carcinoma, chordoma. In the cavernous sinus and superior orbital fissure the IIIrd, IVth, VIth and ophthalmic division of the Vth cranial nerves may all be involved together, e.g. aneurysms (Fig. 7.1), granulomas, meningiomas. More anteriorly at the back of the orbit, mass lesions and granulomas may displace the globe producing diplopia and a proptosis.

Dysthyroid eye disease

An overactive thyroid (hyperthyroidism) may produce abnormal eye signs. These include exophthalmos, a lid lag, conjunctival suffusion and diplopia. The last is most often vertical diplopia from restriction of upgaze or less commonly from limitation of abduction. Dysthyroid eye disease may directly involve the ocular muscles producing thickening, tethering and restricted movements, most often found in the inferior and medial rectus muscles. This is a relatively common cause of diplopia arising in middle age. The affected muscles appear swollen on orbital views of a computerized tomographic (CT) scan. Blood tests will usually confirm the presence of thyrotoxicosis, but sometimes the evidence for thyroid disease is subtle and requires specialized endocrine investigation.

Myasthenia gravis (*see* p. 121)

In any patient with variable diplopia, the diagnosis of myasthenia gravis should be considered. This most commonly is associated with weakness of eye closure, and often involvement of the facial and bulbar muscles. Proximal limb muscles may also be affected. An edrophonium test (Tensilon *see* p. 121) will usually confirm the diagnosis.

Investigation

Patients with ocular motor palsies will require a number of investigations: not all these may be necessary in the same patient. Blood tests should include a full blood count, erythrocyte sedimentation rate (ESR), fasting blood glucose, Wassermann reaction, *Treponema pallidum* haemagglutination (or equivalent), thyroid function tests, autoantibodies and sometimes those for antiacetylcholine receptor antibody (to exclude myasthenia). An edrophonium test may be indicated.

Plain X-rays of the skull, orbits with basal skull views and sometimes sinus films and a chest X-ray should be taken. More specialized imaging studies include CT scan films of the brain and orbits with contrast enhancement, and even magnetic resonance imaging (MRI). Angiography may be necessary to demonstrate an aneurysm. CSF examination will be indicated in patients with a meningitis, subarachnoid haemorrhage, and in those suspected of MS. Evoked potentials and an MRI scan may also be useful in demonstrating multiple lesions in MS.

Cranial nerve V

Trigeminal neuralgia, tic douloureux

This describes episodes of acute neuralgia usually appearing as stabs or jabs of intense pain, lasting seconds, and largely in the territory of the maxillary and mandibular divisions of the trigeminal nerve on one side. The pains are commonly triggered by touch or contact, e.g. washing, shaving, eating, cleaning the teeth, talking or even a cold wind. In many patients there may be severe stabs of pain recurring over weeks or months, followed by periods of remission. In a few there may be no remission but only a grumbling continuation. In some patients after the stab of pain there may be some residual aching. Although these pains usually occur in the day, some patients are disturbed at night.

Between episodes of pain there should be no abnormal signs, in particular intact corneal reflexes, no facial sensory loss, no facial weakness or involuntary movements. The presence of abnormal signs suggests the tic may be symptomatic of some irritative cause.

Persistent trigeminal neuralgia may make some patients so fearful of the next jab that they avoid all contact with the affected part of the face, and even stop eating and speaking. This may leave a very demoralized and depressed patient which may add to the problem.

Trigeminal neuralgia shows an increasing frequency in older patients, around 15 per 100 000, and affects women more than men. It often starts between the ages of 50–60, but it may be found in younger patients where it is more likely to be symptomatic.

Causation

There has been considerable debate about the cause: in many patients it is unknown. However, in those patients who have undergone surgical treatment, at operation a small blood vessel has been found lying in contact with the trigeminal nerve close to the pons. Far less commonly other irritative lesions of the trigeminal nerve have been found; these include aneurysms and cerebellopontine angle tumours. Tic is also found in patients with multiple sclerosis. Some 2–3 per cent of patients with trigeminal neuralgia may have MS. The combination of neuralgic pain with involuntary movements of the face, a hemifacial spasm, may arise from an irritative lesion affecting the trigeminal and facial nerves which lie close together in the pons and cerebellopontine angle.

Investigations

These should be negative unless the tic is a symptom of MS or a cerebellopontine angle tumour. Plain X-rays of the skull with a basal view and sometimes special dental views may prove useful. Special CT scan views may be useful if a basal mass lesion is suspected. Screening for MS may include evoked potential studies, CSF examination and an MRI scan.

Treatment

In over two-thirds of patients the neuralgia can be controlled by drugs. Carbamazepine (Tegretol) is the first choice building the dose up from 100 mg b.d. in the elderly to the smallest dose that gives control of the pain – often 200 mg t.i.d. or q.i.d. The main side-effects of carbamazepine relate to drug toxicity with the appearance of diplopia and ataxia. These are dose related. Less often allergies, marrow depression or hepatic upset may arise. Other drugs that may be effective include the anticonvulsants phenytoin and clonazepam. Baclofen (Lioresal) may also prove helpful in about 60 per cent of patients.

In those patients who fail to respond to medical treatment, are intolerant or upset by it, or cannot countenance their fears of the return of this intense distressing pain, it is possible to destroy the trigeminal nerve or its branches with relief of the pain but at the price of residual facial numbness. Section of peripheral nerve branches will only afford temporary relief as the nerve regenerates. Surgical measures involve either thermocoagulation, or fractional injection of the trigeminal ganglion with aliquots of alcohol, using a probe or needle passed through the cheek into the foramen ovale and the ganglion under

X-ray control, or surgical section of the nerve intracranially by a posterior or middle fossa approach.

The main drawback to destructive measures is the aftermath of facial sensory loss, which may include the cornea with the attendant risks of damage to the vision. In some 5 per cent of patients painful sensations may appear in the anaesthetic face, anaesthesia dolorosa. There may also be technical difficulties in the insertion of the needle or radiofrequency probe into the ganglion. Craniotomy carries the risks of surgery and anaesthesia with a morbidity and mortality which will rise in elderly, frail patients.

Recently, in younger patients, microdecompression of the trigeminal nerve exposed at posterior fossa craniotomy has afforded relief of the neuralgia if a vessel has been found in contact with the nerve, and it has proved possible to separate this from the nerve. In such instances, the neuralgic pain has been relieved without sacrificing the trigeminal nerve and so avoiding sensory loss. However, this procedure carries the risks of a craniotomy and in some patients no vessel is found so that nerve section may be necessary to relieve the pain. In the elderly and frail, thermocoagulation or ganglion injection are the treatment of choice if medical treatment has failed.

Trigeminal neuropathy

This is a condition of unknown aetiology where there is slow progressive loss of sensation involving one or sometimes both sides of the face in the territory of the trigeminal nerve. In some patients paraesthesiae or pain may be the presenting symptoms, however, sensory loss is the relevant sign varying in extent and severity. Usually this spreads very slowly. Facial sensory loss may also arise from a number of lesions involving the pons and lower cranial nerves (e.g. meningiomas, basal tumours, aneurysms, carcinomatous infiltration). Rare toxins, particularly trichlorethylene and stilbamidine, may produce a trigeminal neuropathy. In MS transient facial numbness is common.

In trigeminal neuropathy, investigations usually prove negative and, in a few patients where the nerve has been examined, it has been suggested that it appears thinned and degenerating. There is no specific treatment.

Cranial nerve VII

Bell's palsy

This common condition acutely produces a lower motor neurone facial palsy affecting all the muscles on one side of the face. It has an annual incidence of 23 per 100 000. All ages may be affected including children, although the highest incidence is in patients aged 30–50.

The exact cause is debated. Certain mechanisms are known to produce a lower motor neurone facial paralysis and may be responsible for some of those affected but, in many, the cause is unknown, idiopathic. Theories include:

1. Acute viral infections (e.g. varicella-zoster, mumps).
2. Vascular lesions: the nerve may infarct following damage to the vasa nervorum (e.g. diabetes, hypertension).

3. Inflammatory damage arising from an immunological upset; acute facial weakness may arise in the Gullain-Barré syndrome.
4. Cold exposure: Bell himself proposed this theory and many patients believe a 'cold draught' has been the precipitant. However, this is unlikely as severe degrees of cold are necessary to block conduction in a peripheral nerve in the laboratory.

Pathogenesis

Electrophysiological studies suggest that there is segmental demyelination resulting in a local conduction block proximally. This allows relatively rapid and complete recovery in about 85 per cent. In the others, axonal degeneration occurs which will produce a severe paralysis often leading to incomplete recovery associated with aberrant re-innervation, i.e. fibres from periocular muscles may regenerate and supply muscles to the mouth and vice versa. Such faulty re-innervation may lead to 'jaw-winking'. Where axonal degeneration has occurred, electromyography (EMG) of the facial muscles will show fibrillation and features of denervation. In some instances the pathogenesis is a mixture of axonal degeneration and demyelination.

Symptoms and signs

Many patients present with pain in or behind the ear preceding or appearing with the development of facial weakness. There is inability to close the eye or move the lower face and mouth. The lack of blinking leads to tears spilling out of the eye, which waters to cause complaints of blurred vision. The cheek is flaccid and food may accumulate in it; saliva or fluids may escape from the corner of the mouth. The weakness commonly progresses over 24–72 h to reach a maximum. In many patients there are complaints of numbness in the affected side of the face, although trigeminal sensation is spared and there should be no weakness of jaw movement (supplied by the motor root of the trigeminal nerve).

About 40–50 per cent of patients are aware of disturbed taste on the ipsilateral anterior part of the tongue. This points to a lesion in the distal part of the facial nerve below the geniculate ganglion, but above the origin of the chorda tympani. A significant number of patients may notice hyperacusis because the stapedius muscle in the ear is supplied by a branch of the facial nerve.

If a zoster infection has been the cause, patients may show typical herpetic vesicles on the pinna or in the external auditory canal on the affected side. Ramsay Hunt described a herpetic infection of the geniculate ganglion with the development of an acute facial palsy. In some of these patients the eighth cranial nerve may also be infected producing acute vertigo, deafness and tinnitus.

A few patients may show a bilateral facial palsy of lower motor neurone pattern: this may appear as part of a Guillain-Barré syndrome, from sarcoidosis and even carcinomatous meningitis.

Prognosis

About 80–85 per cent of patients make an excellent recovery over a period of weeks, usually beginning within 6–8 weeks and reaching a maximum over 6–9 months. An incomplete palsy at the onset or signs of recovery within the first 3–4 weeks usually herald a good outlook suggesting the damage is largely demyelination. In the more severely affected where axonal degeneration is the main damage, recovery is much slower and often incomplete with signs of faulty re-innervation. Such patients may be left with facial asymmetry and inability to close the eye. Most often such asymmetry is mild but occasionally this may cause considerable cosmetic distress.

Investigations

These include blood tests to exclude diabetes mellitus, a full blood count and ESR, and often X-rays of the skull and chest. In selected patients a CT scan and CSF examination may be helpful. Examination of the ear is essential. EMG studies may aid the assessment of damage and sometimes predict the outcome. Recurrent facial palsies particularly require further investigation to exclude any compressive lesion in the middle ear, skull base, or for any systemic upset such as sarcoidosis or hypertension.

Treatment

This is debated: many doctors believe a short course of steroids given within 5–7 days of onset may reduce any swelling around the facial nerve and so help to prevent axonal degeneration. Prednisolone 40 mg daily for 5 days, and then tapered off over the next week is a typical regimen. It has been suggested that this regimen be used in all patients with a complete facial palsy at the onset and with impaired taste. Other studies have suggested there is little difference in outcome between steroid-treated and untreated patients.

If herpes zoster is the cause, then a course of acyclovir is appropriate. Zoster-damaged facial nerves recover less well.

Care of the eye is always important if there is incomplete lid closure, but as the cornea is not anaesthetic, the patient will be aware of any foreign body or irritant. Occasionally it may be necessary to suture the lids partially together, a tarsorrhaphy, to protect the eye.

In those patients left with marked residual weakness and asymmetry, a number of surgical measures may be used to try to improve their appearance. These include plastic surgery with implants of soft tissues to restore the contours, or a faciohypoglossal anastomosis where the hypoglossal nerve on the affected side is sacrificed and the proximal end sutured to the distal stump of the degenerated facial nerve. These measures may improve the symmetry of the face at rest but are by no means a 'cure'.

Hemifacial spasm

This is an involuntary twitching of the muscles on one side of the face. The muscles around the eye, in the cheek, or around the mouth are those usually affected. The twitches are irregular clonic movements which may be mild and infrequent, or very prominent and repetitive even leading to closure of the eye. Often the eye muscles appear to wink and the cheek and mouth draw up.

Many patients are aware of considerable variation in the movements: these are worse when tired, physically or emotionally stressed. They may lead to great distress.

EMG studies show synchronous motor discharges in bursts firing rapidly. Rarely, such spasms may reflect irritation of the facial nerve by a cerebello-pontine angle tumour or basilar aneurysm. In a few instances the spasm may follow a facial palsy. Considerable interest has arisen in the last decade from the observation that in many patients with hemifacial spasm, there is a small blood vessel lying in contact with the facial nerve close to its site of exit from the pons. By separation of the vessel away from the nerve under the direct vision of an operating microscope, the spasms may be relieved.

Medical treatment is disappointing. Carbamazepine and clonazepam are drugs that have been tried with usually only limited benefit. Antidepressants and relaxants may sometimes afford a degree of symptomatic relief. Surgical treatment has also been used with selective damage to branches of the facial nerve to produce weakness but relief is not permanent.

Hemifacial spasm may need to be differentiated from *facial myokymia*. In the latter there is a very fine involuntary movement in the facial muscles on one side often in the cheek, like a fine rippling under the skin. This arises from intrinsic pontine lesions, most commonly plaques of demyelination, but also other pathology such as a pontine glioma.

Facial hemiatrophy

The soft tissues, fat and connective tissues on one side of the face, most often in the cheek, may gradually disappear, atrophy. This leads to a curious indenta-tion in the contour of the face. It usually progresses very slowly over many years and is of unknown aetiology.

Attempts at treatment by plastic surgery may be undertaken if the asymmetry is very severe.

Cranial nerve VIII

Deafness

The eighth cranial nerve has two divisions, the cochlear and vestibular components. Disturbances may produce symptoms of deafness, tinnitus and vertigo. In the assessment of hearing loss it is important to determine the onset; whether acute, fluctuating or slowly progressive, also whether this affects one or both ears. Familial (hereditary) forms of deafness may arise and are sometimes associated with other neurological problems. A history of trauma, exposure to noise or to certain drugs e.g. aminoglycosides, may be of relevance. Examination should include particular attention to the cochlear and vestibular function of the eighth nerve (*see* Chapter 3) and to the presence of nystagmus, trigeminal sensory loss or cerebellar disturbance. Fluctuating deafness suggests Ménière's disease, progressive unilateral deafness a possible acoustic neuroma.

Deafness may arise from lesions in the middle ear and is then conductive in type. Such damage may arise in the ossicles, a blocked external canal, from otitis media, a perforated ear drum, otosclerosis, or eustachian tube blockage. These lesions may often be confirmed by a careful examination of the ear. Deafness may also arise from damage to the cochlea or cochlear division of the eighth nerve, sensorineural or nerve deafness. This may be caused by trauma, drugs (e.g. aminoglycosides), Ménière's disease, cerebellopontine angle tumours, hypothyroidism, and presbyacusis. A watch-tick will test high frequency hearing loss: this is impaired in nerve deafness. Audiometry and auditory evoked brainstem potentials allow very accurate and detailed assessment of hearing disorders.

Tinnitus, an hallucination of sound, may be described as ringing, buzzing, hissing or roaring. It is frequently associated with deafness. Occasionally it may reflect a vascular flow murmur from an arteriovenous malformation or abnormal.communication, e.g. caroticocavernous fistula or dural shunt.

Deafness is very common in old age; assessment of such patients may allow provision of a hearing aid or other measures for relief.

Ménière's disease

This is a common disorder, affecting about one per 1000 adults, causing recurrent episodes of severe vertigo associated with fluctuating deafness and tinnitus. In about 40 per cent the symptoms start with deafness, distorted sound and sometimes a sensation of fullness or pressure in the affected ear. This may be associated with a low-pitched tinnitus. In about two-thirds of patients episodic rotational vertigo develops within 6 months of onset usually associated with nausea and vomiting. The vertigo may last minutes to hours and during the attack patients appear unsteady and will fall to the affected side. They prefer to lie down with the affected ear uppermost. During the attack there may be obvious nystagmus. After the attack a sensation of imbalance may last for several days.

Over many years such patients will commonly experience repeated attacks and sometimes long periods of remission. A few patients may end up with positional vertigo, drop attacks or persistent ataxia. There is usually a slowly progressive deafness and some patients develop bilateral disease.

Hearing tests will confirm sensorineural deafness. Initially, caloric tests may be normal but later a canal paresis develops or evidence of directional preponderance. Radiological studies are normal, but it is always important to check the Wasserman reaction (WR), fluorescent treponemal antibody or *Treponema pallidum* haemagglutination (TPHA) as syphilis may cause deafness and vertigo.

It has been suggested that Ménière's disease is due to an endolymphatic hydrops with excess accumulation of fluid in the system which in turn leads to a cochlear degeneration.

Treatment

In the acute attack most patients require bedrest accompanied by an injection of an antihistamine or phenothiazine to relieve the vomiting and vertigo. Cyclizine or dimenhydrinate are useful antihistamines. Prochlorperazine suppositories of 25 mg or injections of 12.5 mg may be used in adults. Frequent attacks of vertigo may be eased by cinnarizine (Stugeron) 15–30 mg t.i.d. or betahistine (Serc) 8–16 mg t.i.d. Acute anxiety and depression engendered by frequent attacks may be helped by benzodiazepines (diazepam, oxazepam) or an antidepressant. Various diets, salt restriction and vasodilator drugs have been suggested. These have limited success.

Surgical measures to drain the endolymphatic sac have been tried and even surgical or ultrasonic destruction of the labyrinth. These will produce deafness but can give relief in selected patients.

Episodic vertigo

Labyrinthine disease is the usual cause for vertigo. The commonest disorder is travel sickness which many people have experienced. The symptoms patients notice well illustrate those found in vertigo, the hallucination of movement, the nausea and vomiting, and the fear and prostration.

Ménière's disease has already been discussed. An acoustic neuroma may cause vertigo (*see* p. 313). Middle ear disease, particular infections, damage following ear surgery, a cholesteatoma or barotrauma may sometimes produce a perilymph fistula. Here episodic vertigo may appear with often the sensation of tilting. This can be provoked by a Valsalva manoeuvre. Other local causes of vertigo include otitis media, drug-induced vertigo and acute alcoholic poisoning, the latter provoking the colloquial 'pillow spin' described by patients as they lie down.

Positional vertigo

Here patients complain of acute episodes of vertigo provoked by changes of position, most usually lying down or sitting up quickly. Vertigo may also be provoked by acute head turning or neck extension. Most frequently such positional vertigo is produced by otolith damage (*see* p. 78). This may follow a head injury, vascular lesion or a viral infection but the cause may be uncertain.

It must be emphasized that many types of vertigo may be aggravated by positional changes or head turning. These include vertigo of both peripheral and central causes.

Benign positional vertigo

This is the most common cause of positional vertigo and the diagnosis can be easily confirmed by bedside testing (*see* p. 78). A positive response will elicit transient acute vertigo accompanied by rotatory nystagmus directed to the undermost ear. The nystagmus appears after a latent interval and usually lasts a few seconds. Sitting up will elicit the same symptoms but of lesser degree and if the test is repeated it will show fatigue, i.e. it will lessen and disappear. Patients are often distressed by this test but it will confirm that the symptoms are identical to those they experience. The affected otolith lies in the undermost ear.

Management rests in explanation and vigorous reassurance. The condition usually subsides spontaneously over a number of months but may recur.

Vestibular sedatives, such as cinnarizine, prochlorperazine or betahistine, may help in the acute phase. Some patients may benefit from vestibular balancing exercises of Cooksey-Cawthorne type to re-educate the faulty balance mechanism.

A much less common form of positional vertigo may appear with central brainstem lesions as in multiple sclerosis, cerebellar tumours, basilar territory vascular disease. Here, on testing for positional nystagmus there is no latent period, no fatigue, variable nystagmus and often far less severe vertigo. Furthermore, such patients will show other signs of brainstem disease.

Acute vestibular failure

In many instances where acute vertigo develops, the cause is undetermined but it appears to arise from an acute loss of labyrinthine function on one side. Such patients complain of acute prostrating vertigo accompanied by nausea and vomiting but without hearing loss or tinnitus (cochlear symptoms). During the attack most patients will lie on one side with the affected ear uppermost. Nystagmus is usually present, the fast phase away from the affected ear, and caloric tests will demonstrate a canal paresis on the affected side. Attempts at walking will elicit prominent ataxia. Such acute vertigo will usually settle within 2–3 weeks.

The cause is unknown: some may arise from a vascular disturbance perhaps from occlusion of the vestibular division of the internal auditory artery, others perhaps from a viral infection and the term *vestibular neuronitis* may then be used. This latter feature is most often seen in young adolescents and sometimes may follow an infection. There are symptoms of acute vestibular failure as described above without hearing upset. Again the symptoms and signs usually settle within weeks or 2 months. In the acute phase rest, vestibular sedatives, and antiemetics are the mainstay of treatment. Later balance exercises and some-times vestibular sedatives for a few weeks, may be necessary to rehabilitate the patient's faulty balance.

Cranial nerves IX, X, XI and XII

The glossopharyngeal and vagus nerves supply the bulbar muscles concerned with articulation and swallowing. Damage to the innervation of the soft palate will allow nasal regurgitation of fluids and if the laryngeal muscles are paralysed the voice becomes hoarse and weak (*see* p. 85).

Common lower motor neurone lesions may arise acutely in the Guillain-Barré syndrome, and with a slow progression in the bulbar palsy of motor neurone disease. In the differential diagnosis of an acute bulbar palsy it is always important to exclude thyrotoxicosis, polymyositis and myasthenia gravis, all potentially treatable conditions.

The jugular foramen syndrome

Damage to the IXth, Xth and XIth cranial nerves may arise from lesions at the skull base centred in and around the jugular foramen. Tumours of the skull base include metastases, a chordoma, glomus jugulare tumour, and meningioma. These may spread to involve the hypoglossal nerve and the cervical sympathetic nerves (producing an ipsilateral Horner's syndrome). If there is intracranial involvement long tract signs may appear with features of brainstem compression.

Good quality skull X-rays with basal views, CT scans and MRI scans will usually demonstrate such tumours.

The *glomus jugulare tumour* is a highly vascular mass arising from paraganglioma cells (like carotid body tumours) in the jugular bulb which lies just below the floor of the middle ear. As the tumour expands slowly it may produce deafness, bulbar problems (cranial nerves IX and X), weakness and wasting of one side of the tongue (cranial nerve XII). Later there may also be facial weakness, numbness, a Horner's syndrome and cerebellar ataxia. A red vascular polyp may be visible in the external ear and sometimes a palpable mass in the neck. There is sometimes a bruit. Basal skull X-rays will show bone erosion and a CT scan will confirm the presence of a mass. Treatment is usually by surgery and radiotherapy.

Glossopharyngeal neuralgia

This has many similarities to trigeminal neuralgia with brief intense stabs of pain experienced at the base of the tongue, at the angle of the jaw, in the throat, ear or side of the neck. The pain may be triggered by eating, swallowing, touch or even cleaning the teeth. During the jabs of pain which may be repetitive some patients cough or attempt to clear their throat. In a few patients a profound bradycardia (vagal slowing) or even syncope may arise indicating involvement of the vagus nerve.

Patients show no abnormal signs although glossopharyngeal neuralgia may sometimes by symptomatic particularly of a nasopharyngeal carcinoma, a tonsillar carcinoma or lymphoma.

Treatment is by carbamazepine as for trigeminal neuralgia (*see* p. 165). If medical treatment fails, surgical section of the glossopharyngeal nerve and upper two rootlets of the vagus through a posterior fossa craniotomy, is usually effective.

Polyneuritis cranialis

Multiple cranial nerve palsies may sometimes appear, often with patchy involvement of a number of cranial nerves. In some the cause may be from carcinomatous invasion or cuffing of the cranial nerves by tumour cells. This may also occur with leukaemia and lymphomas. A nasopharyngeal carcinoma may locally erode the skull base and compress a number of cranial nerves. Other causes may be inflammatory as from sarcoidosis, or from an arteritis (e.g. polyarteritis nodosa). Infective causes include tuberculous meningitis, and glandular fever. In some patients, particularly the elderly, no cause may be found.

Often two or three cranial nerves may be affected and in some the diagnosis of cranial nerve involvement is easily recognizable (e.g. a left abducens palsy, right optic nerve lesion and right lower motor neurone facial weakness). However, in some instances it may be difficult to determine whether the pathology is within the brainstem or extrinsic. The presence of long tract signs in the limbs suggests an intrinsic lesion.

The diagnosis rests on careful examination and in particular a search for any primary neoplasm; breast and bronchus being the most common causes of carcinomatous meningitis. The nasopharynx should be examined by an otolaryngologist, under anaesthetic if necessary, and tests carried out to exclude a lymphoma. Extensive radiological studies, CT scanning and CSF examination are important. Cytospin preparations of the CSF may show the presence of tumour cells which will confirm a diagnosis of carcinomatous meningitis. This pattern of neoplastic meningitis may also give a very low CSF sugar and this should be considered if no bacterial or fungal infection has been found.

The treatment is that of the underlying cause. Carcinomatous meningitis has a very poor outlook despite attempts at treatment with cytotoxic drugs.

8

Spinal diseases

In this chapter emphasis will be placed on the recognition and assessment of those spinal diseases which commonly involve neurologists and neurosurgeons. No attempt has been made to make an exhaustive study of all possible disorders. The discussion on symptoms and signs should give sufficient information to ensure that patients with relevant lesions will be recognized, investigated and when appropriate referred to a specialist.

The presentation and clinical features of any disorder of the spine depend on the pathological process and the site primarily involved, e.g. intervertebral synovial joints, discs, dura or the nervous system. Destructive lesions whether due to trauma, infection or neoplasia produce pain, deformity and loss of supportive function of the vertebral column. When the normal anatomy and integrity of the vertebral column is deranged, the nervous elements within the spinal canal and/or the intervertebral foramina may become involved secondarily. Certain diseases develop within the nervous elements and only secondarily disorganize the normal spine.

Symptoms and signs

Pain

Pain from lesions of the vertebral column is felt in the midline posteriorly and located near the affected part of the spine. When the spinal nerves are involved pain is referred to the distribution of those nerves. Associated muscle spasm may be present. Only rarely will involvement of the cord itself produce pain.

Acute inflammatory disease is characterized by severe pain with marked associated muscle spasm causing spinal rigidity. There is local tenderness and an associated systemic disturbance. Generally there is a recognizable source of infection present or evidence of one in the short history.

Chronic infection (e.g. tuberculous or chronic staphylococcal) produces pain of more insidious onset with features akin to neoplasia. The pain is less acute, especially in the earlier stages, although as the disease process advances it can become very severe with marked muscle spasm and local tenderness. Clinical evidence of systemic illness may be absent, although in children this is unusual. Chronic pyogenic infection is almost always associated with the debilitation of age or immunocompromised states.

Pain produced by tumours varies greatly both in its duration and severity. It depends on the particular pathology, the tissue in which it arises and the site. Generally speaking pain due to tumour has a gradual and insidious onset. When the tumour is slow growing, as in the case of spinal meningioma, minor back pain is often dismissed as fibrositis and even when weakness of the lower limbs develops, back pain may not be mentioned spontaneously by the patient. Tumours arising within the spinal cord itself (e.g. astrocytoma, ependymoma) do not produce pain until the cord is enlarged to occupy fully the vertebral canal, by which time there is ample evidence of cord dysfunction. On the other hand, extradural tumours (usually malignant) arising in the epidural space or in the bone of the vertebral column produce local spinal pain with a radicular radiation as nerve roots become involved. Local pain and tenderness are a good guide to the site of the compression, especially if deformity and a corresponding sensory level are present. This contrasts with primary tumours of the spinal cord which rarely produce a clear sensory level and local pain. Tumours within

Table 8.1   Upper limb roots

5th cervical root	
Pain and/or paraesthesiae	Neck, top of shoulder, outer aspect of arm and forearm
Sensory loss	Outer upper arm
Weakness	Deltoid, supraspinatus and brachioradialis
	Shoulder abduction and elbow flexion
Reflex reduction	Biceps and supinator jerks
6th cervical root	
Pain and/or paraesthesiae	Neck, shoulder, outer arm, forearm, thumb and index finger
Sensory loss	Thumb and index finger
Weakness	Biceps, brachioradialis and extensor carpi radialis longus
	Elbow flexion and radial wrist extension
Reflex reduction	Supinator and biceps jerks
7th cervical root	
Pain and/or paraesthesiae	Neck, shoulder, arm and forearm to middle and index finger
Sensory loss	Predominantly middle and index fingers
Weakness	Triceps and majority of the muscles on the dorsum of the forearm
	Elbow extension, wrist and finger extensors
Reflex reduction	Triceps jerk
8th cervical root	
Pain and/or paraesthesiae	Neck, shoulder, inner arm, little and ring fingers
Sensory loss	Little and ring fingers
Weakness	Forearm flexors
Reflex reduction	Finger jerk
1st thoracic root	
Pain and/or paraesthesiae	Neck, axilla, medial aspect of the arm and forearm, ring and little fingers
Sensory loss	Little finger and medial arm
Weakness	Small muscles of the hand
Reflex reduction	Finger jerk

(After R.S. Maurice-Williams, *Spinal Degenerative Disease*. Wright 1981)

the dural envelope and involving the cauda equina, such as a neurofibroma in a young adult, may produce very severe pain in the legs with a virtual absence of signs in the early stages. Such patients may find it more comfortable to sleep in a chair rather than go to bed in the normal manner.

Spinal pain following injury must always be taken very seriously. The history of the circumstances of injury will provide some indication of the forces which may have acted on the spine. Spinal injuries are often missed when there is clouding of consciousness and are very easily overlooked in the comatose patient.

The slow degenerative process of ageing is generally painless even when radiological examination of the spine shows extensive changes to be present. When pain occurs the symptoms remit and relapse, are relieved by rest and increased by activities which increase the mechanical stresses on the spine. In a healthy individual, a clear relationship to mechanical factors, with remissions and a long history, characterizes pain due to wear and tear.

Clinical features of nerve root involvement

Anatomically the anterior and posterior roots emerging from the cord join before leaving the spinal canal through the intervertebral foramen. Thus in clinical practice nerve root compression, so frequently present in the vicinity of the exit foramen, will result in both motor and sensory disturbance in the myotome and dermatome (*see* Fig. 3.11). While pain may be felt over a large area, the extent of objective sensory loss is usually small. The motor nerves in the root are distal to the anterior horn cells of the spinal cord so the disturbance will be of 'lower motor neurone' character; weakness, wasting, reduced tone, loss of tendon reflexes and fasciculation may be present. Tables 8.1 and 8.2 set out the main characteristics of lesions affecting the spinal nerves to the limb girdles. Lesions above the second lumbar vertebra often produce signs of cord compression in addition.

Spinal compression

It is imperative that reversible causes of cord compression are recognized as quickly as possible. An accurate pathological diagnosis is essential and generally an operation is required. However, the speed with which the clinician must act depends on the nature of the underlying pathology. Most benign tumours present with long histories and few signs and there is no need to act with unseemly haste. On the other hand, compression from pyogenic infection (rare), of the cauda equina due to a giant disc prolapse (not uncommon), secondary deposits and reticuloses are emergencies requiring the immediate attention of a neurosurgeon so that urgent diagnostic and therapeutic measures can be undertaken to preserve as much function as possible. Failure to relieve spinal cord compression will condemn the patient to permanent paraplegia.

Clinical features of compression

Although there are many causes of spinal cord compression, the effects on the nervous system are the same and the clincal picture similar irrespective of the

Table 8.2   Lower limb and lower sacral roots (see p. 154)

2nd and 3rd lumbar roots

Pain and/or paraesthesiae	Anterior thigh, groin (and testicle)
Sensory loss	Anterior thigh
Weakness	Quadriceps and hip flexors
Reflex reduction	Knee jerk

4th lumbar root

Pain and/or paraesthesiae	Anteromedial aspect of the leg
Sensory loss	Anteromedial aspect of leg
Weakness	Quadriceps, tibialis anterior and posterior
Reflex reduction	Knee jerk

5th lumbar root

Pain and/or paraesthesiae	Buttock, posterolateral thigh and anterolateral leg across dorsum of foot
Sensory loss	Dorsum of the foot and anterolateral aspect of the leg
Weakness	Extensor hallucis longus, extensor digitorum longus, peroneus longus and hamstrings
Reflex reduction	Extensor hallucis longus (difficult)

1st sacral root

Pain and paraesthesiae	Buttock, back of thigh, calf, and lateral border of the foot
Sensory loss	Lateral border of the foot
Weakness	Plantar flexors, extensor digitorum brevis, peroneus longus and hamstrings
Reflex reduction	Ankle jerk

Lower sacral segments

Pain and paraesthesiae	Buttock and back of thigh
Sensory loss	Perianal/saddle
Weakness	
Reflex reduction	Anal

pathological process. Certain intrinsic cord diseases, notably multiple sclerosis can also produce a similar clinical picture. On rare occasions, an intracranial lesion involving both cerebral hemispheres in the parasagittal regions will produce a clinical picture which is difficult to differentiate from a spinal lesion.

Lesions of the spinal cord above the level of the conus produce a progressive loss of all cord functions at and below the level of compression. There will be a spastic weakness of the limbs with exaggerated tendon reflexes and extensor plantar responses, signs which characterize an 'upper motor neurone lesion'. Sphincter disturbance is characterized by precipitancy culminating in retention of urine. If paraplegia is complete automatic bladder emptying will be possible if the sacral segments are preserved.

The cauda equina commences at the termination of the spinal cord usually at the level of the second lumbar vertebra. The pattern of moter upset is that of a 'lower motor lesion', weakness with flaccidity, loss of tendon reflexes, wasting and perhaps fasciculation. The exact pattern will depend, in part, on the vertebral level. Sphincter disturbance is characterized by retention with overflow. In the event of permanent paraplegia automatic bladder emptying is not possible.

Lesions of the conus produce a mixture of signs, some characterizing an 'upper motor' and others a 'lower motor' lesion.

A tumour growing within the substance of the cord produces loss of function partly through infiltration and partly by distortion. In the early stages, intra-dural but extramedullary tumours which grow in the subdural space displacing CSF are often clinically silent. As the tumour enlarges, ultimately the spinal cord is compressed to produce syndromes which to some extent reflect the part of the cord receiving the greatest pressure from the tumour. Extradural compressive processes produce a progressive loss of all functions below the level of the lesion, for the most part without significant asymmetry of signs. Medical causes of paraplegia should not be forgotten, demyelination (*see* p. 345), degeneration (*see* p. 353) and vascular (*see* p. 406).

Investigations

The history and clinical examination usually make it possible to suggest a differ-ential diagnosis and a treatment plan. However, at this stage, full under-standing will be incomplete and investigations are generally necessary. The differential diagnosis will determine the choice. If an operation is contemplated then the age, past medical history, general health, feasibility of rehabilitation and social circumstances are among the factors which will have to be taken into account and may have an important influence on the type and extent of investigation.

The choice of haematological and biochemical investigation is determined by the differential diagnosis, but will normally include estimation of the haemo-globin, full blood count, sedimentation rate and perhaps serum calcium, phos-phate, alkaline phoshatase (liver function tests), serology and vitamin B12. The possibility of rheumatological diseases will require special consideration and the appropriate tests. Evoked potential studies may suggest anatomical localization and support a local lesion. Examination of the urine should be part of the general examination and when operation is planned on patients aged over 50 a chest X-ray and electrocardiogram should be performed even in the absence of specific indication.

Examination of the CSF is of limited value but may be required to establish diagnoses such as polyneuritis (signs of a generalized peripheral neuropathy, CSF revealing high protein and no cells); myelitis (evidence of a cord lesion with evidence of systemic disturbance and CSF revealing increased cells, raised protein and oligoclonal bands), etc. These diseases are discussed elsewhere (*see* p. 351). If a tumour is suspected the CSF should not be examined because (currently) myelography will be required and a recent lumbar puncture makes it difficult for a radiologist to re-enter the subarachnoid space. Contrast media in the subdural space produces images impossible to interpret accurately. Furthermore, patients with critical compression from an intradural tumour may deteriorate rapidly after lumbar puncture; if the tumour is in the lumbar theca, CSF is not obtained.

Imaging techniques

Plain X-rays reveal the bony architecture but give little information about the soft tissues. They will reveal congenital bony abnormalities; new bone forma-tion around the facet joints and disc margins with loss of disc height as occurs in

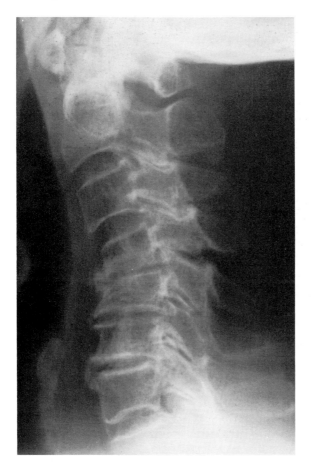

Fig. 8.1. Severe cervical spondylotic degeneration. There is loss of lordosis, loss of disc height between the fourth, fifth, sixth and seventh vertebrae and new osteophytic bone formation

degenerative disease (Fig. 8.1); bone destruction, scalloping of vertebral bodies and enlargement of the vertebral canal, as may occur with spinal tumours; healing fractures, etc; ligamentous calcification in ankylosing spondylitis; loss of bone calcium either general, as occurs in severe osteoporosis, or local, as the result of neoplastic infiltration or infection (Fig. 8.2); soft tissues shadows present in close association with bony abnormalities.

Tomography blurs shadows produced by X-rays not in the plane of the cut, but the thinner the slice the higher must be the difference in the X-ray absorption characteristics between the structure to be demonstrated and its surroundings. Better information is now generally obtained from a computerized tomography (CT) scan (Fig. 8.3).

Radioactive isotope techniques are a sensitive method for detecting inflammatory and neoplastic processes in bone before changes are demon-

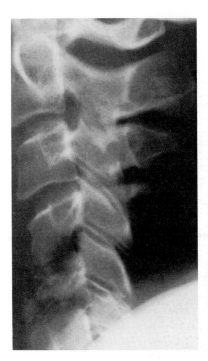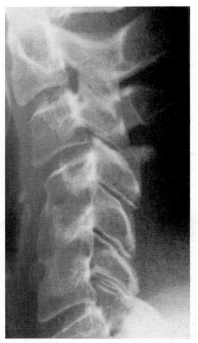

Fig. 8.2. Spinal infection. (a) Two disc spaces and three vertebral bodies are eroded. The extent of the soft tissue shadow anteriorly has been obscured by the bars of the Stryker turning frame. No preoperative plain X-rays and an extensive laminectomy (?unwisely) have been performed. (b) Complete interbody fusion between third, fourth and fifth cervical vertebrae has taken place. The pharynx and trachea have resumed their normal position with the resolution of the soft tissue mass

strable using plain radiographic techniques where approaching 60 per cent of the mineral content must be lost before changes become visible. Isotope scanning is particularly useful for detecting widespread cancerous deposits (Fig. 8.4).

Myelography gives evidence of the site of cord compression and the pattern will often give a good indication of the pathological process. It should be used in all instances of a progressive paraparesis where a compressive lesion needs to be excluded. Myelography remains the most commonly used and available means of investigating spinal diseases where the neural structures are involved. Modern contrast media are water soluble and carry small risk. Nonetheless, myelography is an invasive procedure and is not totally without any discomfort or hazard (Figs. 8.5, 8.6, and 8.7).

CT scanning may be used to show soft tissues, but the proximity of bone limits its usefulness in this respect. Generally CT scanning of spinal conditions is combined with myelography (Fig. 8.8). It is also possible to reconstruct the axial images and obtain alternative views. However, the resolution of such reconstructions falls short of that of the original axial pictures (Fig. 8.8 and 8.9).

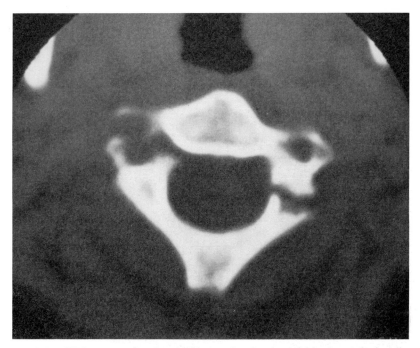

Fig. 8.3. CT demonstrating that the fracture has involved the lamina at the junction with the pedicle on the left and on the right passes through the canal for the vertebral artery. The spinal cord is surrounded by CSF and there is no evidence of compression or damage to this structure

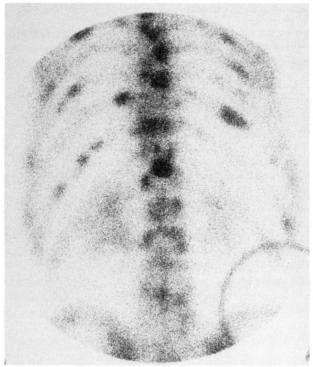

Fig. 8.4. Isotope bone scan of the lower thoracic and lumbar spine. There are multiple metastases present in the spine and ribs

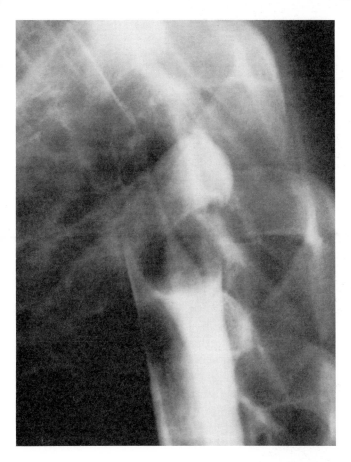

Fig. 8.5. Neurofibroma. The myelogram shows the typical crescentic shadow and displacement of the spinal cord anteriorly by the posteriorly placed tumour.

Magnetic resonance imaging (MRI) is similar to CT in that the image is generated from a matrix of calculated values. Proximity of bone to soft tissue does not produce artefacts and tissue contrast can be varied to some extent by 'weighting' T_1 and T_2. High quality images may be produced in several planes. In some respects MRI is superior to CT scanning. MRI is proving a very powerful diagnostic tool with the potential to replace myelography and it is already recognized as the best imaging technique available for the cranio-cervical junction (Fig. 8.10).

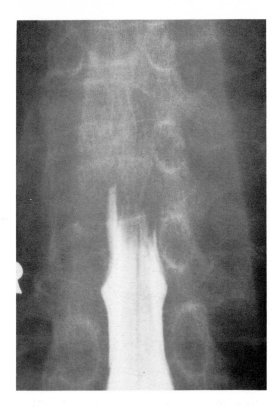

Fig. 8.6. Spinal metastatic cancer. There is a complete ragged obstruction to the contrast medium in the subarachnoid space and erosive destruction of two pedicles

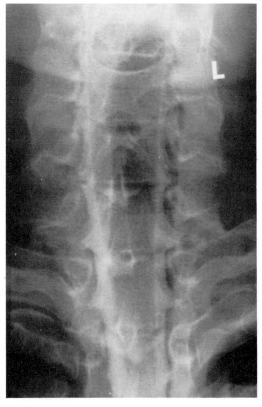

Fig. 8.7. Astrocytoma of the cervical cord, anteroposterior view. There is a fusiform expansion of the cervical cord in an enlarged vertebral canal

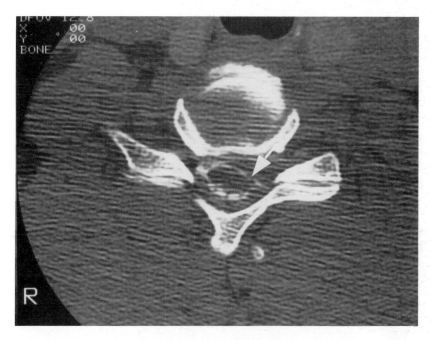

Fig. 8.8. Cervical disc. CT myelogram showing the spinal cord outlined by contrast and displaced by a large soft lateral disc protrusion

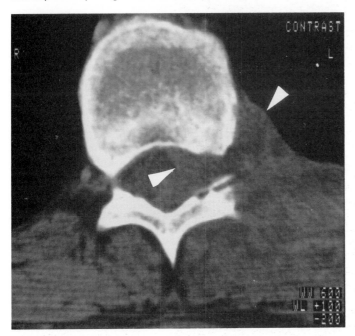

Fig. 8.9. Spinal metastatic cancer. The CT scan shows increased tissue mass in relation to the left intervertebral foramen, displacement of the spinal cord to the right and some early erosion of bone. CT myelography would have emphasized the boundary between the tumour within the vertebral canal and the spinal theca and its contents

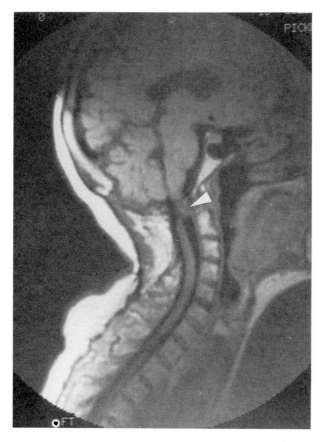

Fig. 8.10. Meningioma. The MRI reveals a small recurrent meningioma (arrowed) at the craniocervical junction just lateral to the midline displacing spinal cord which as a result appears thin in this section

Principles (benefits and hazards) of surgical treatments

Certain factors favour surgical solutions: a good correlation between the patient's complaint, physical findings and the demonstrated abnormality; a single well circumscribed lesion and a pathology of benign (controllable) character; and a patient in sufficiently good general health able to withstand the stresses of an operation. Other factors mitigate against success, e.g. multiple lesions, as in metastatic cancer, clearly make a total surgical solution impossible. Surgical exploration may be justified to provide an accurate histological diagnosis when it will affect further management. Osteoarthritis of the spine is also a diffuse process which may produce compression of the spinal cord or nerve roots, which if localized may respond to surgery. In chronic diffuse disorders the search for a clear correlation between the 'surgical' abnormality and the patient's complaint is the vital part of the assessment. Sometimes spinal instability may be present and caution will thus be required when planning any surgical intervention. If the relationship between demonstrated pathology, clinical complaints and physical signs is not clear then the outcome from operation will be poor. A clear understanding of the pathology and the mechanism producing a patient's symptoms is an essential prerequisite for the planning of successful treatment.

The operations

The contents of the vertebral canal may be approached from a number of directions. Laminectomy is a posterior approach and the one most commonly used. Costotransversectomy is a lateral approach used primarily for the removal of thoracic disc lesions. The cervical spine is easily reached anteriorly between the carotid sheath and midline structures as in the Cloward operation for removal of cervical discs and interbody fusion. Most of the thoracic and upper lumbar spine can be approached anterolaterally, either through the chest or retroperitoneally, giving access for the treatment of thoracic disc lesions, osteomyelitis and fractures.

Such procedures permit decompression of the contents of the vertebral canal through the removal and biopsy of tumours, evacuation of pus and the excision of disc sequestra. The limited procedures are directed at specific small lesions, e.g. microdiscectomy for cervical and lumbar disc prolapse, and foraminotomy for the decompression of nerve roots in the cervical and lumbar regions. In the cervical spine the anterior approach is commonly used for disc lesions and fusion is often carried out at the same time (Cloward's operation). When there is destruction of the vertebral body surgical exploration must generally be accompanied by procedures to stabilize the spine either by bone grafting or an implanted mechanical device.

Commoner causes of compression of the contents of the vertebral canal

The causes of compression of the contents of the spinal canal are conveniently classified according to the pathology and site (Table 8.3).

Tumours: some important features

Malignant extradural tumours

Malignant extradural tumours are the commonest spinal neoplasms encountered in clinical practice. They can arise in the extradural tissue and/or bone. In many patients involvement of the spine and cord compression are the presenting features. The primary tumour which usually has its origin in lung, breast, prostate, kidney or thyroid often defies detection. Myeloma may also present with a single spinal deposit.

It requires emphasis that while the course of the illness may be influenced by surgery, radiotherapy, chemotherapy and endocrine manipulations, the nature of the tumour determines prognosis. Nonetheless, involvement of the spine

Table 8.3 Causes of cord compression

Tumours
  Extradural
    secondary carcinoma
    reticuloses including myeloma
    neurofibroma
    chordoma
    primary sarcoma
  Intradural
    extramedullary
     neurofibroma
     meningioma
     dural angioma
    intramedullary
     ependymoma
     astrocytoma
     angioma
  Mixed
    lipoma and dermoids
Infection
  Extradural
    staphylococcal
    tuberculosis
  Intradural
    infected dermoid
Intervertebral disc lesions and sequestra
Haematoma
  extradural
    (defects of blood coagulation)
Deformity
  Congenital
    spondylolisthesis
    craniovertebral anomalies
    kyphoscoliosis
    diastematomyelia
    other faults in skeletal development
  Acquired
    degenerative disease (spondylosis)
    rheumatoid disease
    Paget's disease of bone
'Cysts'
  Intradural
    syringomyelia
    arachnoid

---

often has two important consequences, namely irreversible neurological damage and spinal instability, which only too often represent a terminal event in an incurable disease.

Secondary carcinoma usually arises in the body or pedicles of the vertebrae. Local pain is an early feature and it indicates involvement of the periosteum, either directly or through stresses arising in it from loss of mechanical strength. The signs of cord compression usually herald vertebral collapse and irreversible paraplegia.

Persistent spinal pain with root involvement without evidence of disease elsewhere should be an indication for CT scanning or MRI imaging. It is possible that early treatment may prevent death through paraplegia even though cure of the underlying condition is not possible.

The surgical issues are complex. While most deposits arise with a particular relationship to the cord, at operation they seem to surround the dural envelope. If the vertebral body has been destroyed laminectomy increases instability which may make an incomplete paraplegia complete. Laminectomy should be combined with a stabilization procedure, or an increasingly popular anterior approach considered. Early and precise diagnosis is now possible. Treatment which decompresses the neural elements, maintains the stability of the spine and halts the progress of the tumour can now prevent paraplegia. Radiotherapy or medication are essential adjuvants for the successful management of malignant spinal disease.

Intradural extramedullary tumours

Neurofibromas occur at any level, but meningiomas are commonly located in the midorsal region of middle-aged and elderly women. They are benign tumours. Pain at the level of the lesion is a usual but not invariable feature. These tumours may present with the partial cord syndromes depending on the relationship to the spinal cord (*see* Fig. 8.5). When the tumour is located between foramen magnum and fifth cervical level diagnosis may be difficult. Postural and discriminatory sensory loss in the hand in excess of other signs of cord compression should suggest the diagnosis. Meningiomas situated at the foramen magnum were often difficult to demonstrate until the advent of MRI scanning (*see* Fig. 8.10). Neurofibromas arise from nerve roots and the lumbar canal is a frequent site and in the early stages symptoms exceed signs. Neurofibromas may extend into the intervertebral foramen and beyond as 'dumb-bell' tumours with characteristic changes on the plain X-ray. Most neurofibromas and meningiomas are effectively cured by removal through a laminectomy exposure. The sacrifice of the sensory nerve root on which a neurofibroma arises rarely causes significant disability unless a major limb plexus root is involved. The neurofibromas associated with von Recklinghausen's disease present difficulty and often insoluble problems as they may be multiple and extensive.

Intramedullary tumours

Intramedullary tumours fall into two main groups, ependymomas and the astrocytomas, in approximately equal proportion and varying degrees of malignancy. They may occur in any part of the spinal cord but are commonly located in the cervical region where they produce a progressive tetraparesis. Ependymomas are generally well circumscribed, are associated with cysts and do not infiltrate the neural elements to any great extent. Slow growing tumours often enlarge the vertebral canal, a change demonstrable on plain film radiology. It is often possible to carry out an effective surgical removal by making an incision in the posterior aspect of the cord and separating the dorsal columns to expose the tumour. In contrast astrocytomas are frequently not well demarcated and usually surgical excision must be limited to avoid risk of inflicting severe damage to the functioning neural tissue.

Other tumours involving the spine are rare. These include primary sarcoma of bone, chordoma, dermoids, lipoma, enterogenous cysts, seeding of primary brain tumours through the CSF pathway (medulloblastoma) and so on.

Angiomas

Angiomas are not strictly tumours in the sense of their capacity to produce cord compression. However, they may present as a progressive paraplegia, although the mechanism is obscure. In the event of haemorrhage this usually takes place into the subarachnoid space. Haemorrhage into the cord creates a haematomyelia and may also interfere with the normal blood supply leading to sudden loss of function at and below the level of the lesion. Characteristically myelography reveals curvilinear defects due to dilated vessels. Spinal angiography is

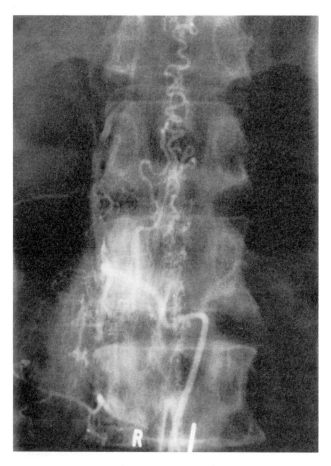

Fig. 8.11. Spinal angiogram demonstrating dilated vessels. Further serial pictures with subtraction techniques were used to define the site of the fistula

the definitive test, but is not without dangers for it requires catheterization of the feeding vessels (Fig. 8.11). Successful surgical treatment depends on the excision or obliteration of the fistula without inflicting damage to the cord or its blood supply. A significant number of angiomas primarily involves the dura. The assessment is complex and requires close collaboration between neurosurgeon and neuroradiologist.

Spinal infection

The clinical effects and natural history of spinal infections depend on the structures primarily involved, the organism and the host's response modified by any treatment the patient may have received. Infection may reach the spine by contiguous spread, the bloodstream or directly through a penetrating injury or a dermal sinus. The dura usually forms an effective barrier to local spread unless it is breached, e.g. by lumbar puncture. The neurological deficit is produced by a mixture of compression and vasculitis. Those patients whose immunity is compromised through age, debility or disease present with atypical pictures usually of chronic character when organisms of low virulence take hold.

Infection within the dural envelope

Abscess, solitary or multiple within the dural envelope is very rare and may be located within the spinal cord, in the subdural space or among the roots of the cauda equina, when it is usually associated with a dermal sinus. These infections are distinguished from meningitis by the fact they are localized. Patients have a short history, often with clear evidence of the source of infection, are systemically ill, and have a bad prognosis with high mortality. Those with chronic infection present like an intramedullary tumour and respond better to surgical drainage of the pus and antibiotic treatment.

Infection in the epidural space

Infection usually reaches the epidural space through the bloodstream from an identifiable source, commonly a staphylococcal skin infection. Characteristically the illness is acute with intense spinal and root pain with a rapidly advancing loss of neurological function at and below the lesion. Generally there is clear evidence of a systemic disturbance, local tenderness and muscle spasm complemented by varying degrees of spinal cord or cauda equina dysfunction. This is an acute surgical emergency. Once neurological deficits are well established in which vascular damage plays an important part recovery is unusual. Plain X-rays of the spine are usually normal. Lumbar puncture (for myelography) is usually safe below the level of the lesion but it is customary to aspirate on reaching the epidural space to exclude pus before entering the subarachnoid space. A cervical myelogram may be required to define the upper level. MRI, if available, will provide the information necessary to plan treatment without the risks of lumbar puncture. Surgical decompression usually by laminectomy, by an appropriate approach, often posterior, is essential to drain pus and provides the opportunity to identify the infecting organism and rationalize antibiotic treatment.

Infection of bone and cartilage

Osteomyelitis is uncommon in healthy individuals but must be considered in the immune compromised, diabetics, the debilitated elderly and those with rheumatoid arthritis who present with local spinal and root pain of short duration. The onset is insidious but progress depends on the organism and the host's response. There is local tenderness particularly to percussion of the spines at the level of infection, muscle spasm, and if vertebral collapse has occurred, a kyphus. While systemic disturbance is usual in children it may well be absent in the elderly. In the early stages cord compression is unusual because infection is largely prevented from spreading to the epidural space by the strength and rigidity of the posterior longitudinal ligament. In the event of vertebral collapse extrusion of pus and granulation tissue into the vertebral canal usually produces cord compression with rapid loss of all functions below the level of the lesion. As in the case of early carcinoma, there often are no changes demonstrable on plain film radiology. Over a period of 4–12 weeks demineralization and the loss of the bony trabeculae become sufficient to be visible on a plain X-ray. By this time vertebral collapse is imminent. Unlike carcinoma which leaves the disc space intact, infection characteristically destroys the disc space and the two adjacent vertebrae. Investigation with the CT scanner will show early bone destruction and evidence of a paravertebral abscess and will be more informative than a plain X-ray. Needle biopsy is required to obtain pus for culture and look for tuberculous infection. When the spinal canal is not compromised treatment consists of immobilization and the appropriate antibiotic. Patients with extensive bone destruction and a compromised vertebral canal will require debridement and bone grafting. Most patients will obtain a solid fusion in 6–12 months. For pyogenic infection antibiotics will be required for at least 6 months and for tuberculosis at least one year. Where vertebral collapse is present and laminectomy is indicated for the treatment of an associated epidural abscess an additional stabilization procedure may be necessary.

Disc rupture and degenerative diseases of the spine

Acute mechanical derangements and degenerative disorders of the spine are numerically the most important and also present the clinician with some of the most difficult problems in management. Two factors, trauma and the degenerative process of ageing, influenced by lifestyle or occupation, operate on the spine to varying degree. Sciatica due to a ruptured lumbar disc precipitated by a sudden strain in a young adult contrasts with the process of attrition of diffuse degenerative spondylosis in the elderly compressing the cervical cord or cauda equina, yet the presenting constellation of symptoms have many features in common.

Acute disc rupture may be the result of a sudden major event, but more commonly it is the end result of repeated minor stresses which predispose to rupture of the annulus and sequestration of disc material. Stresses of this kind predominantly affect the lumbar spine.

The cervical section is the most mobile segment of the spine and degenerative change is a normal part of the ageing process. Acute disc rupture with sequestration is rare, but narrowing of the intervertebral foramina and the reduction in the size of the vertebral canal which occurs as a result of the degenerative process is responsible for myelopathy and nerve root symptoms.

The clinical syndromes fall into three categories singly or in combination: spinal, radicular (*see* Tables 8.1 and 8.2) and cord or cauda equina compression. Acute disc rupture, lumbar or cervical, often follows a history of recurrent bouts of lumbago or neck pain respectively. The pain is exacerbated by mechanical factors and relieved by rest. Eventually a further episode of spinal pain is accompanied by or quickly followed by radicular pain. Sequestration usually takes place laterally into the vertebral canal because the posterior longitudinal ligament is strongest in the midline. Occasionally sequestration of the content of the disc space enters the central part of the vertebral canal and then the spinal cord or cauda equina is in peril. Central disc prolapse with neurological involvement is a neurosurgical emergency. On the other hand, radicular syndromes often respond to conservative methods but the persistence of severe radicular pain or increasing neurological signs are indications for operation.

Cervical spine

Cervical spondylosis is almost a normal part of the ageing process. Characteristically there is loss of disc space height, and reactive/osteoarthritic changes at the edges of the vertebral bodies and around the facet joints. Eighty per cent of people over the age of 55 years show changes at C5/6 and C6/7 on a lateral radiograph but few will have any symptoms. The osteophytes around the disc margin, the thickening of the soft tissues, the hypertrophy of the facet joints and the loss of disc height which leads to a buckling of the ligamentum flavum all contribute to a narrowing of the normally capacious vertebral canal. In some patients this results in pressure on the cord itself and/or adjacent nerve roots.

Immobilization of the neck in a firm collar should be the initial treatment of symptomatic patients. It is believed that the degenerate joints and tissues, just like other arthritic joints in the body, will easily become swollen as a result of movement and stresses across them. By immobilizing them and thus stopping the aggravating effect of repeated movement, the swelling and inflammation will settle and so reduce the pressure on the adjacent neural structures. This will be beneficial to the patient, frequently relieving pain and other symptoms and is the main rationale behind advising patients to rest and wear a collar (or corset for lumbar problems). Additional relief may be gained from prescribing nonsteroidal anti-inflammatory medication or simple analgesics.

In some patients the degenerative process is also accompanied by myelopathy which may be relieved by a decompressive procedure. If the compressive lesion is over several segments then a posterior decompression (laminectomy) is generally favoured. Localized lesions at one or two levels are best tackled by the anterior route, excising the degenerate disc with or without fusion. There are circumstances where the degenerative process is so far advanced that the operative goals cannot be reached.

Acute disc prolapse in the cervical spine with brachalgia usually resolves with conservative treatment within 3 months. Unremitting pain with neurological signs is an indication for investigation, CT myelography being the investigation of choice, and considering microdiscectomy.

Thoracic spine

The thoracic spine is the least mobile part of the spinal column and symptomatic degenerative disease is rare. Thoracic disc protrusion is exceedingly uncommon and is usually diagnosed when some other condition is suspected. Because the lesion lies anterior to the spinal cord where the vertebral canal is narrow removal by a posterior approach is hazardous. Careful neurosurgical evaluation is required, but generally these discs may be safely removed either by a lateral approach, costotransversectomy or anteriorly through the chest. Pain in a thoracic root distribution may present as chest pain and even be misdiagnosed as pleurisy. It can often be reproduced by rotation of the thoracic spine. As with cervical spondylosis, the pain often settles spontaneously over a few days or weeks. Simple analgesics and reassurance may be all that are required.

Lumbar spine

Acute back pain, the result of a sudden or repeated mechanical stress, is probably one of the most common afflictions of mankind. Fortunately most episodes resolve with rest and simple analgesics. Sometimes, despite all kinds of conservative measures, pain persists. Plain X-rays are usually uninformative but are carried out to exclude more sinister causes. MRI may reveal one disc at fault and it may be tempting to remove the abnormal disc or fuse the spine at that level.

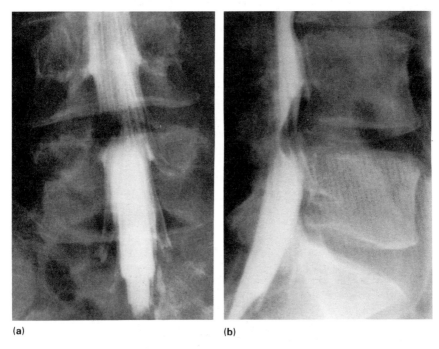

(a)   (b)

Fig. 8.12.   Lumbar disc rupture. Myelogram showing a large disc rupture 'amputating' the nerve root on the right side at the fourth lumbar interval on (a) the posteroanterior film and (b) lateral film

Sciatica which follows a history of mechanical back pain is likely to be the result of a lumbar disc disorder and in a young adult a soft disc protrusion with or without sequestration is the most likely explanation. The majority of acute disc protrusions occur at the fourth and fifth lumbar intervals. Acute rupture with sequestration is rare at higher levels and these patients have symptoms which relate to the relevant nerve roots (*see* Table 8.2). Loss of spinal movement, muscle spasm and limitation of straight leg raising with those of root compression are the cardinal signs.

Similar symptoms in patients in their 50s or 60s are more likely to be the result of hypertrophy of a facet joint. When a disc protrusion is present this is often small but causes severe symptoms as there is less available space for the nerve root due to the hypertrophied facet joint.

Before the annulus ruptures there is often a stage when a bulging deformity is present. This may be sufficient to produce physical signs of nerve root irritation. Complete rest at this stage will generally relieve sciatica. A plaster jacket is

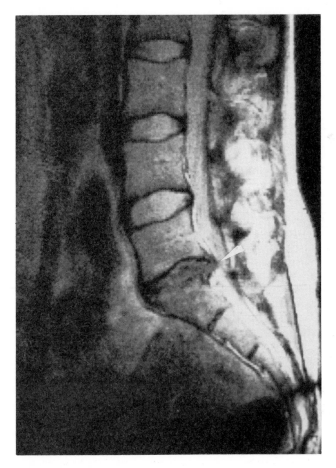

Fig. 8.13. Lumbar disc lesion. MRI showing a large disc rupture and degenerative disc at the fifth lumbar interval

less effective but keeps the patient mobile. Once disc material has sequestrated into the vertebral canal or exit foramen symptoms are unlikely to resolve until the sequestrum is removed. Myelography (with or without CT) is the most commonly used method for confirming the clinical diagnosis (Fig. 8.12). However, MRI (Fig. 8.13) may replace myelography because it is non-invasive; the patient can be examined as an outpatient. The use of the operating microscope and improved instruments has made it possible to remove sequestrated discs with relatively little disturbance to the normal structures.

Bilateral sciatica especially if accompanied by root signs (loss of ankle jerks, foot drop and particularly perianal sensory loss) should alert the clinician to the possibility of a central disc prolapse and cauda equina compression. Any suggestion of sphincter disturbance or perianal sensory loss is reason for immediate referral to a surgeon with a special interest in spinal surgery.

Lumbar spondylosis is almost an inevitable consequence of ageing. Like the cervical spine the osteophytes around the disc margins, the hypertrophy of the facet joints and loss of disc height with kinking of the ligamentum flavum, narrow the lumbar canal. In most people the process remains symptomless but, in some, the nerve roots or the cauda equina become compromised. Characteristically these patients, frequently in their 60s, complain of weakness and bilateral sciatica-like discomfort or pain brought on by exercise. Signs are often minimal though muscle wasting may be present and loss of reflexes is unusual. Myelography usually reveals a near or complete block at the fourth, fifth and/or the third lumbar intervals (*see* Fig. 8.12). When there is a clear correlation between the history, the signs and the myelographic findings, relief of symptoms can be anticipated from a decompressive laminectomy. However, the duration of relief depends in part on the extent of the disease and its rate of progress.

Syringomyelia

Syringomyelia is a rare disorder, affecting the sexes equally, usually in the fourth of fifth decade, in which there develops a progressive cystic cavitation in the spinal cord. The process generally begins in the cervical cord but, as the cavity expands, the brainstem and distal cord also become involved. Patients present with stiffness and weakness of the legs and many have pain in the neck and arms associated with numbness in the hands. Congenital anomalies of the nervous system and sometimes of the bone structures at the level of the foramen magnum are common. There is cerebellar ectopia through the foramen magnum and cavitation of the cord in a typical case. The content of the cavity of the syrinx is similar if not identical to CSF. At the level of the syrinx the grey matter of the anterior horn cells is lost producing weakness and atrophy of the muscles with loss of tendon reflexes in the upper limb, signs of a 'lower motor neurone lesion'. The syrinx interrupts the central decussating fibres of the spinothalamic tracts, producing dissociated loss of thermal sensibility and pain sensation in a characteristically cuirasse-like distribution. The loss of spinothalamic function is associated with the development of neuropathic arthropathies and other trophic changes. Particularly in the early stages the symptoms and signs may not be symmetrical. Below the level of the syrinx there are signs of paraparesis. Sphincter function is usually well preserved.

Pathology

It has been postulated that the syrinx fills from the ventricular system through a patent medullary-cervical communication promoted by the ectopic tonsillar obstruction to the normal drainage of the CSF from the fourth ventricle into the basal cisterns. Cavitation of the cord can occur in other circumstances, e.g. in association with arachnoiditis around the foramen magnum (another type of obstruction to the CSF pathway). Rarely a syrinx develops as a late sequel to spinal injury and should be suspected when a patient with a traumatic paraparesis or paraplegia develops a painful ascending myelopathy. Spinal arachnoiditis is a very rare cause of spinal cord cavitation.

Syringomyelic-like syndromes may occur in association with intra- (and very rarely with extra-) medullary spinal tumours but the cavities are better considered as cystic (fluid unlike CSF) extensions of the tumour.

Investigations

X-rays of the spine, commonly normal, may reveal anomalies at the foramen magnum or an enlarged vertebral canal. The skull X-ray is usually normal but may reveal evidence of arrested hydrocephalus. MRI is the definitive investigation which provides a clear and unequivocal picture of the syrinx, any craniocervical anomaly or ventricular enlargement. If syringomyelia is seriously suspected MRI should be undertaken before any other investigation.

Management

Management must in part depend on the aetiology and therefore each group should be considered separately. As a general principle, treatment must be directed at the primary cause and sometimes the syrinx itself. Where there is an association between an Arnold-Chiari malformation (p. 372) and a syrinx, the aim is to relieve the pressure by removing the lower central part of the occipital bone and the spines and arches of the atlas and axis at the craniocervical junction to restore normal CSF dynamics and prevent further extension of the syrinx. The dura may be opened and a fascial graft inserted to enlarge the dural envelope. Headache, neck and arm pain, and signs of recent and progressive character are most likely to be relieved by operation. Surgical decompression of the structures at and adjacent to the foramen magnum seems to give some benefit in about two-thirds of cases and may prevent further deterioration. However, the extent of the improvement may be disappointing.

Patients with basal arachnoiditis, without the anomaly of tonsillar descent, are not improved by decompressive procedures. Drainage of the syrinx into the subarachnoid space or into the pleural or peritoneal cavities may give some relief and in particular prevent further deterioration. Direct drainage of the syrinx into the subarachnoid space has been used with some benefit in patients with post-traumatic cavitation.

Spinal injuries

Most spinal injuries are managed by orthopaedic surgeons but neurosurgeons and sometimes neurologists become involved when the nervous system is damaged. There are about 35 cases of spinal injury with neural damage per million of the population annually. A small number are instantly fatal but, without complications, life expectancy is not shortened. Motor vehicle accidents and sport account for the majority.

Most spinal injuries do not damage the spinal cord or the nerves. When the cord or nerves are damaged there is usually a fracture-dislocation involving one of the more mobile sections of the vertebral column, namely the cervical or thoracolumbar junction. However, it must be stressed that devastating neurological injury can result without an obvious fracture and routine X-rays may appear 'normal'. A person with a narrow cervical canal from cervical spondylosis may be rendered paraplegic by a trivial blow, without a fracture.

In common with head injuries, the two major management concerns are: first, the prevention of further damage to the spinal cord and nerves; and second, to provide the best conditions favouring recovery. Both spinal cord and nerves are usually damaged at the site of the injury.

In the conscious patient local neck or back pain and limb paralysis or paresis should be recognized but many patients suffer a head injury at the same time so that when first seen consciousness is clouded and limb paralysis may be missed. While the maximum displacements generally occur at the time of injury, excessive movements of the neck, as can occur during unskilled endotracheal intubatoin, may render a partial lesion complete. All injured patients should be handled with gentleness and whenever a fractured cervical spine is a possibility the neck should be protected with a collar as a first aid measure.

A good lateral cervical X-ray is crucial but it must be examined carefully. Major displacements present at the time of injury may spontaneously reduce leaving a small avulsed fragment of bone and retropharyngeal swelling as the only clues to the severity of the injury. The whole cervical spine including the cervicothoracic junction must be examined and the clinician aware of this fact will assist the radiographer depressing the shoulders if necessary at the moment of exposure to ensure that the X-ray examination is successful.

Cervical lesions may cause difficulty with respiration which depends on the integrity of the phrenic nerves. Loss of normal autonomic control leads to vasomotor instability. Blood gas measurements are an important part of the initial assessment. Many patients have other major injuries to the trunk and limbs which will need treatment. Skull traction on a Stryker frame simplifies nursing and protects the spine from secondary injury.

Transient concussive loss of function of the cord may show signs of recovery within 6 h; if none has occurred within 48 h then the lesion is complete and no recovery can be expected. In this connection it is essential to distinguish between spinal cord and nerve root damage as may occur at the thoracolumbar junction, the site of the conus medullaris. Good recovery is possible with the mixed lesions that occur at this site.

Retention of urine will require catheterization with meticulous aseptic technique. Intermittent regular catheterization commencing as soon as practical after injury favours early return of normal control or automatic bladder voiding in complete paraplegia.

Paralysed limbs must be put through a full range of movements regularly and as spasticity develops splints will be required to prevent the development of contractures.

Rehabilitation is best carried out in specialized spinal units where the question of operative stabilization can be considered. There is some evidence that such procedures may reduce the incidence of late spinal pain. Surgical procedures are almost never required in the acute phase.

9

Movement disorders

The field of movement disorders comprises two main categories:

1. *Akinetic-rigid syndromes*, characterized by slowness of voluntary movement and muscular rigidity, often called the parkinsonian syndrome. The most important cause of an akinetic-rigid syndrome is Parkinson's disease.
2. *The dyskinesias* characterized by abnormal involuntary movements. Most dyskinesias can be included within five main types:
   a) tremor
   b) chorea
   c) myoclonus
   d) tics
   e) dystonia.
   These are not diseases, but clinically identifiable syndromes with many causes.

Parkinson's disease

Parkinson's disease is a slowly progressive, degenerative disease of the basal ganglia, producing an akinetic-rigid syndrome, usually with rest tremor, and accompanied by many other motor disturbances including a flexed posture, a shuffling gait and defective balance.

Epidemiology

Parkinson's disease is a common illness of advancing years. The prevalence rate in the UK is about 100/100 000 of the population, rising progressively and steeply over the age of 50 to about 500/100 000. There are about 100 000 patients with Parkinson's disease in the UK. Both sexes are affected approximately equally, and the illness occurs in all races. Accurate epidemiological data are difficult to obtain, because the onset is insidious making early diagnosis a problem, and minor degrees of the disease may be indistinguishable from the changes of senility in the elderly. While there are no striking differences in the various populations of the world, the incidence may be somewhat less in Africa and China.

Pathogenesis

The main pathological finding in Parkinson's disease is loss of the pigmented neurones in the brainstem, particularly those in the substantia nigra.

The substantia nigra pars compacta projects to the striatum (the caudate nucleus, putamen and related structures) via the nigrostriatal pathway, which utilizes dopamine as its neurotransmitter. Parkinson's disease is associated with a considerable loss of striatal dopamine content, 80 per cent or more, proportional to the loss of substantia nigra neurones. Striatal dopamine deficiency is thus the cardinal biochemical feature of Parkinson's disease. This discovery led to the introduction of treatment with levodopa, the amino acid precursor for dopamine synthesis in the brain. However, the dopamine concept of Parkinson's disease is an over-simplification, for other brain regions and neurotransmitters also are affected.

Other dopaminergic neuronal systems degenerate, including those projecting to the cerebral cortex from the ventral tegmental area adjacent to the substantia nigra, and those in the hypothalamus. The dopaminergic projection from the diencephalon to the spinal cord may be spared.

Degeneration of the locus coeruleus leads to the loss of noradrenergic pathways to cerebral cortex and other brain regions. There is also degeneration of cells in the raphe complex which leads to deficiency of serotonin neurotransmission, and of cells in the substantia innominata, which project acetylcholine-containing pathways to the cerebral cortex.

In all areas of cell loss, surviving neurones contain eosinophilic inclusions known as Lewy bodies.

Aetiology

The cause of Parkinson's disease is not known. In the 1920s, an outbreak of a pandemic infection, encephalitis lethargica, was followed by many cases of post-encephalitic parkinsonism. This led to the suggestion that Parkinson's disease itself might be due to some virus, but none has been found, and the pathology of post-encephalitic parkinsonism is quite different from that of Parkinson's disease.

A sizeable number of patients, perhaps 10–15 per cent, give a history that another family member was affected by Parkinson's disease, suggesting that the illness might be inherited. However, careful studies of twin pairs, one of whom has Parkinson's disease, have shown that the risk of the second identical twin developing the illness is no different from that of non-identical twins, and no different from that among the general population. Accordingly, heredity plays little or no part in the cause of Parkinson's disease. The family incidence merely reflects the high frequency of the disorder in the population.

If heredity is not involved, then some environmental agent might be responsible. Recently, a small outbreak of an illness indistinguishable from Parkinson's disease occurred among drug addicts on the west coast of America. This was traced to a highly selective contaminant, MPTP (1-methyl-4-phenyl-1, 2, 3, 6-tetrahydropyridine) produced in a designer-drug aimed at replacing heroin. MPTP is not the active poison, but is converted in the brain, by mono-amine-oxidase B in glia, into the toxic species MPP^+. MPP^+ is then taken up into dopaminergic neurones, by the normal dopamine re-uptake mechanism, where it is trapped by binding to neuromelanin. MPP^+ then poisons mito-chondria to cause death of pigmented dopaminergic neurones in the brain. This remarkable model of Parkinson's disease suggests that environmental toxins may be the cause, but none have been definitely identified. However, MPTP is one of a number of toxic species, and there have been tentative suggestions that the incidence of Parkinson's disease may be higher in populations exposed to pesticides or contaminated well water. Such hypothetical exposure to an environmental toxin could occur cumulatively throughout life. Alternatively, exposure early in life could be followed by the effects of natural ageing in dopa-minergic systems in the brain, the combination of the two leading to the appea-rance of the illness with increasing frequency in old age.

The nature of the characteristic intracellular inclusion, the Lewy body, is also unknown. The Lewy body contains cytoskeletal elements such as neurofila-ments and mitochondria.

Main clinical features

There is no laboratory test for Parkinson's disease, so the diagnosis depends on clinical judgement. Characteristic features are tremor, rigidity, postural abnormalities, and akinesia.

Tremor is the initial complaint in about two-thirds of those with Parkinson's disease, and occurs eventually in most patients. The characteristic tremor is present at rest at a frequency of 4–6 Hz; it is most common in the upper limbs, to produce the typical 'pill-rolling' movement. The jaw, head and legs may shake as well. The tremor is intensified by mental or emotional stress but disappears during deep sleep. Many patients also exhibit a tremor of the outstretched hands on posture, at a faster frequency of 6–8 Hz.

Rigidity of muscles is detected clinically by resistance to passive manipula-tion of the limbs and trunk. The examiner encounters uniform resistance throughout the range of passive movement, equal in agonists and antagonists (hence the terms 'plasticity' or 'lead-pipe' rigidity). When tremor is also present, rigidity is broken up ('cog-wheel' rigidity). In the early stages of the illness, rigidity is often best detected in the axial muscles, such as those of the neck and shoulder.

Postural abnormalities are typical of Parkinson's disease. Rigidity contri-butes to the characteristic flexed posture, with the chin towards the chest, the back bent, and the limbs flexed at the elbows and knees. Many patients, espe-cially later in the illness, also exhibit postural instability. They have a tendency to fall, and when they do, they do not throw out their arms to protect themselves.

The gait of Parkinson's disease is diagnostic. The patient walks without swin-ging the arms in the typical flexed posture. The feet shuffle with small steps, and there is a tendency to fall forward with the result that the steps become increasingly fast to catch up (festination). Often the patient cannot initiate gait, but may shuffle on the spot. Frequently the patient freezes during walking and becomes rooted to the spot, particularly when passing through doorways or in a narrow passage.

Akinesia is the most important disabling feature of Parkinson's disease so far as the patient is concerned. Strictly speaking akinesia means an inability to move, while bradykinesia refers to slowness of movement, and hypokinesia means reduced amplitude of movement. Akinesia, bradykinesia and hypokinesia are independent of rigidity, although the latter contributes to the patient's problems. Typically, there is a slowness of initiation and execution of all movement, and a general poverty of spontaneous and automatic or associated movements. The more complex the movement, the greater the impact of akinesia. Akinesia accounts for many of the characteristic features of Parkinson's disease – the masked expressionless face, the loss of blinking, the absence of arm-swing when walking, the small cramped handwriting, the soft monotonous speech, and the difficulties with walking.

Other symptoms and signs

Patients with Parkinson's disease frequently exhibit additional symptoms and signs. Many are due to the illness itself, but the side-effects of drug therapy and intercurrent illness in this aged population must be taken into account.

Mental disturbances are common. Although the intellect and senses are often preserved, at least in the initial stages, many patients develop some degree of intellectual deterioration as the disease progresses. A certain slowness of thought and of memory retrieval (bradyphrenia), and subtle changes in personality occur in about two-thirds of cases. Frank global dementia appears in some 15–20 per cent. Depression affects one-third. Acute toxic confusional states are often precipitated by intercurrent infections or by drug therapy.

Sensory complaints are common in Parkinson's disease, although sensory examination is normal. Discomfort in the limbs, often amounting to pain, is frequently mentioned and sometimes is associated with an unpleasant restlessness of the legs and an urge to move (akathisia). Curious feelings in the skin described as itching, creeping or burning, are also common.

Apparent skeletal deformities of the hands and feet resemble those seen in rheumatoid arthritis. These are due to rigidity, not contracture, and can be relieved by drug treatment. Osteoporosis is common in this age group and may be a cause of pain.

A number of ocular abnormalities are recognized. Blepharospasm and fluttering of the closed eyelids (blepharoclonus) are common. Paralysis of convergence and limitation of upgaze may occur, as well as a break up of voluntary horizontal and pursuit eye movements into jerky saccades.

Gastrointestinal disturbances include constipation, which is almost universal. Weight loss is very common, and sometimes severe. Some 75 per cent of patients are below their optimum weight. Drooling of saliva is frequent in severe cases, as is dysphagia.

Urinary difficulties may be caused by Parkinson's disease itself, which produces an irritable bladder with frequency, urgency and urge incontinence.

Prostate enlargement is common in elderly males and contributes to the overall problem.

Assessment of the significance of many of these complaints may be difficult. For example, constipation may be due to a combination of immobility, reduced food intake, dysphagia, and anticholinergic medication, or may indicate the incidental development of a large bowel neoplasm. As a general principle it is wise to investigate such complaints on their own merits before accepting them as due to the disease or to therapy, although frequently no other pathology is discovered.

Diagnosis

Typical Parkinson's disease is not difficult to recognize. The mask-like, immobile, staring face, infrequent blinking, flexed posture, rest tremor and rigidity, poverty and slowness of movement, small spidery handwriting, and typical gait can be easily recognized by the layman. However, the diagnosis is often missed in the early stages of the disease, especially if tremor is absent.

The onset is frequently unilateral, with the patient complaining of minor clumsiness of an arm, a change in handwriting, or dragging of a leg. In these circumstances, a hemiparesis can be closely simulated, although the tendon jerks are not exaggerated, and the plantar responses remain flexor.

Sensations of pain or numbness in the affected limbs may be the presenting complaint, and give rise to suspicion of musculoskeletal disorders such as a frozen shoulder or sciatica. If generalized, such complaints may suggest rheumatism or polymyalgia rheumatica.

Fatigue is a common problem, and may be generalized or limited to one limb, or even deceptively to a single task. Thus, progressive difficulty with handwriting accompanied by stiffness and discomfort in the forearm muscles may simulate writer's cramp. The picture of a general loss of vitality, aches and pains, and slowing-up may simply be dismissed in the elderly as the result of 'growing old'.

Depression is one of the most difficult presentations. The patient is aware that they have slowed down and that life has become weary and difficult. The loss of facial expression may be attributed to a depressive illness, which may indeed be present in response to the patient's appreciation of their changing physical state.

Differential diagnosis

Parkinson's disease must be differentiated from other causes of the akinetic-rigid syndrome (*see* Table 9.1), brief descriptions of which are given below. Parkinson's disease is unlikely to be the diagnosis if the patient was taking drugs at the onset that may cause parkinsonism, if there is a history of encephalitis or oculogyric crises (p. 207), if there is a severe disturbance of eye movements including impairment of downgaze, or if obvious autonomic neuropathy, ataxia, or severe dementia occur early in the course of the illness. A common mistake is to confuse the tremor of Parkinson's disease with that of essential tremor, although the latter is a postural tremor and such patients have no rigidity or akinesia.

Treatment

A range of drugs is available to relieve the symptoms of Parkinson's disease. The most powerful is levodopa, which crosses the blood–brain barrier and is converted in the brain into dopamine. The efficacy of levodopa replacement therapy has been enhanced by combination with a peripheral inhibitor of dopa decarboxylase. The latter prevents the metabolism of levodopa to dopamine outside the brain, but itself does not enter the brain so that cerebral dopamine can be replenished. Two such extracerebral decarboxylase inhibitors are available: carbidopa, which is combined with levodopa in Sinemet, and benserazide, which is combined with levodopa in Madopar. Both Sinemet and Madopar are available in a variety of dosages and there is little to choose between the two. The advantage of such combined therapy over levodopa alone is a reduction of those side-effects caused by peripheral metabolites of levodopa, in particular nausea and vomiting and some cardiovascular problems.

Levodopa does not alter the underlying pathology of the illness, and does not cure the disease. Many patients on long-term levodopa therapy run into problems (*see* below), and it is a complicated treatment. Accordingly, for the newly diagnosed patient with mild disability, levodopa therapy can often be held in reserve and other treatments employed.

Amantadine is an antiviral agent which was found by chance to be of benefit in Parkinson's disease. Its complete mode of action is not understood, although it does release stored dopamine. It is less potent than levodopa, but easy to use in a dose of 100 mg b.d. or t.d.s. About two-thirds of patients gain benefit from amantadine in the early stage of the illness, but its effect often disappears with the passage of time. Side-effects include ankle oedema and skin changes, in particular a rash on the legs, livedo reticularis; in high doses it can cause a toxic confusional state and fits.

The original drugs used to treat Parkinson's disease before levodopa was available were the anticholinergics. There are many anticholinergic preparations, including benzhexol, orphenadrine, and benztropine. These give modest benefit, again in about two-thirds of patients. Unfortunately, they cause a high incidence of unwanted side-effects, including those of peripheral cholinergic blockade (dry mouth, blurred vision, constipation and urinary retention), as well as those due to their central actions (memory impairment, personality change and acute toxic confusional states). Because of the cognitive changes present in a large proportion of elderly patients with Parkinson's disease, anticholinergics are best avoided in older patients.

The judgement as to when to begin levodopa therapy depends upon an individual's disability and needs. When the patient is incapacitated by his disease, treatment should be started with Sinemet or Madopar, beginning in a small dose and gradually increasing over a matter of weeks to the optimum.

Levodopa benefits the great majority of patients with Parkinson's disease. Initially, most gain considerable benefit. However, about two-thirds of patients report some loss of efficacy after 5–10 years of therapy, probably due to progression of the underlying disease. Typically, the relief from each dose of levodopa lasts for shorter and shorter periods, resulting in fluctuations in disability throughout the day in relation to the timing of levodopa intake. With time, these fluctuations become increasingly frequent, prolonged, and erratic (the 'on-off' phenomenon). In addition, with time, and often because of an increase in dosage required to overcome these fluctuations, patients begin to develop abnormal involuntary movements or dyskinesias. These may occur at the peak time of action of each dose of the drug (peak-dose dyskinesias), when they are usually choreiform in nature. Alternatively, they may occur as the drug begins to work, and as it effect begins to wear off (biphasic dyskinesias), when they are often dystonic in nature. These various dyskinesias may in themselves cause disability such as difficulty with speaking, using the hands or walking.

Levodopa also may cause psychiatric side-effects such as an acute toxic confusional state, isolated hallucinations or even frank psychotic episodes. Both dyskinesias and psychiatric problems remit if the dosage of levodopa is reduced.

Other side-effects of levodopa treatment include nausea and vomiting, which may be controlled by the addition of an antiemetic such as domperidone (which itself dose not penetrate into brain), postural hypotension, and urinary difficulties.

There are no absolute contraindications to levodopa therapy, but the drug should not be given to those on monoamine oxidase A inhibitors, or to those with a recent history of myocardial infarction.

The art of levodopa treatment for Parkinson's disease is to titrate each patient to their optimum, using the smallest dosage. Initially Sinemet or Madopar are given three or four times a day. As fluctuations appear, the frequency of dosage may have to be increased. If fluctuations break through, the duration of each dose of levodopa may be prolonged slightly by the addition of the monoamine oxidase B inhibitor, selegiline. If this is insufficient, then the directly-acting dopamine agonist bromocriptine may be added to levodopa therapy. It seems likely that the long-term problems of levodopa treatment may be avoided or delayed by the early introduction of bromocriptine treatment, so there is now a tendency to give both Sinemet or Madopar with bromocriptine as soon as signs of fluctuations begin to appear.

While specific drug treatment is the mainstay of therapy for Parkinson's disease, many patients also gain benefit from an exercise programme, or from physiotherapy and speech therapy. Careful attention to aids to assist toileting, eating and mobility is important. Depression may require treatment with a tricyclic antidepressant drug. Surgical treatment by stereotactic thalamotomy is now employed infrequently, being reserved for the occasional young patient with predominantly unilateral drug-resistant tremor.

Prior to the levodopa era, Parkinson's disease was relentlessly progressive and the majority of patients were severely disabled or dead within 10 years of the onset. Mortality was increased threefold compared to age-matched controls. With modern levodopa treatment, and other therapy, life expectancy is now more or less the same as that of a similar age-matched population. The majority of patients can remain gainfully employed and lead active lives for many years.

Other akinetic-rigid syndromes

Many other illnesses may cause an akinetic-rigid syndrome (Table 9.1).

Table 9.1   Causes of akinetic-rigid syndrome in adults

Pure parkinsonism	*Parkinsonism plus*
Parkinson's disease	Progressive supranuclear palsy
Drug-induced parkinsonism	Multiple system atrophy
Post-encephalitic parkinsonism	olivo-ponto-cerebellar degeneration
MPTP toxicity	strionigral degeneration
Other toxins	progressive autonomic failure (Shy-Drager)
	Basal ganglia calcification

Drug-induced pseudoparkinsonism

The neuroleptic drugs employed to control psychotic illness, in particular schizophrenia, all block dopamine receptors in the brain. Such drugs include the phenothiazines, butyrophenones such as haloperidol, thioxanthines such as flupenthixol, and benzamides such as sulpiride and metoclopramide. About two-thirds of those taking neuroleptics exhibit some signs of drug-induced parkinsonism, whose symptoms and signs include all those seen in Parkinson's disease itself. Such drug-induced parkinsonism usually remits in weeks or months after the offending neuroleptic drug is withdrawn or its dosage is reduced. If it is necessary to continue the neuroleptic to control the psychotic illness, then the addition of an anticholinergic may be beneficial.

These drugs are also used commonly to treat vertigo and a variety of gastrointestinal disturbances; such patients also may develop drug-induced parkinsonism.

Encephalitis lethargica

This disease was endemic throughout the world in the 1920s, but virtually disappeared by the 1930s. Occasional sporadic cases still probably occur today. Eighty per cent of patients with post-encephalitic parkinsonism developed their symptoms within 10 years of the infection. In addition to the characteristic features of the akinetic-rigid syndrome, many patients with post-encephalitic parkinsonism exhibited behavioural disturbances, other dyskinesias especially dystonias, and oculogyric crises. The latter consists of spasms of eye deviation, usually upwards or laterally, often accompanied by compulsive thoughts, lasting for a matter of hours.

Steele-Richardson-Olszewski disease

This is an uncommon non-familial progressive disease of middle and late life, characterized by akinesia, predominantly axial rigidity especially of the neck, often marked bradyphrenia, and a characteristic abnormality of eye movements termed a supranuclear gaze palsy (the illness is sometimes called progressive supranuclear palsy because of this). The latter consists of an inability voluntarily to shift gaze or follow a moving object, particularly in the vertical plane and always involving downgaze. With time, lateral gaze also becomes affected. Although the patients cannot voluntarily move their eyes, a full range of eye movements can be produced by the 'dolls-head' manoeuvre of passive neck rotation, which evokes normal brainstem reflex eye movements. Unfortunately, this condition does not respond to the usual treatments for Parkinson's disease.

The multiple system atrophies

The multiple system atrophies consist of a variety of syndromes. All present in middle or late life, and a family history is rare.

Strionigral degeneration presents as a progressive akinetic-rigid syndrome, unresponsive to levodopa, and usually without tremor. Pathologically there is degeneration not only of the substantia nigra (without Lewy bodies), but also of the striatum itself. Olivo-ponto-cerebellar degeneration presents with prominent cerebellar ataxia, with the subsequent development of an akinetic-rigid syndrome. Pathologically there is degeneration of the olives, pons and cerebellum. The Shy-Drager syndrome presents with a severe autonomic neuropathy with symptomatic postural hypotension, loss of sweating, impotence, and sphincter disturbances. Such patients with progressive autonomic failure may go on to develop signs of an akinetic-rigid syndrome. Pathologically the autonomic failure is due to loss of the intermediolateral columns of the spinal cord which contain preganglionic sympathetic outflow neurones, as well as the parasympathetic neurones in the brain.

These three conditions overlap clinically and pathologically, hence their designation as the multiple system atrophies.

Diffuse brain disease (Table 9.2)

Whatever its cause, diffuse brain disease may produce an akinetic-rigid syndrome (without tremor), in addition to other signs of brain damage such as dementia, fits and pyramidal deficit. Elements of parkinsonism may be seen in those with diffuse cerebral vascular disease (either as part of multi-infarct dementia, or Binswanger's disease), Alzheimer's and Pick's diseases, and other presenile dementias. Severe head injury or cerebral anoxia, due to cardiac

Table 9.2 Diffuse brain diseases causing multifocal dementia in adults, in which elements of parkinsonism also may occur

Common	Rare
Alzheimer's disease (including senile dementia)	Corticobasal degeneration
Multi-infarct dementia	Pick's disease
Binswanger's disease	Creutzfeldt-Jakob disease
Congophilic angiopathy	Manganese poisoning
Head injury (e.g. boxers)	Neurosyphilis
Cerebral anoxia	Cysticercosis
	Communicating hydrocephalus

arrest or carbon monoxide poisoning, may also leave elements of the akinetic-rigid syndrome as well as other multiple brain deficits.

Juvenile parkinsonism

Juvenile parkinsonism in a child or young adult poses a different diagnostic problem (Table 9.3). Parkinson's disease is rare under the age of 40 years, and almost unknown in childhood. At this age other conditions must be considered, in particular Wilson's disease (*see* below). Huntington's disease may also present in this fashion in this age group, as may variety of other childhood degenerations of the basal ganglia including the primary pallidal atrophies and Hallervorden-Spatz disease.

Table 9.3 Causes of an akinetic-rigid syndrome in childhood

Hereditary	Other
Wilson's disease	Drugs
Hallervorden-Spatz disease	Athetoid cerebral palsy
Progressive pallidal atrophy	
Juvenile Huntington's disease	
Pelizaeus-Merzbacher disease	
Ataxia telangiectasia	
Lesch-Nyhan disease	

Wilson's disease

This is a rare, often familial illness inherited as an autosomal recessive trait, which produces progressive disease of the central nervous system and liver due to retention of copper in the body. It is important, because it is treatable.

Pathogenesis

The primary abnormality of Wilson's disease is a failure to excrete copper normally in bile. As a result, copper accumulates in the body, initially in the liver. Progressive liver damage occurs due to copper toxicosis, and gradually the liver cannot contain excess copper which spills over into the circulation. Copper then accumulates in many other organs throughout the body, in particular in the brain. The most vulnerable area in the brain to copper toxicosis appears to be the basal ganglia. The striatum and globus pallidus are destroyed by copper poisoning, but the cerebral cortex and other brain structures are also damaged.

In addition to the failure to excrete copper in bile, the majority of patients with Wilson's disease also exhibit a deficiency of the copper-carrying plasma protein ceruloplasmin.

Clinical features

Onset usually is in childhood or adolescence, but may be delayed as late as the age of 50. Wilson's disease presents in childhood usually to hepatologists with the complications of liver disease, and in adolescence and adult life to neurologists with a variety of psychiatric and movement disorders.

Initial hepatic manifestations may mimic acute hepatitis (often with a haemolytic anaemia), or chronic progressive cirrhosis with all its complications. Sometimes the disease is discovered accidentally by the finding of abnormal liver function in patients investigated for other conditions.

Wilson's disease presents to neurologists as a behaviour disturbance, often a deterioration in school performance, or as a variety of movement disorders. These include an akinetic-rigid syndrome, a picture of generalized dystonia, or a picture reminiscent of a cerebellar ataxia, or a compilation of all three. Any child, adolescent or young adult presenting with an unexplained movement disorder must be investigated to exculde Wilson's disease.

Without treatment the disease is invariably progressive with increasingly severe dysarthria and dysphagia, akinesia and rigidity with dystonia, leading to contractures and immobility. Dementia supervenes in a proportion of cases, and occasionally fits occur. Sensory deficit and paralysis, however, are not features of Wilson's disease.

Clinical evidence of liver disease may or may not be present in those with neurological symptoms and signs, but abnormalities of liver function are usually found upon investigation. A history of hepatitis or jaundice may be obtained, there may be hepatomegaly or hepatosplenomegaly, and hepatic precoma and gastrointestinal haemorrhage due to varices may occur.

A characteristic clinical finding in Wilson's disease is the presence of a Kayser-Fleischer ring in the cornea. This consists of a ring of greenish-brown copper pigmentation around the margin of the cornea in Descemet's membrane. It may be visible to the naked eye, but frequently requires examination with a slit-lamp by an experienced observer to be detected.

Diagnosis

Any child or young adult presenting with any form of movement disorder, or with unexplained liver disease, should be investigated to exclude Wilson's disease. In an established case, relatives must be screened to detect homozygotes who require treatment to prevent the appearance of the disease. Heterozygotes, carrying one gene of the illness, will not develop Wilson's disease, although they may have minor abnormalities of copper metabolism.

The crucial investigations are to examine the cornea by slit-lamp for a Kayser-Fleischer ring, and to measure the serum concentration of ceruloplasmin, which is reduced in about 95 per cent of patients with Wilson's disease. The total copper content in serum may also be reduced, in proportion to the reduction of ceruloplasmin, although free serum copper content is increased, as is the urinary excretion of copper. The Kayser-Fleischer ring and a low serum ceruloplasmin concentration are not specific for Wilson's disease. However, a patient with liver disease or a movement disorder who has both Kayser-Fleischer rings and a low serum ceruloplasmin level has this illness. If there is doubt about the diagnosis, a liver biopsy to measure the content of copper in liver tissue and to look for pathological evidence of liver damage is decisive.

Treatment

Without treatment the disease is fatal in about 5–15 years from the onset. The mainstay of treatment for Wilson's disease is to promote excretion of copper from the body. Penicillamine is the drug of choice. Penicillamine chelates with copper to form a complex that is excreted in the urine. Penicillamine treatment can effectively remove excess copper stores from the body and reverse or halt both liver and brain damage. The response to treatment may take weeks or months to appear, but the majority of patients can be maintained healthy by such therapy, which has to be taken for life.

The dyskinesias

The first step in analysis of patients with abnormal involuntary movements is to decide which category of dyskinesia they exhibit.

Tremor is easily recognized as a rhythmic sinusoidal movement. It is useful to distinguish between tremor at rest (typical of Parkinson's disease), tremor most obvious when maintaining a position, e.g. holding the arms outstretched (commonly seen in the entity essential tremor), and tremor occurring on movement as intention tremor (typical of cerebellar ataxia). The chief diseases causing tremor are listed in Table 9.4.

Chorea consists of a continuous flow of irregular, jerky and explosive movements, that flit from one portion of the body to another in random sequence. The limbs, trunk, gait and facial features are continually disturbed by unpredictable short-lived movements. Each muscle contraction is brief, often appearing as a fragment of what might have been a normal movement, and quite

Table 9.4 Causes of tremor

Rest tremor
   Parkinson's disease
   Post-encephalitic parkinsonism
   Drug-induced parkinsonism
   Other extrapyramidal diseases
Postural tremor
   Physiological tremor
   Exaggerated physiological tremor
      thyrotoxicosis
      anxiety states
      alcohol
      drugs (sympathomimetics, antidepressants, lithium)
      heavy metal poisoning (e.g. mercury – the 'hatter's shakes')
   Structural brain disease
      severe cerebellar lesions ('red nucleus tremor')
      Wilson's disease
      neurosyphilis
   Benign essential (familial) tremor
Intention tremor
   Brainstem or cerebellar disease
      multiple sclerosis
      spinocerebellar degenerations
      vascular disease
      tumour

Table 9.5   Causes of chorea

Sydenham's chorea: variants include chorea gravidarum, chorea caused by
   contraceptive pill
Huntington's disease: variants include senile chorea, juvenile chorea, Westphal variant
Benign hereditary chorea
Hereditary chorea with acanthocytosis (neurocanthocytosis)
Symptomatic chorea
   Thyrotoxicosis
   Systemic lupus erythematosus
   Polycythaemia rubra vera
   Encephalitis lethargica
   Hypernatraemia
   Hypoparathyroidism
   Subdural haematoma
Drug-induced chorea
   Neuroleptic drugs
   Phenytoin
   Alcohol
Hemiballism (hemichorea)
   Stroke
   Tumour
   Trauma
   Post-thalamotomy

---

unpredictable in timing or site. The chief causes of chorea are shown in Table 9.5.

Myoclonus describes brief, shock-like muscle jerks, similar to the effect of stimulating the muscle's nerve with a single electric shock. The muscle jerks differ from those of chorea in that they are intermittent with distinct pauses between each movement. The timing of the jerks may be irregular or rhythmic, and they may occur repetitively in the same muscle. Myoclonus may be confined to one part of the body (focal myoclonus), or affect many different parts at different times (multifocal myoclonus), or consist of a whole body jerk (generalized myoclonus). The chief causes of myoclonus are shown in Table 9.6.

Tics resemble myoclonus since they consist of brief muscle contractions, but differ in that they are repetitive and stereotyped, they can be mimicked by the observer, and they can usually be controlled through an effort of will by the patient, often at the expense of mounting inner tension. Typical tics involve the face (e.g. blinking, sniffing, lip smacking), or the upper arms and neck (shrugging of the shoulders with inclination of the head). The chief causes of tics are shown in Table 9.7.

Dystonia (athetosis) consists of sustained irregular muscle spasms, lasting longer than the individual movements of chorea, myoclonus or tics. These prolonged muscle spasms occur repetitively as dystonic movements, and often distort the body into characteristic postures, which may be sustained. Thus, the neck is twisted to one side (torticollis), or extended (retrocollis), or flexed (anticollis); the trunk is forced into excessive lordosis or scoliosis; the arm is commonly extended and hyperpronated, with the wrist flexed and the fingers extended; the leg is commonly extended with the foot plantar flexed and

Table 9.6 Causes of myoclonus

GENERALIZED MYOCLONUS
Progressive myoclonic encephalopathies *
With demonstrable metabolic cause
    Lafora body disease
    GM_2 gangliosidosis (Tay-Sachs disease)
    Ceroid lipofuscinosis (Batten's disease)
    Sialidosis (cherry red spot myoclonus syndrome)
Hereditary myoclonus with no known metabolic cause
    Familial myoclonic epilepsy (Unverricht-Lundborg disease)
    Myoclonus associated with spinocerebellar degenerations (Ramsay Hunt syndrome)
Other sporadic diseases
    Encephalitis lethargica
    Subacute sclerosing leucoencephalitis
    Creutzfeldt-Jakob disease
    Alzheimer's disease
    Metabolic myoclonus
        uraemia
        hyponatraemia
        hypocalcaemia
        hepatic failure
        CO_2 narcosis
        drug-induced myoclonus
        alcohol and drug withdrawal
Static myoclonic encephalopathies †
Post-anoxic action myoclonus (Lance-Adams syndrome)
Post-traumatic myoclonus
Myoclonic epilepsies **
First year of life
    infantile spasms
    'dancing eyes' syndrome
Two to six years:
    Lennox-Gastaut syndrome
Older children and adolescents (and adults)
    photosensitive epileptic myoclonus
    myoclonic absences
    morning myoclonus – primary generalized epilepsy
Benign essential (familial) myoclonus
FOCAL MYOCLONUS (segmental)
    spinal
    tumour
    infarct
    trauma
Palatal myoclonus
Hemifacial spasm
Cortical reflex myoclonus
Epilepsia partialis continua

*Obvious myoclonus (with or without fits) clearly as part of a progressive encephalopathy
†Obvious myoclonus after some acute and now static cerebral insult
**Obvious epilepsy as the main problem, with myoclonus

Table 9.7 Causes of tics

Simple tics
transient tic of childhood
chronic simple tic
Complex multiple tics
chronic multiple tics
Gilles de la Tourette syndrome
Symptomatic tics
encephalitis lethargica
drug-induced tics
Post-traumatic
Neuroacanthocytosis

inturned. Initially, these dystonic muscle spasms may occur only on certain actions, so that the patient may walk on his toes or develop the characteristic arm posture only on writing (action dystonia). In progressive dystonia, however, the abnormal muscle spasms and postures become apparent at rest and cause increasing movements and deformity. Such dystonic spasms and postures are often called athetoid, although the term athetosis is best restricted to a particular form of cerebral palsy that may produce dystonia. Dystonia may be confined to one part of the body, as in isolated spasmodic torticollis (focal dystonia), affect adjacent segments of the body, e.g. the neck and one or both arms (segmental dystonia), the limbs on one side (hemidystonia), or the whole body (generalized dystonia). The chief causes of dystonia are shown in Table 9.8.

While most patient's abnormal movements may be categorized into one of these five major types, it must be admitted that many exhibit a combination of dyskinesias. In these circumstances, it is best to concentrate on the most obvious abnormal movement.

Having categorized the predominant dyskinesia in an individual patient, the next step is to consider the differential diagnosis of that particular form of abnormal movement. The common causes of each of the categories of dyskinesias are shown in Tables 9.4–9.8. Descriptions will now be given of those diseases which typically are characterized by abnormal involuntary movements.

Benign essential (familial) tremor

Essential tremor is about 20 times more frequent than Parkinson's disease. Its cause is not known, but a positive family history is obtained in over one-half of the patients, and the pattern of inheritance indicates an autosomal dominant trait.

Pathogenesis

No pathological or biochemical abnormality has been identified in the very few cases that have come to necropsy. The condition maybe due to some instability in the many feed-back neuronal loops that control the posture of the hands, head and other parts of the body. There are two separate mechanisms which cause a postural tremor.

Table 9.8 Causes of torsion dystonia

Generalized dystonia
Idiopathic dystonia musculorum deformans
  autosomal recessive
  sex-linked recessive
  autosomal dominant
  sporadic
Drug-induced dystonia
  acute dystonic reactions
  chronic tardive dystonia
Symptomatic dystonia
  various lipid storage diseases and leucodystrophies
  acidosis
  ataxia telangiectasia
  mitochondrial encephalopathies*
  athetoid cerebral palsy
  encephalitis lethargica
  Wilson's disease*
  juvenile Huntington's disease
  Hallervorden-Spatz disease
Paroxysmal dystonia (paroxysmal choreoathetosis)
  paroxysmal kinesogenic choreoathetosis
  paroxysmal dystonic choreoathetosis
  dystonia with marked diurnal fluctuations
Focal dystonia
Spasmodic torticollis
Axial (truncal) dystonia
Dystonic writer's cramp (and other occupational cramps)
Oromandibular dystonia
Blepharospasm
Cranial dystonia
Hemiplegic dystonia (hemidystonia)
  stroke*
  tumour*
  A-V malformation
  trauma*
  encephalitis
  post-thalamotomy

---

*May cause low-density lesions in basal ganglia on CT scan

1. *Enhanced physiological tremor*: everyone has a physiological tremor of the outstretched hands at about 8–12 Hz. Physiological tremor is exaggerated by adrenergic overactivity as in anxiety, thyrotoxicosis, and due to sympathomimetic drugs. In these circumstances, loop delay in the operation of the stretch reflex arc is such as to cause an exaggerated tendency to oscillate at around 10 Hz.

2. *True essential tremor*: this is usually of a slower frequency at 6 Hz. Most evidence suggests that it is due to abnormal discharge of an oscillator in the central nervous system, although this is modulated by peripheral feedback.

Essential tremor in the vast majority of cases is not associated with any other evidence of damage to the nervous system. However, a few cases are found to have a peripheral neuropathy, spinal muscular atrophy, or a cerebellar degeneration. A similar postural tremor is also seen in Parkinson's disease.

Clinical features

Tremor is present in one or both hands on maintaining a posture, as when holding a cup or glass. Handwriting becomes untidy and tremulous. Anxiety makes matters worse. There is no tremor at rest, but a rhythmic oscillation develops when the patient holds the arms outstretched. On movement, as in finger-nose testing, the tremor continues, but does not become strikingly worse. Tremor of the head (titubation) and jaw is present in about 50 per cent of cases, and tremor of the legs occurs in about one-third. Despite the tremor, tests of coordination are usually performed normally, walking is unaffected, and there are no other neurological abnormalities. In particular, there are no signs of parkinsonism.

A small or moderate dose of alcohol characteristically suppresses the tremor. A large sherry, or gin and tonic, may be sufficient to 'steady the hands'.

Generally the illness is only slowly progressive in most patients, causing predominantly a social disability, but individuals dependent upon manual skills may be severely disabled by the tremor. The condition may become more severely progressive in later years.

Some variants of the syndrome of essential tremor are occasionally encountered. Thus isolated inherited head tremor may occur, and tremulous 'writer's cramp' (primary writing tremor), are recognized.

Treatment

Although alcohol may suppress the tremor effectively, and can be of value if used wisely, there is the risk of alcoholism. About one-half of patients respond satisfactorily to a beta-adrenergic receptor antagonist such as propranolol. Primidone, in standard anticonvulsant dosages, has been reported to help some patients. Antiparkinsonian drugs have no effect.

Sydenham's chorea

Rheumatic fever, the cause of Sydenham's chorea (St Vitus' dance), is now a rare disease. The chorea appears up to 3 months after a bout of rheumatic fever due to Group A streptococcal infection. It affects children and adolescents. It may recur in adult life, particularly in pregnant women (chorea gravidarum) or in those taking the contraceptive pill. Pathologically, the brain shows a diffuse inflammatory encephalitis.

Clinical features

The onset is usually gradual, but may be abrupt. The initial symptoms are often irritability, agitation, disobedience, and inattentiveness. A frank organic confusional state occurs in about 10 per cent of patients. Generalized chorea then appears and may get worse for a few weeks. Headaches, fits and sensory change are not features of the illness. The chorea may be unilateral, and in severe cases may be accompanied by flaccidity and subjective weakness. Although cardiac signs may be found, the child usually has no fever or other manifestations of rheumatic disease. The erythrocyte sedimentation rate characteristically is normal and the antistreptolysin titre is not raised. The chorea and psychological disturbance slowly recover over one to 3 months, but recurrences occur in about one-quarter of patients over the next few years. About two-thirds of patients develop chronic rheumatic heart disease.

Treatment

Treatment as for rheumatic fever is necessary, with bedrest and sedation. The chorea may be controlled with diazepam, tetrabenazine or a phenothiazine. A course of penicillin should be given, and prophylactic oral penicillin should be continued until the age of about 20 years to prevent further streptococcal infection.

Huntington's disease

Huntington's disease is a rare, dominantly inherited, relentlessly progressive illness, usually of middle life, characterized by chorea and dementia. It occurs worldwide and in all ethnic groups with a prevalence of about 1 in 20 000. The gene is fully penetrant, so that the children of an affected parent have a 50 per cent risk of the disease, which never skips a generation. New mutations are almost unknown, but relatives frequently conceal the family history. Recent studies have shown the abnormal gene to lie on the short arm of the fourth chromosome. The DNA probe G8 identifies a restriction fragment length polymorphism linked to the Huntington's disease gene.

Pathogenesis

The brain is generally atrophic with conspicuous damage to the cerebral cortex and corpus striatum. The cortical gyri are atrophic, as are the caudate nucleus and putamen which show extensive loss of small neurones.

These pathological changes result in a profound reduction in the neurotransmitters associated with striatal neurones including gamma-aminobutyric acid and acetylcholine.

Clinical features

The onset is insidious usually between the ages of 30 and 50 years. The initial symptoms frequently are those of a change in personality and behaviour, but chorea may be the first sign of the illness. The family may begin to notice a blunting of drive and depth of feeling, irritability and truculence, a tendency to uncontrolled aggressive or sexual behaviour, all indicating coarsening of the personality. As the disease progresses, dementia becomes more pronounced and the chorea more severe and grotesque. Rigidity and akinesia may appear and begin to dominate the picture. Finally, the patient becomes bedridden and emaciated. Death occurs on average about 14 years from the onset.

A number of variants are recognized. About 6 per cent present not with chorea but with an akinetic-rigid parkinsonian syndrome (the Westphal variant), which is commonest in children. Dementia is profound in those with early onset, and epilepsy may occur. Huntington's disease in old age may present as senile chorea when it may be difficult to obtain a family history of the illness.

Diagnosis is not difficult if the characteristic and unique family history is available. However, often such a family history is not known, or is hidden. In the absence of a family history, such patients require full investigation to exclude other (and sometimes treatable) causes of chorea.

Treatment

There is no cure for the disease. The chorea may be reduced by a phenothiazine or other neuroleptic, but these drugs commonly cause disabling side-effects. The mental complications of the illness often pose particular problems for the family, and eventually chronic hospital care may be required.

Genetic counselling of all family members is necessary. This difficult problem is likely to be aided by the advent of new gene markers which will allow accurate premorbid diagnosis.

Hemiballism

Hemiballism refers to wild flinging or throwing movements of one arm and leg. They are like those of chorea but predominantly involve the large proximal muscles of the shoulder and pelvic girdle. The syndrome is usually seen in elderly hypertensive diabetic patients as a result of a stroke affecting the contralateral subthalamic nucleus or its connections. In this case, the onset is abrupt. The intensity of the movements varies from mild to severe enough to cause injury. It usually gradually remits spontaneously over 3–6 months. Treatment with a neuroleptic may be required to control the hemiballism.

Generalized myoclonus

Generalized or multifocal myoclonus occurs in a wide variety of primary diseases of the nervous system, or as a manifestation of metabolic or toxic encephalopathy. In many of these conditions, myoclonus arises from spontaneous or reflex-triggered discharges in the cerebral cortex. Such cortical myoclonus is closely related to epilepsy.

Epileptic myoclonus is a feature of primary generalized epilepsy, or may be symptomatic of progressive brain disease as in the progressive myoclonic epilepsies. These conditions are discussed further in Chapter 11.

Myoclonus may dominate the clinical picture in a number of cerebral diseases. In these conditions, myoclonus may occur spontaneously, on movement (action myoclonus), or in response to visual, auditory or somatosensory stimuli (reflex myoclonus). Severe myoclonus may be the major residual deficit after cerebral anoxia (postanoxic myoclonus), whatever the cause. Myoclonus may be the characteristic feature of a number of degenerative dementing illnesses, such as Alzheimer's disease, and is characteristic of Creutzfeldt-Jakob disease. Myoclonus, with occasional seizures may occur in conjunction with a progressive cerebellar ataxia in the Ramsay Hunt syndrome. Myoclonus may also follow a variety of viral illnesses (postinfectious myoclonus). In all these conditions there are likely to be other signs of damage to the central nervous system.

Benign essential myoclonus is a familial disease, inherited as an autosomal dominant trait, in which myoclonus is the only physical abnormality. Onset usually is in childhood or adolescence with multifocal myoclonus affecting all four limbs, the trunk, neck and face, occurring at 10–50 min, and enhanced by action and sensory stimuli. Disability is usually mild, there is no progression, intellect is normal, fits do not occur, and no other neurological deficit appears. Some patients report that alcohol helps their jerks, and many respond to a beta-adrenergic antagonist such a propranolol.

Focal myoclonus

There are a number of conditions in which myoclonic jerking is restricted to one part of the body. Such focal myoclonus may be due to discharges occurring anywhere from the cerebral cortex (epilepsia partialis continua), the brainstem (palatal myoclonus), the spinal cord (spinal myoclonus), or even peripheral nerves and roots.

Such focal myoclonus is often repetitive and rhythmic. For example, in the entity of palatal myoclonus there are rhythmic contractions of the soft palate at 60–180/min, persisting throughout the day and night. Sometimes this rhythmic myoclonus spreads to involve the pharynx and larynx, the intercostal muscles and diaphragm, and even the external ocular muscles. The commonest identifiable cause is an infarct involving the brainstem, in particular in the region of the olive, dentate nucleus and red nucleus.

Gilles de la Tourette syndrome

Many children exhibit simple tics transiently during development. Typically these consist of eye blinks, grimaces, a sniff, or a hand gesture. Usually these transient tics of childhood disappear, but sometimes they persist into adult life as chronic simple tics.

In a proportion of patients, these chronic tics are accompanied by vocalization, when the condition is known as Gilles de la Tourette syndrome.

The illness begins between the ages of 5 and 15 years with tics affecting particularly the upper part of the body, especially the face, neck and shoulders. Their severity and distribution tend to wax and wane with time, and one tic may be replaced by another. Sooner or later, such patients begin to make involuntary noises, such as grunting, squealing, yelping, sniffing or barking. In about 60 per cent of cases these noises become transformed into swear words (coprolalia). One third of patients also exhibit obsessive-compulsive rituals.

Formal neurological examination reveals no abnormality, and the intellect is preserved. The illness tends to be life-long, although its severity usually decreases in adulthood. The condition appears to be inherited as an autosomal dominant trait with variable penetrance.

The tics and vocalizations may cause considerable distress to the child or adolescent. Drugs such as haloperidol or pimozide may control the involuntary movements and noises, although the effective dose requires careful and gradual titration in each individual patient.

Torsion dystonia

Torsion dystonia may affect the whole body (generalized dystonia or dystonia musculorum deformans) which typically has an onset in childhood. Alternatively, it may affect only one part of the body (focal dystonia), typically with onset in adult life. Such adult-onset focal dystonias include spasmodic torticollis, writer's cramp, blepharospasm and the related oromandibular dystonia (cranial dystonia).

Torsion dystonia may be due to some identifiable brain disease (secondary or symptomatic dystonia), in which case there are likely to be other signs and symptoms of damage to the nervous system. Alternatively, torsion dystonia may be the only manifestation (primary or idiopathic torsion dystonia). Many patients with primary dystonia give a family history, most commonly suggesting inheritance as an autosomal dominant trait. No consistent pathology has been identified in those with primary torsion dystonia.

Primary generalized dystonia

This illness with onset in childhood usually commences with dystonic spasms of the legs on walking, or sometimes of the arms, trunk or neck. Typically the affected child begins to walk on the toes, or develops a writer's cramp or torticollis. The illness is usually progressive when it commences in childhood. The spasms spread to involve all body parts leading to severe disability within about 10 years. The intellect is preserved and there are no signs of pyramidal or sensory deficit. A spontaneous remission occurs in about one in 20 patients, usually in the first 5 years of the illness. A family history is often evident.

Primary generalized torsion dystonia is distressing and difficult to treat. About 5 per cent of patients respond dramatically to a levodopa preparation (dopa-responsive dystonia). Often these individuals may describe variation in the severity of their dystonia in the course of the day (diurnal dystonia). Typically the child or adolescent is normal in the morning, but develops increasing dystonia as the day wears on which is relieved by sleep.

If the affected individual does not respond to levodopa, the most successful treatment employs high dose anticholinergic therapy, usually in the form of benzhexol. The aim is to start with a low dose and gradually increase to the maximum the patient can tolerate, dictated by side-effects, over a matter of many months. About 50 per cent of patients with primary generalized torsion dystonia may respond to such treatment. Occasionally, stereotactic surgery may be justified in those severely affected. A unilateral thalamotomy may suppress dystonia in the contralateral limbs. However, in those with generalized dystonia, bilateral lesions are required, with a high risk of damage to speech.

Spasmodic torticollis

Isolated spasmodic torticollis usually occurs in the middle-aged or elderly. The onset is insidious often with initial pain, and sometimes precipitated by local injury. The head turns to one side (torticollis), or occasionally extends (retrocollis), or flexes (anticollis). The spasms may be repetitive to cause tremulous torticollis, or sustained to hold the posture fixed.

The illness is usually life-long, but remissions occur in about one-fifth of cases, often transiently. Patients are otherwise normal apart from their torticollis, although some may exhibit a postural tremor similar to that of benign essential tremor.

Drug treatment is often unrewarding, although a minority may respond to an anticholinergic drug. The injection of botulinum toxin into the affected neck muscles may give satisfactory relief, but requires repeating every 2–4 months.

Dystonic writer's cramp

A specific complaint of inability to write (or to type, to play a musical instrument, or to wield any manual instrument) may be due to a variety of causes. These include local joint disease, carpal tunnel syndrome, a spastic or ataxic hand, Parkinson's disease or benign essential tremor. However, there are some patients with such complaints in whom no other neurological deficit can be found. Typically they develop a dystonic posture of the arm when gripping the pen, which is driven into the paper with force. Other manual acts such as wielding a knife or screwdriver may be similarly affected. Isolated dystonic writer's cramp usually appears in middle or late life and does not progress to involve other parts of the body. It occasionally responds to treatment with an anticholinergic drug.

Blepharospasm and oromandibular dystonia (cranial dystonia)

Blepharospasm refers to recurrent spasms of eye closure. The periocular muscles forcibly contract for seconds or minutes, often repetitively, and sometimes so frequently as to render the patient functionally blind. Such eye spasms are commonly precipitated by reading or watching television, or bright lights. Oromandibular dystonia refers to similar recurrent spasms of muscles of the mouth, tongue and jaw. Blepharospasm and oromandibular dystonia commonly coexist. Some patients with cranial dystonia may also exhibit torticollis or writer's cramp. Otherwise the individuals are normal.

Blepharospasm and oromandibular dystonia occasionally respond to treatment with an anticholinergic drug. Botulinum toxin may be injected into the periocular muscles three or four times a year to relieve functional blindness.

Drug-induced movement disorders

The many neuroleptic drugs used to treat psychiatric illness (*see* above under Drug-induced parkinsonism) can cause a wide range of movement disorders.

Acute dystonic reactions

Some 2–5 per cent of those given such drugs may develop acute dystonia within 24–48 h. Typically this consists of spasms of the jaw, mouth and tongue, with torticollis, and sometimes more widespread dystonia affecting the limbs. Such acute dystonic reactions are often accompanied by considerable distress. They can be abolished by the intravenous administration of an anticholinergic drug.

Drug-induced parkinsonism

This appears after some months of neuroleptic therapy, and has been discussed in detail (p. 207).

Akathisia

This refers to a sense of motor restlessness, and the inability to sit still. Such patients are driven to stand up and walk about to gain relief. When sitting, they often exhibit restless movements of the legs and hands in the form of stereotypies. Akathisia is linked to drug-induced parkinsonism and even occurs in Parkinson's disease itself. It may be relieved by a benzodiazepine or propranolol.

Tardive dyskinesias

These are abnormal involuntary movements which appear after many months or years of neuroleptic treatment. The commonest is a choreiform orofacial dyskinesia consisting of repetitive movements of the mouth and tongue. It occurs particularly in the elderly. In younger patients, the abnormal movements of tardive dyskinesia may be dystonic (tardive dystonia). Treatment of tardive dyskinesias is difficult. About 60 per cent will remit if the offending neuroleptic drug can be withdrawn. However, if neuroleptic therapy is required to prevent relapse of schizophrenia, this may be impractical. The orofacial dyskinesias may respond to treatment with tetrabenazine. Tardive dystonias may benefit from treatment with an anticholinergic drug.

10

Dementia

Intellectual decline associated with old age had been recognized from earliest times but it was not until the early nineteenth century that dementia was distinguished from insanity and mental retardation. Increasing clinical skills of physicians in the fields of psychiatry and neurology led to the demonstration of different clinical syndromes, but although syphilis was recognized as a cause, the aetiology of dementia was generally unknown and was usually assumed to be due to chronic underperfusion of the brain. The first attempt at classification, therefore, resulted in the separation into presenile and senile dementia, the two groups being thought to have the same aetiopathogenesis and differing only in the age of onset. For many years a more satisfactory classification failed to emerge. The majority of cases arose in old age and full investigation was costly, not without risk and often inconclusive. In particular, ethical controversy surrounding cerebral biopsies ensured that neuropathological examination was usually undertaken on post-mortem specimens which, since they reflected advanced disease states, were less than ideal. As effective therapy did not exist the need for a more vigorous classification was not clearly recognized. Thus lacking the means of successful research and lying uneasily between the realms of the psychiatrist, geriatrician, physician and neurologist, dementia remained for many years in the backwaters of medical interest.

Within the last 20 years, however, attitudes have changed, induced by a substantial increase in the prevalence of dementia and the availability of new investigative techniques. Improvements in public health and medical care have brought about an explosion in the size of the elderly population. Dementia is predominantly a condition of the elderly, and a fourfold rise in dementia compared with 1950 can be predicted on epidemiological grounds. The consequent impetus given to research has arisen at a time when remarkable advances have been made in neurobiological investigation. Brain imaging has evolved so rapidly that it is now moving away from structural definition to demonstration of function, while the successful identification and replacement of the missing neurotransmitter in Parkinson's disease has raised hopes of a similar neurochemical approach to primary degenerative dementias. Despite these encouraging advances, however, our understanding is handicapped by a lack of knowledge of the natural history of dementia within the population and problems of definition and classification.

Problems of definition and classification

Difficulties arise in constructing a definition which adequately encompasses the different clinical syndromes. Dementia is a socially defined disorder in which diagnosis and management depend on more than medical criteria. The term implies an acquired syndrome of chronic widespread impairment of intellect, behaviour and personality associated with a normal level of consciousness and due to an organic cause. That it is acquired distinguishes it from mental retardation while its persistence and full consciousness exclude a confusional state. It must have an organic cause since psychiatric states can result in pseudo-dementia. Impairment of personality and emotional response are inevitable, indeed may be the predominant clinical feature, but can be trivial initially. Intellectual impairment must involve more than one of the basic faculties of language, memory and perceptuospatial function since patients with focal lesions such as stroke-induced aphasia have otherwise normal cognitive abilities. The rate at which cognitive and emotional responses are generated is as important as their quality and the degree of cognitive deficit must be considered in the context of the patient's background, since cultural factors will determine social competence.

No fully satisfactory definition exists, but for practical purposes it has been suggested that dementia can be considered as an acquired persistent impairment of intellectual function with compromise in at least three of the following aspects of mental activity: language, memory, perceptuospatial skills, emotion, personality and cognition (abstraction, judgement, sequencing and calculation).

The brain is vulnerable not only to intrinsic neuronal disorders but, because of its specialized metabolism and high energy demands, it is susceptible to circulatory and metabolic disturbances. It is not surprising, therefore, that there is a long list of conditions characterized by or associated with dementia, (Table 10.1) and that such a diverse aetiology makes classification on this basis unsatisfactory. However, the older distinction between senile and presenile dementia is misleading, particularly since dementias in the elderly may arise from a number of causes. Moreover, any classification of dementia must take into account the neuropathological relationship between normal ageing and Alzheimer's disease as well as the clinical features of the different dementia types. Normal senescence is accompanied by cortical atrophy which, histologically, is associated with limited development of cortical senile plaques and neurofibrillary tangles confined to the hippocampus. Young patients developing Alzheimer's disease have the same but more extensive changes, particularly affecting the frontal and temporal lobes with abundant tangles present throughout the cortex. Older patients with the clinical syndrome have similar but less marked changes. Thus Alzheimer's disease and senile dementia of the Alzheimer type (SDAT) appear to be similar expressions of a common disorder which may have its origins in the acceleration and distortion of the normal ageing process, becoming apparent when a neuropathological threshold of change is reached. Furthermore it has been suggested that the limited findings in the normal ageing brain represent a subclinical Alzheimer state which may become apparent when another disease process associated with cognitive

Table 10.1 Disorders causing or associated with dementia

---

1. Dementia due to primary neuronal damage (dementia inevitable and progressive)
    *Senile dementia of Alzheimer type (SDAT)
    *Alzheimer's disease
    *Parkinson's disease
    Pick's disease
    Huntington's chorea
    Steele-Richardson syndrome
    Striatonigral degeneration
    Olivo-ponto-cerebellar degeneration
    Subacute sclerosing panencephalitis
    Progressive multifocal leucoencephalopathy
    Creutzfeldt-Jakob disease
2. Dementia secondary to disease process elsewhere (dementia variable and not necessarily progressive)
    Vascular
    *Multi-infarct dementia
    Other dementias associated with cerebral atheroma
    Vasculitides
    Cerebral anoxia
    Trauma
    *Non-penetrating head injuries
    Subdural haematoma
    Structural
    Primary and secondary tumours, e.g. frontal meningioma, corpus callosum glioma, metastases
    Cerebral lymphomas
    Inflammatory
    Multiple sclerosis
    Encephalitides including non-metastatic effects of malignancy
    Syphilis
    AIDS
    Sarcoid
    Whipple's disease
    Metabolic and toxic
    Chronic renal failure
    Portosystemic encephalopathy
    Alcohol
    Wilson's disease
    Heavy metal poisoning
    Endocrine and vitamin deficiencies
    Hypothyroidism
    Cushing's disease
    Addison's disease
    Panhypopituitarism
    B12 deficiency
    Pellagra
    Thiamine deficiency
    Hydrocephalus
    Communicating
    Non-communicating

---

*Common

impairment such as Parkinson's disease or a cerebrovascular accident super-venes. The hypothesis is unproven but provides an attractive explanation for the occurrence of mixed forms of dementia in the elderly.

The recent demonstration of dementias which predominantly involve the subcortical nuclei has led to a classification based on the site of maximum cognitive and anatomical involvement. Cortical dementias such as Alzheimer's disease, SDAT and Pick's disease are marked by focal involvement of temporal, parietal and frontal lobe function. Since the subcortical mechanisms for maintaining concentration are maintained, alertness remains intact and apart from cognitive function there is little involvement of the central nervous system. This contrasts with subcortical dementias where focal deficits such as amnesia or aphasia are less apparent, but there is a global psychomotor retardation with slowing of all aspects of cognition and personality. The subcortical localization of pathology causes widespread neurological dysfunction with prominent disturbance of posture, gait, eye movements and coordination.

There is considerable functional overlap between the cortical and subcortical structures due to the influence of the abundant subcortical projections on the frontal lobes. Separation of dementias into cortical or subcortical categories is therefore incomplete. For instance, Huntington's chorea may present either as a subcortical or frontal dementia, while many disorders such as multiple sclerosis or those due to slow viruses may be widespread throughout the nervous system.

The epidemiology of dementia

Understanding the natural history is necessary in order to plan the allocation of health resources, but problems in diagnosis and classification pose considerable difficulties in surveillance. The world-wide rise in the numbers of elderly is reflected in changes in the population of Britain with OPCS predictions of nine million people over the age of 65, nearly half being 75 or over, by the turn of the century. Since there are no agreed criteria for diagnosis, studies to determine prevalence have given conflicting results, but it is suggested that 1 per cent of the population over 65 will develop dementia, rising to 10 per cent in those over 75 years. When this prediction also takes into consideration those with early onset causes, it is likely that within 15 years there will be half a million patients suffering from dementia in Britain.

The majority of cases of dementia are due either to senile dementia of the Alzheimer's type or multi-infarct dementia (MID), but prevalence of each type is not easy to determine. Surveys suggest that MID may account for up to 40 per cent of cases of elderly dementia, with SDAT and mixed or undifferentiated causes both occurring in 30 per cent; but there is wide variability in these studies and more accurate estimates await improvements in diagnosis.

Age is clearly associated with intellectual impairment but, despite the greater longevity of women, it is unclear whether sex constitutes a risk factor over and above this. Family history of dementia and a previous family history of cerebro-vascular disease, and its precursors such as hypertension or diabetes are causally associated, but studies have not demonstrated a clear association of dementia with social class or geographic location. Risk factors for Alzheimer's disease and SDAT have been subjects of considerable interest. Families have been described in which the disorder is inherited as a Mendelian dominant factor and familial incidence is common.

The assessment of dementia

Investigation aims at determining whether intellectual impairment has an organic or functional basis, demonstration of its clinical and neuropsychological characteristics, and whether it is due to a primary degenerative process or secondary to a structural or multisystem disorder.

History

Intellectual deterioration may present in a variety of ways: as a complaint of impaired performance or personality, in association with neurological or psychiatric symptoms, or as a part of a widespread disease process. Of these, the first is the most common. It is characteristic of this form of presentation that it is described by relatives or friends. Patients who complain that they are dementing are less likely to be than those who do not. Reports of forgetfulness in the house, difficulty in planning complex tasks such as cooking a meal, or impaired work performance are common as are minor changes in personality. Early complaints of language and perceptuospatial dysfunction are unusual, although clumsiness and difficulty in naming common objects (anomia) may be described. A general slowing of intellectual and motor function may be apparent, sometimes misdiagnosed as Parkinson's disease. Similarly, a poor response of personality disturbance to psychiatric treatment may herald the development of Pick's disease. However, it should be appreciated that while dementia can present as psychiatric disturbance the converse is much more common, particularly in the elderly where depression can masquerade as pseudodementia.

The mode of onset and progression is important to the diagnosis. A gradual onset with steady evolution implies degeneration or a structural cause while abrupt onset and stepwise progression suggests a cerebrovascular origin. In the previous history, the occurrence of major or minor head injury, meningitis, exposure to toxins and nutritional changes should be sought, as well as the more commonly occurring conditions such as diabetes, ischaemic heart disease and malignancy. A detailed history of drugs and alcohol consumption should be taken. A family history of mental disturbance, institutionalization or unspecified neurological illness is as important as determining the pedigrees associated with inherited defects such as Wilson's disease or Huntington's chorea, particularly since in the latter, patients and relatives may go to considerable lengths to conceal the truth.

Examination

Examination should attempt to answer three questions.

1. Are the findings outside the nervous system related to the diagnosis?

2. Are there abnormalities in the nervous system apart from dementia?
3. What is the nature of the cognitive impairment?

In the general examination a careful search for endocrine dysfunction, vasculitic disorders, and malignancy should be combined with a clinical assessment of the patient's vascular status. Neurological examination without significant abnormalities suggests a cortical dementia, but many of the diagnostic clues are easy to overlook. Olfactory function may be deficient in frontal lobe syndromes due to head trauma or subfrontal meningioma. Abnormal findings when testing visual fields usually result from impaired concentration but can imply specific parietal or occipital lobe dysfunction. In testing extraocular movements, gaze response to passive head movements as well as to command should be noted, as differential impairment is a feature of early subcortical dysfunction. A pseudobulbar palsy is most common in multi-infarct states, but can occur whenever the brainstem is affected, as in Wilson's disease. In the limbs, upper motor neurone signs predominate, although peripheral neuropathies may complicate commoner causes of dementia like alcoholism, as well as the rare varieties such as metachromatic leucodystrophy. Fasciculation with wasting occasionally occurs in Creutzfeldt-Jakob disease, while asymmetrical long tract signs are suggestive of cerebrovascular disease. Early chorea can be seen when the patient is walking or lying relaxed on the bed, when minor twitches of the fingers and toes become apparent. Observation of gait is one of the more revealing examinations in dementia but the most difficult to quantify. The bent posture and shuffling gait of the parkinsonian patient contrasts with the ramrod stance caused by axial rigidity in progressive supranuclear palsy, or the equine trotting found in striatonigral degeneration. The apraxic gait of communicating hydrocephalus can be almost impossible to describe but the description 'feet glued to the floor' is as good as any.

Evaluation of cognitive function

Even a brief review of current literature on dementia reveals a wealth of schemes designed to evaluate intellectual impairment. This variety suggests the importance of measurement of cognition and the impossibility of fulfilling all the requirements of neuropsychological testing with one approach. At one end of the spectrum, simple reproducible formats such as the Mini-Mental State Evaluation provide a screen for cognitive impairment (*see* p. 64) and such tests, particularly when used with a standardized assessment of daily living, provide a measure of the practical problems. However, they cannot detect minor impairment nor exclude delirium and affective disorders. At the other end of the neuropsychological spectrum it has become increasingly apparent that, in skilful hands, full assessment of cognitive function surpasses most commonly available neuroradiological procedures as a diagnostic tool. Measurement is time consuming and may require the expertise of a clinical psychologist if the results are to be interpreted correctly.

Investigation of dementia

Clinical assessment of the dementing patient is diagnostically far more useful than an unconsidered battery of tests. Investigations are resource dependent. To achieve a balance between benefit and cost, testing should only include procedures which are clinically indicated and those screening tests which are justifiable on the grounds that the condition sought is a real diagnostic possibility and could be otherwise overlooked. Over 75 per cent of elderly demented patients will have either SDAT or MID but the diagnostic possibilities in younger onset dementia are more varied and are, as a general rule, likely to require more extensive investigation. A list of justifiable screening tests is given in Table 10.2.

Table 10.2   Routine screening tests in dementia

Full blood count and ESR
Urinalysis
Biochemical profile: urea, calcium, liver function
Serum B12
Thyroid function (TSH)
Wasserman reaction, *Treponema pallidum* haemagglutination, etc
Chest X-ray
Other tests may be indicated
  Psychometry
  CT brain scan
  EEG
  ECG

A raised erythrocyte sedimentation rate (ESR) may imply an underlying malignancy or vasculitic disorder, including giant cell arteritis, causing intellectual impairment but sparing the superficial temporal arteries. Anaemia may imply poor nutrition. A normal mean corpuscular volume (MCV) cannot exclude B12 deficiency but a low folate, like other vitamin deficiencies, is more likely to be a consequence than a cause of dementia and should be sought only if there is a history of nutritional disturbance. Two per cent of demented patients have abnormal thyroid function tests and although 'myxoedema madness' is rare it should be excluded. Abnormalities in the biochemical profile may suggest a metabolic cause. Hepatic or renal failure may be obvious clinically, but disorders of calcium metabolism or ADH secretion may only come to light this way. Syphilis, although uncommon, is increasing and is so protean in its manifestations that serology should be included in the assessment. Tests for more complex inflammatory, endocrine or metabolic causes of dementia should be undertaken only where clinically indicated.

Lumbar puncture cannot be regarded as an automatic investigation. It is non-contributory in the commonest forms of dementia and may cause coning in the presence of a space-occupying lesion, or subdural haematoma. However, in global dementia an elevated CSF protein or pleocytosis may be the only available evidence of organic dysfunction.

Because of the limitations of early neuroradiology, electroencephalography was regarded as an essential tool. However, in most dementias the findings are non-specific, while the ability to locate structural lesions has been superseded by computerized tomography (CT) scanning. In certain circumstances the EEG can be very revealing, as in subclinical epilepsy which may be severe enough to cause intellectual failure. Severity of abnormalities correlates well with the degree of dementia and serial tracings have, therefore, a predictive value. Loss of normal rhythms with diffuse slowing indicate a widespread or metabolic cause while in unusual dementias such as those due to cerebral lymphomas focal slow and sharp waves may precede structural changes.

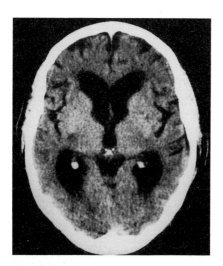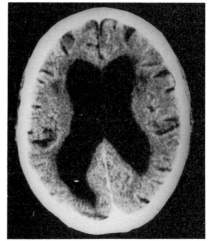

Fig. 10.1. (a) and (b). CT scan showing cerebral atrophy. The ventricles are enlarged, the cisterns and surface sulci widened

Imaging techniques

The value of a simple skull X-ray in the demonstration of raised intracranial pressure or ectopic calcification has become neglected in the enthusiasm for more sophisticated neuroradiology. CT scanning and more recently with a different technique, magnetic resonance imaging (MRI) both provide a detailed picture of intracranial neuroanatomy. However, it should be appreciated that although cerebral atrophy can be convincingly displayed (Fig. 10.1), this does not correlate with intellectual function and cannot be used by itself as evidence of primary cortical degeneration. Both methods are more diagnostically useful in the assessment of structural disturbance such as tumours (Fig. 10.2), or the development of hydrocephalus (Fig. 10.3). In dementia due to cerebrovascular disease multiple infarcts may be seen (Fig. 10.4), although lacunar strokes may not be visible even on high resolution CT scans.

The measurement of cerebral blood flow by inhalation of radioactive tracers and cerebral angiography have only a strictly limited role in investigation of

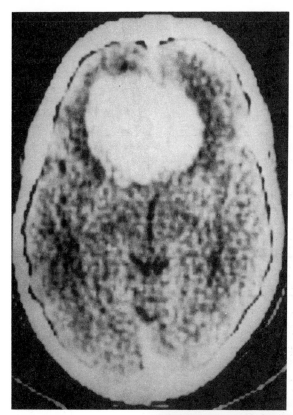

Fig. 10.2. CT scan showing a very large frontal meningioma. The patient gave an 18-month history of irrational behaviour and incontinence

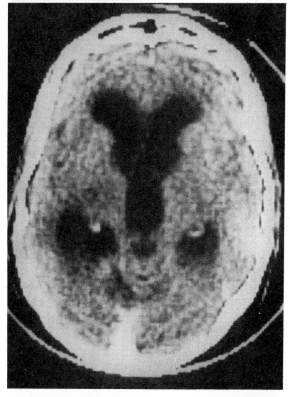

Fig. 10.3. CT scan showing hydrocephalus with enlargement of the lateral and third ventricles from obstruction of the aqueduct

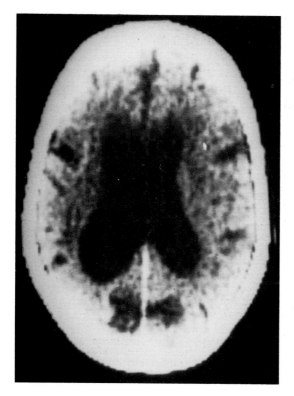

Fig. 10.4.   CT scan showing multi-infarct damage. Note the low density patches in the occipital lobes and the enlarged ventricles

dementia, but they do represent a shift from simple demonstration of structure to evaluation of function. The importance of this approach is demonstrated by positron emission tomography in which positron emitting ions are tagged to cerebral metabolic analogues to measure cerebral blood flow, the ability of tissue to extract oxygen and glucose metabolism. Using this technique regional deficiencies can be demonstrated in a number of conditions. This complex investigation is confined to a few centres. Although image definition is less precise than CT or MRI scanning, this technique represents an exciting advance in the measurement of cerebral function. Simple radionuclide scans have always had a place in the assessment of CSF dynamics in hydrocephalus, but only recently have improvements in image resolution enabled regional cerebral perfusion to be assessed using single photon emission tomography (SPET). Focal deficits are demonstrable in cortical and subcortical dementias (Fig. 10.5), and can be shown to correlate well with patterns of cognitive impairment.

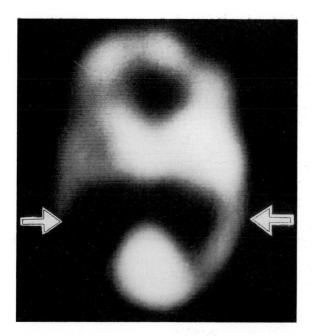

Fig. 10.5. The SPET scan is obtained by injecting a radioisotope tracer which delineates cerebral perfusion. The marked decrease in concentration in the parietal regions, especially on the left (arrowed), is characteristic of Alzheimer's disease. (Picture courtesy of Dr Testa, Manchester Royal Infirmary)

Types of dementia

The cortical degenerative dementias

Alzheimer's disease

Since its description in 1907, Alzheimer's disease has become recognized as the most typical of the primary degenerative dementias. The selective involvement of the cortex with the brunt falling on the junction of the temporal, parietal and occipital lobes with sparing of the motor and somatosensory cortex as well as most of the frontal and occipital lobes gives rise to a characteristic clinical pattern which can be divided into three stages. The first phase lasting between one and 3 years is marked by progressive loss of memory and topographical sense with relative preservation of speech, minor personality changes and normal locomotor function. Household tasks become more difficult and are exacerbated by the increasing difficulty in spatial orientation so that the patient becomes lost in unfamiliar, then familiar surroundings and exhibits impairment of constructional skills. Vocabulary is restricted but language is otherwise normal early on.

As the disease progresses the features of the second stage become more apparent. Memory impairment increases with severe disorientation so that the patient is lost in time and space. Speech becomes empty (fluent aphasia) and although elementary motor skills and coordination are preserved even simple constructional skills decline. Insight is lost being replaced by indifference and irritability. Although in younger patients the final phase may be reached within 3 or 4 years of onset, up to double this is more usual. This stage is marked by almost complete loss of intellectual function with incontinence and emergence of primitive reflexes and severe motor disabilities with spasticity developing terminally.

There is no clear clinical cut-off between the early and late presentation of Alzheimer's disease, but the distinction between the two forms is sufficient for presentation after 65 to be identified as senile dementia of the Alzheimer type or SDAT. This presentation is more common, and has a female preponderance with longer life span, while speech disorders and early spatial disorientation are less marked than in younger patients.

Neurochemically, both types show a loss of neurotransmitters, particularly in the presynaptic cholinergic system with reduction of acetylcholine, choline acetyltransferase and acetylcholine esterase. Loss of these enzymes is more pronounced in early onset cases. Identification of this deficit has prompted attempts at treatment with acetylcholine precursors such as choline and lecithin or physostigmine, but so far none has demonstrated a satisfactory response and at present treatment is supportive. The aetiology is unclear with aluminium and viruses both proposed as causes. The association with Down's syndrome, chromosome aneuploidy and lymphoproliferative disease has suggested that microtubular dysfunction may play a part in the pathogenesis. Recent work has suggested that the gene conferring susceptibility in familial Alzheimer's disease is mapped to chromosome 21 as well as to a region responsible for the cerebral beta amyloid protein found in both elderly Down's patients and Alzheimer's disease.

Pick's disease

Pick's disease, the other major primary cortical dementia, is 15 times less common than Alzheimer's disease and SDAT. Cortical atrophy is confined to the frontal and temporal lobes and while the age of onset and duration are similar to Alzheimer's disease, this distribution results in a different clinical picture. Disturbance of judgement and personality are prominent early features with antisocial behaviour and emotional blunting sometimes becoming sufficiently pronounced to resemble the Kluver-Bucy syndrome (loss of emotional response, altered sexual activity, bulimia and apparent visual and sensory agnosia). Memory, mathematical abilities and parietal function are otherwise relatively preserved but speech deteriorates with circumlocution, vocabulary restriction and other features of empty speech, progressing to mutism with widespread pyramidal signs. As in the other cortical dementias laboratory investigations are non-contributory. Neuropathological examination reveals frontal and or temporal atrophy within the microscopic features of Alzheimer's disease, although 60 per cent show enlarged disorganized cells, 'inflated neurones', and in about 30 per cent characteristic dense structures known as Pick's bodies are found within the neuronal cytoplasm of the affected cortex.

Dementia due to cerebrovascular disease

Cerebrovascular disease is well recognized as a cause of intellectual failure usually by causing neuronal loss from infarction. This may arise from embolic or thrombo-occlusive events, but although dementia may complicate most diseases states characerized by cerebrovascular involvement, the major causes are cerebral atheroma and hypertension. However derived, the effects of infarction depend on size, location and number. Cerebral infarcts over 100 ml in size may be associated with dementia, and although smaller single lesions do not cause widespread cognitive deficit, a strategically placed lesion affecting the dominant angular gyrus may simulate Alzheimer's disease demonstrating the importance of location. Intellectual function is more susceptible to multiple minor vascular insults causing multi-infarct dementia (MID). The type of dementia depends on the location of the damage. Multiple cortical infarcts cause defects of cortical function but, unlike Alzheimer's disease, the motor strip and visual pathways are vulnerable with resulting long tract signs and visual field loss. Such changes can be seen on CT scan but in vascular disease, particularly associated with hypertension, subcortical infarcts known as lacunes may occur which are too small, 2–15 mm, to be detected. Lacunar predilection for the basal ganglia and upper pons results in a subcortical picture with slowing, dysarthria, clumsiness, gait disturbance (*marche à petit pas*) and extra-pyramidal features.

In most cases features of cortical and subcortical involvement are apparent and both types are characterized by abrupt onset, stepwise deterioration and fluctuating course. These features form the basis of the Hachinski ischaemic score which can be used to identify a vascular origin in some cases of dementia. Such identification is valuable since, although there is little justification for the use of cerebrovasodilators, the control of blood pressure, and other treatable risk factors for cerebrovascular disease, with the use of low dose aspirin would be expected to be as useful in MID as in other forms of stroke.

Dementia due to trauma and structural lesions

Head injury

Cognitive dysfunction following trauma while not uncommon is often neglected as a cause of dementia. It is a frequent cause of severe intellectual impairment with a UK incidence of 1600 cases per annum usually resulting from road traffic accidents. Most commonly a non-penetrating injury causes multiple contusions and shearing lesions of the white matter, the frontal and temporal poles being particularly at risk. The length of retrograde amnesia, the extinction of memories prior to injury and post-traumatic amnesia, the inability to lay down new information subsequently, indicates its extent. The vulnerability of the frontal lobes is reflected in the frequency of personality change due to the development of the frontal lobe syndrome. This is marked by increased rigidity in thinking, reduction in powers of concentration, abstraction, planning and problem solving with loss of fluency and an inability to change rapidly from one task to another. This is associated with emotional blunting, loss of insight and facile or apathetic mood. Such disturbance may be difficult to quantify, particularly in previous 'high flyers' and may not be easy to separate from secondary affective responses caused by insight into the consequences of the injury.

Although dementia usually results from a single episode, recurrent trauma, as in boxing, results in a characteristic picture (dementia pugilistica) of progressive ataxia, dementia, extrapyramidal features, dysarthria and personality impairment.

Structural causes

Surveys have suggested that in between 5 and 10 per cent of patients with dementia this may be due to intracranial neoplasms. Impairment of cognition may result from focal compression or infiltration, oedema or impairment of CSF circulation causing hydrocephalus. Development may be very slow as with a subfrontal meningioma, but is usually less than 12 months in duration. Tumours causing lateralizing deficits are normally easy to identify, but those in unusual sites such as the corpus callosum may present with mental change only.

Subdural haematomas have such varied presentations that they may mimic other causes of dementia even causing a metabolic encephalopathy due to inappropriate ADH secretion. They are most commonly seen in the elderly and investigation is sometimes misleading. Suspicion of a subdural haematoma should always be aroused by fluctuations in cognitive and neurological findings (*see* p. 287).

Subcortical dementias

The principal cognitive features of subcortical dementia, forgetfulness, slowness of thought, depression or apathy and impairment of the ability to manipulate acquired knowledge, were first identified in the intellectual decline associated with progressive supranuclear palsy, an uncommon condition with progressive axial rigidity, pseudobulbar palsy and supranuclear gaze paresis. Subsequently this pattern of coigntive deficit was recognized in other conditions marked by extrapyramidal phenomena including Parkinson's disease, Huntington's chorea, some multi-infarct states and Wilson's disease. However, although the concept of subcortical dementia is a useful advance in categorization, it is far from fully developed. The extent and type of dementia in Parkinson's disease is debatable since with such a common disorder co-existing Alzheimer's disease may complicate assessment while the influences of the subcortical nuclei on the frontal lobes is far from clear. This is well illustrated in Huntington's chorea (*see* p. 217).

Dementia due to infectious and inflammatory causes

Infectious causes

Infections cause relatively few cases of dementia but are important because some cases are responsive to treatment. The brain may be affected in a number of ways. Dementia may arise from the development of a chronic meningitis with secondary damage to the brain often associated with impaired immunity. *Cryptococcus neoformans* is the most common infection, but *Candida, Aspergillus,* toxoplasmosis and *Plasmodium falciparum* malaria have all been implicated. Some causative agents cause a more extensive meningovascular response such as tuberculous meningitis, while others additionally involve the brain parenchyma, e.g. Whipple's disease which causes a chronic meningoencephalitis. These conditions evoke an inflammatory response which may also cause cerebral infarction or hydrocephalus from thickened basal meninges. Syphilis may cause dementia through any of these mechanisms as well as rarely from the mass effect of a gumma (*see* p. 341).

In contrast in subacute sclerosing panencephalitis (SSPE) the parenchyma of the brain is damaged by a chronic reaction to measles virus in children. The progress from behavioural changes through intellectual deterioration and widespread neurological changes with prominent myoclonus to death, may occur within months. Direct destruction of the grey and white matter without an inflammatory response may also cause dementia. In *Creutzfeldt-Jakob disease,* a spongiform encephalopathy due to a transmissible agent, there is a brisk evolution from a stage of non-specific confusion with unsteadiness to the development of frank widespread neurological abnormalities terminating in a vegetative state. This is normally fatal within 12 months; in some patients more rapid progression over a number of weeks may occur. Although there may be a variety of extrapyramidal and long tract signs, diagnostically the presence of startle myoclonus is the most useful sign, while typical EEG findings occur ultimately in 75 per cent of patients (Fig. 10.6). The disorder is rare, 121 cases being confirmed in the UK between 1970 and 1979, and is unresponsive to

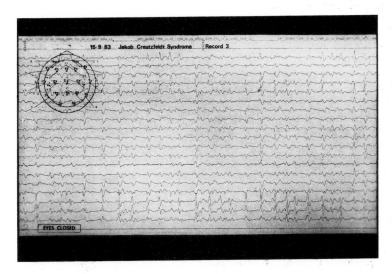

Fig. 10.6. The characteristic changes of periodic synchronous sharp waves superimposed on an isoelectric background are seen in this tracing from a patient with Creutzfeldt-Jakob syndrome. A few weeks earlier the EEG only showed non-specific slowing

treatment. Clinically it resembles kuru, a dementia said to be associated with cannabalism in New Guinea and has affinities with degenerative conditions in animals caused by slow viruses. Increasing interest has been aroused by the demonstration of transmission to primates, and this has been supported by examples of accidental surgical transmission in man.

Progressive multifocal leucoencephalopathy is due to viral infection of the brain. The causative agent is a papova virus which in the presence of chronic disturbed immunity causes widespread progressive cortical and subcortical neurological and cognitive abnormalities. Visual disturbance due to occipital involvement is more evident than in other dementias. Antiviral treatment is unconvincing and death can be expected within a year.

Human immunodeficiency virus (HIV) may cause brain disorder through a variety of mechanisms. Dementia is common in AIDS (greater than 65 per cent) and may precede other manifestations. It may result from direct infiltration of the brain with HIV, giving a mixed cognitive picture which proceeds to tetraplegia, mutism and death and in one-fifth of patients it may be rapidly progressive. Where immunodeficiency is established, dementia may be secondary to chronic infection with a variety of opportunistic infections. (*see* p. 337).

Inflammatory and granulomatous conditions without an infective cause may also result in dementia. Mood disturbance is common in multiple sclerosis and although euphoria is rarer than described, it suggests widespread frontal demyelination, the extent of the cognitive impairment reflecting the underlying severity of the disease. Rarely malignancies, particularly oat-cell carcinoma of the lung may be associated with a paraneoplastic inflammatory process (limbic encephalitis) without obvious cause. Vascular disorders such as Behçet's disease and systemic lupus erythematosus cause neuronal damage secondary to microcirculatory impairment, while granulomatous disorders, notably sarcoid, can affect cerebral function through the development of basal meningitis or strategically placed granulomas, especially in the hypothalamus.

Metabolic, nutritional and toxic causes

Chronic disturbance of electrolyte balance, particularly hyponatraemia from any cause may disturb brain activity through the development of cerebral oedema while cognitive function is sensitive to the accumulation of toxic metabolites in chronic renal failure and portosystemic encephalopathy. These conditions are marked not only by neuropsychiatric disturbance but also a variety of movement disorders such as myoclonus and asterixis. Constructional apraxia is said to be specifically disturbed in hepatic failure but probably reflects overall cortical deterioration rather than a specific parietal dysfunction. Uraemic encephalopathy should be distinguished from dialysis dementia which occasionally occurs after several years treatment of any form of renal failure with haemodialysis (*see* p. 418). It causes a distinctive picture of personality disturbance and prominent disturbance of articulation and language formation, myoclonus, epilepsy, incoordination and a characteristic EEG. The cause is unknown, although aluminium deposition has been suggested and improvement only rarely follows transplantation.

Endocrine dysfunction

Thyrotoxicosis may cause behavioural disturbance resembling an anxiety state but may present in the elderly as an apathetic form with widespread psychomotor slowing, while 5 per cent of hypothyroid patients also have non-specific slowing of cognition and lethargy. Similar patterns of dysfunction may complicate Cushing's disease, and hypopituitarism from any cause. The means is unknown but probably reflects electrolyte disturbance. Hypercalcaemia may result in reversible neuropsychiatric disturbance while hypocalcaemia when associated with basal ganglia calcification in hypoparathyroidism is sometimes associated with subcortical dementia having extrapyramidal features.

Vitamin deficiencies

Thiamine deficency causes a specific type of amnesia rather than dementia, and while neuropsychiatric disturbance may follow B12 deficiency this is very much rarer than subacute combined degeneration of the cord. The dementia of pellagra, niacin deficiency, is more conspicuous with pathological changes in the Betz cells and brainstem nuclei giving rise to extrapyramidal rigidity and primitive reflexes as well as cognitive dysfunction.

Toxic causes

A variety of therapeutic agents have been implicated in dementia. Immuno-suppressants permit the development of opportunistic CNS infections while most drugs are toxic in excess. Some may exacerbate an underlying dementia process, particularly hypotensives, tranquillizers and antiparkinsonian therapy. Anticholinergics and industrial organophosphates may affect CNS neurotransmission. A number of drugs cause inappropriate ADH secretion while some anticonvulsants, especially phenytoin and barbiturate, in long-term high dosage can cause intellectual impairment which may not be reversible.

Alcohol abuse causes intellectual deterioration in several ways and is an appreciable cause of dementia, a mild to moderate frontal lobe syndrome being the commonest form of encephalopathy (*see* p. 410). Alcohol in rare instances may cause subacute demyelination in the corpus callosum (Marchiafava Bignami disease). More commonly it results in dementia indirectly through dietary deficiency, cerebral trauma and increased incidence of infection. Heavy metal poisoning although rare, causes intellectual deterioration. The effect of chronic inhalation of lead on intelligence in children is currently a matter of concern and 'hatter's shakes' and 'mad as a hatter' describe the mental disturbance, ataxia and restlessness found in workers who dressed hats with mercury. Contaminated seafood and mercury treated seed corn have more recently been reported as sources of dementia.

Miscellaneous conditions

There is a large number of inherited disorders sometimes with a demonstrable biochemical or enzyme defect which affect the brain often as part of a multi-system disorder. For instance porphyria and homocystinuria may be associated with variable intellectual deficits, while storage diseases such as metachromatic leucodystrophy result in a progressive picture of dementia and neurological abnormality. Pathologically the white matter is particularly vulnerable to abnormal lipid deposition. Mild diffuse intellectual impairment often accompanies the muscular dystrophies and spinocerebellar degenerations and may be pronounced in dystrophia myotonica. The association of dementia with epilepsy is varied. In some conditions such as Unverricht's disease (progressive myoclonic epilepsy) dementia is an essential part of the syndrome while in symptomatic epilepsies it may be an epiphenomenon. In severe chronic epilepsy, dementia may arise through repeated anoxic or traumatic insults, although the effects of long-term anticonvulsants are a far more common cause of intellectual deterioration.

Hydrocephalus

Hydrocephalus (*see* p. 295), whether communicating or non-communicating, can cause dementia. The typical picture is of a progressive disturbance of gait, incontinence and cognitive changes.

Management of dementia

In some 15 per cent of patients with dementia there may be a treatable cause, e.g. B12 deficiency, benign cerebral tumour, but in the majority there is no obvious cause and the process will progress. Such patients remain severe management problems for their families and medical attendants.

Ideally patients are best kept in familiar surroundings with support, if necessary, from attendance at day centres or from home visits by health visitors and nurses. Further help at home may be provided by the local Social Services, e.g. meals on wheels, home helps, incontinence laundry service. Attention to correctable deficits may give further aid, e.g. hearing aids, correct spectacles. It is important to discuss the likely outcome with the family to help them plan the future. As the patient's condition deteriorates an increasing number will be admitted to psychogeriatric wards or long-stay units.

Demented patients are particularly prone to develop acute toxic confusional states. These may be precipitated by an intercurrent infection, e.g. chest, urine, by heart failure or a stroke, by the medicines they take (often polypharmacy), or by trauma, e.g. after a fall. The cause of such deterioration should be elicited by careful inquiries and some tests. These should include:

1. Inquiry about all medication, and any history of alcohol abuse.
2. Details about hydration and nutrition.
3. Urine analysis and culture.
4. Blood tests for a full blood count, ESR, urea and electrolytes, glucose, liver function tests and, if not already checked, thyroid function, B12 level and Wasserman reaction or *Treponema pallidum* haemagglutination.
5. Chest X-ray.
6. Severely ill patients may need admission to hospital and if febrile may require blood cultures and even CSF examination.

Acute confusion may need sedation. The smallest effective dose should be used. Phenothiazines, e.g. promazine 25–50 mg or thioridazine 25–50 mg b.d. or t.i.d., may be useful. In very disturbed patients injections of haloperidol 2.5–5 mg intramuscularly can be given, increasing the dose until the desired clinical effect is reached.

In any demented patient where depression may be present, a trial of anti-depressant treatment is always justified.

As yet there is no effective therapy for the majority of dementia syndromes and management problems brought about by rising numbers are becoming increasingly acute as attitudes in society evolve. Traditionally the extended family provided support for the aged, but although 60 per cent of the demented elderly remain at home, changes in family structure mean that domestic care has become more problematical.

Permanent institutional care remains a last resort, and the majority of patients will continue to be managed at home. The family burden that this entails is considerable, and recognition of this specialized form of support has evolved within the NHS and Social Services (Fig. 10.7), with the formation of multidisciplinary teams and the development of psychogeriatrics as a speciality. The extent of this support varies throughout the country, and even under optimum conditions still demands a substantial family commitment. Never-theless, the contribution made by Social Services, sedation for restlessness, adaption of the house to safeguard the patient, and most importantly the provi-sion of regular breaks in caring, makes the difference between coping at home and institutional care. There are substantial economic consequences arising from this support. Identification of the proportion of the DHSS budget spent on the elderly demented is inadequate, but it has been assumed that at least one-quarter of resources devoted to the elderly are associated with dementia, consumption increasing with age.

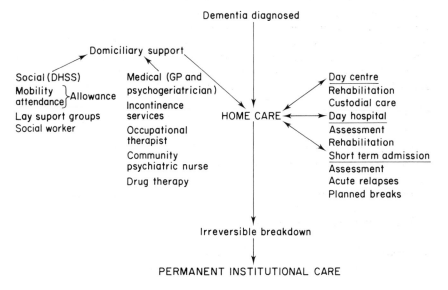

Fig. 10.7. Practical management of dementia

11

Epilepsy and sleep disorders

Epilepsy

Epilepsy is not a disease: it is a symptom of which the patient may or may not complain. The manifestations are protean and the consequences may vary from very little or no problem to major social, psychological and physical disability. This is what makes management so difficult: a firm statement that a patient suffers from epileptic attacks inevitably carries with it certain legal restrictions with regard to driving, and other restrictions about work which are often due to ignorance or prejudice.

Classical grand mal generalized tonic-clonic seizures are the best known manifestation of epilepsy, the 'falling sickness' of antiquity. However, there are many varieties of epilepsy which produce merely a transitory alteration in awareness of an aspect of the internal or external environment with little or no loss of control. Yet other forms exist which occur only in response to specific stimuli, flicker is the commonest; but reading, loud noises, immersion in water, or even listening to a particular verse of one 'pop song' have all been reported to trigger attacks. Patients find it hard to accept that these forms of attack, which cause them little or no disability, should carry the same legal and employment restrictions as major seizure disorders.

Even after many years of research it is still very difficult to define the underlying pathophysiological mechanisms of an epileptic attack. We know that in animals experimental seizures can produce an increase in cerebral metabolic rate two to three times above normal. Cerebral blood flow rises and with it glucose and oxygen utilization. If the seizure is prolonged, the demand may outstrip the supply so that large reductions in cerebral glucose and accumulations of lactate and cyclic nucleotides occur, together with an inhibition of regional protein synthesis. The exact trigger which starts an attack remains elusive. Genetic predisposition at least plays a part; in those with primary generalized seizures the convulsive threshold is lowered so that attacks occur more easily in response to a given stimulus. Ounsted (1971) has suggested that it is unnecessary to think of epilepsy in terms of pathology, and it is more useful to see it as part of a spectrum of paroxysmal behaviour to which man is prone. A sneeze for example has a prodrome, a phase of involuntary muscular activity, and a recovery phase; so do hiccups, yawns, coughs, certain forms of laughing, even orgasms. Some paroxysmal behaviour may in certain circumstances be dangerous, e.g. repetitive sneezing or epileptic attacks when driving, and some may not. Some, like coughing and sneezing, are socially acceptable in public: others, like yawning, orgasms, and epilepsy are not.

Incidence of epilepsy: the scale of the problem

Because of problems with classification and diagnosis, incidence and prevalence figures vary widely. Studies based on hospital series inevitably ignore the fact that not all patients with epilepsy attend hospital. Studies based on general practice cannot include those individuals who never consult a doctor at all. In most studies (excluding febrile convulsions) incidence figures for new cases of established epilepsy are about 50/100 000 per year; for single seizures they are about 20/100 000 per year. The prevalence of epilepsy is about 5/1000, and the life-time prevalence, i.e. the prevalence of established cases plus cases of single seizures is 20/1000. From the above figures it must be clear that in most individuals the tendency to have seizures remits.

Classification

No classification of seizures can be entirely satisfactory because of the infinite variety of clinical manifestations and causes. A seizure may arise for no known reason or it may be symptomatic of an underlying metabolic or structural abnormality, e.g. hypoglycaemia, cerebral anoxia, brain infection or neoplasm. Table 11.1 gives a simplified version of Chadwick's summary of the 1981 International classification of seizures (excluding infantile and childhood epilepsies). This classification is descriptive and takes little account of possible underlying pathology.

The manifestations of *simple partial seizures* depend on the area of the brain from which they arise. If their origin is in the motor strip the classical jacksonian march occurs: e.g. rhythmic twitching of the foot spreading to involve the leg and then even the arm; often this is followed by a period of weakness (Todd's paralysis) which may last for several hours and may be mistaken for a stroke unless the initial history of clonic movements is obtained. If seizures arise in the sensory cortex, transient brief paraesthesiae of sudden onset and lasting minutes may occur; these are easily mistaken for transient ischaemic attacks (which tend to last rather longer). With an origin in the temporal lobe various psychic or autonomic symptoms occur, feelings of extreme fear, usually arising in the stomach; illusions of intense familiarity with a strange environment (dèjà vu); and hallucinations (those of taste and smell are the commonest). If awareness is lost the seizure becomes a *complex partial seizure*. During this phase bizarre complex acts occur like taking things out of a purse, dancing, walking round and picking up objects aimlessly, or uttering meaningless and sometimes obscene words or phrases. Frequently, if such a seizure is observed in the initial phases, the patients smack their lips and make swallowing movements as if tasting someting. In adults, partial seizures, particularly of the jacksonian or sensory type, are often indicative of underlying structural brain disease and always need further investigation if the cause is not immediately clear.

Table 11.1   Classification of seizures

1. *Partial seizures beginning locally*
    (a) Simple (consciousness not impaired)
        i)   With motor symptoms
        ii) With somatosensory or special sensory symptoms
        iii) With autonomic symptoms
        iv) With psychic symptoms
    (b) Complex (consciousness impaired)
        i) Beginning as a simple partial seizure (and progressing to loss of consciousness)
        ii) Impairment of consciousness only, with or without automatism
    (c) Partial seizures becoming generalized
2. *Generalized seizures*
    (a) Absence
        i) Simple (petit mal)
        ii) Complex
    (b) Myoclonic
    (c) Clonic
    (d) Tonic
    (e) Tonic-clonic (grand mal)
    (f) Atonic
3. *Adolescent epilepsies*
    (a) Early morning myoclonus associated with tonic-clonic seizures
    (b) Myoclonus plus simple absence
4. *Progressive myoclonic epilepsies* (due to inherited metabolic disorders, or other, often genetic, syndromes)

The two classic forms of generalized seizure are the simple absence (petit mal) and the generalized tonic-clonic seizure (grand mal).

Simple absences occur in childhood and adolescence and by adulthood have disappeared in 80 per cent of cases, or have been replaced by generalized tonic-clonic seizures. They do *not* occur de novo in adults. In an attack, the child or teenager abruptly ceases what he is doing as if frozen; the eyes stare straight ahead and the upper eyelids on occasions flicker slightly. A few seconds later normal behaviour returns. Frequent attacks can cause learning difficulties at school because of gaps in attention. Attacks can often be provoked by getting the patient to hyperventilate for one to two minutes. As a corollary, such attacks sometimes present as loss of consciousness after exercise because of the hyperventilation this entails.

Generalized tonic-clonic seizures usually occur without warning although in some patients brief myoclonic jerks herald the loss of consciousness. The patient may give a cry and then fall to the floor like a felled tree. A tonic phase then occurs when rigidity and cyanosis are followed by generalized clonic twitching of all four limbs, usually for one to 10 min. Patients are then unrousable for a brief period after which responses return but in a confused fashion. The final phase is of deep sleep from which patients wake, usually with a bitten tongue, aching muscles and frequently headache. Single or double incontinence sometimes accompanies attacks.

In teenagers there is a syndrome, which on occasions persists into early adulthood, of morning myoclonus associated with tonic-clonic seizures. Attacks usually occur after a late night. The patient will rise at the normal time, perhaps getting up more quickly than usual having overslept, and while dressing or making breakfast he is overcome by uncontrollable jerks which may proceed to a generalized convulsion.

A proportion of teenagers and children may have generalized seizures of the absence, tonic-clonic, or myoclonic variety in response to specific stimuli; flicker from television sets or computer games is the commonest. Children may find the experience pleasurable and be driven to induce an attack by putting their faces to the television screen, staring at patterns or passing hands with outstretched fingers back and forth across their faces while staring at the light. Reflex complex partial seizures are much rarer but have been reported.

Diagnosis

The only way to diagnose an epileptic attack with any degree of certainty is on the history from the patient, and an account from a witness. There are no short cuts.

Particular questions to be asked of the patients are:

1. The circumstances of the attack – what they were doing, where they were, the time of day, and what exactly are their memories prior to loss of awareness.
2. Immediate memories after return of consciousness.
3. Whether injury or incontinence occurred.

This information should then be correlated and corroborated if possible with an account from a witness who can tell of events during the period of loss of

Table 11.2 Clinical diagnosis of epilepsy

1. *History*
   (1) Details of event from patient and if possible from a witness
   (2) Birth details
   (3) Febrile or teething convulsions?
   (4) Blackouts as a child?
   (5) Previous head injury: duration of loss of consciousness, any post-traumatic seizures
   (6) Previous intracranial infection?
   (7) Family history: epilepsy or any neurological disease
   (8) Alcohol or drugs?
2. *Examination*
   (1) Skin: signs of neurofibromatosis, tuberous sclerosis
   (2) BP: standing and lying. Any evidence of postural drop?
   (3) Pulse: if irregular consider emboli
   (4) Heart sounds: emboli, valvular disease, atrial myxoma (rare)
   (5) Liver and spleen: alcohol, glycogen storage, lymphoma
   (6) Limb asymmetry: underdevelopment of one side suggests a long-standing fault, ?hemiatrophy
   (7) Cranial bruits: AVM if young, atheroma if elderly
   (8) Sense of smell: subfrontal meningioma
   (9) Optic discs: papilloedema due to intracranial mass
   (10) Visual fields: intracerebral lesion
   (11) Limb weakness: intracerebral lesion
   (12) Reflex asymmetry: intracerebral lesion
   (13) Plantar responses: intracerebral lesion

awareness. Details of past and family history should be sought, with particular reference to birth, febrile or teething convulsions, previous intracranial infections or head injuries, epilepsy or neurological disease in relatives. The possibility of excess alcohol consumption and/or drugs as a precipitating cause should also be explored. A scheme for history and physical examination is set out in Table 11.2.

It cannot be emphasized enough that a diagnosis of epilepsy (or an epileptic attack) made on inadequate grounds may do a patient a great disservice. If the diagnosis is wrong, the long-term consequences in terms of job prospects and lifestyle can be very serious. Remember that an isolated epileptic attack does *not* constitute a diagnosis of 'epilepsy'. A diagnosis of epilepsy can only be made when more than one attack has occurred, or where, taking into account the type of the attack, the family history, and the underlying cause of the attack (if known) there is a significant risk that further attacks will occur.

Differential diagnosis

A list of differential diagnoses for attacks of loss of consciousness and 'funny turns' is set out in Table 11.3.

Metabolic causes of loss of awareness tend to have a much longer warning, although this is not invariable. For example a man with a previous history of

Table 11.3   Causes of transient loss of consciousness and 'funny turns'

1. *Neurological*
   (a) Epilepsy: all types
   (b) Vertigo: note may rarely be the aura of an epileptic fit
   (c) Other causes of paroxysmal behaviour, e.g. paroxysmal dystonia, kinesiogenic spasm (rare)
   (d) Mechanical: intermittent obstructive hydrocephalus
   (e) Vascular: transient global amnesia, basilar migraine, vertebrobasilar insufficiency
   (f) Cataplexy and narcolepsy
   (g) Causes of myoclonus other than epilepsy
   (h) If epilepsy is confined to sleep, other paroxysmal sleep disorders
2. *Cardiac*
   (a) Dysrhythmias
   (b) Complete heart block
   (c) Atrial myxoma (rare)
3. *Psychiatric*
   (a) Pseudoseizures
   (b) Periodic disinhibition syndrome
4. *Metabolic*
   (a) Hypoglycaemia
   (b) Dumping syndrome
   (c) Phaeochromocytoma
   (d) Hyponatraemia
   (e) Hypocalcaemia
   (f) Renal failure
   (g) Hepatic failure
   (h) Drugs and alcohol
5. *Syncope*

gastrointestinal surgery abruptly lost consciousness after three bites of a Mars bar: his blood sugar at that point was 0.3 mmol/litre. The faint possibility of hypoglycaemia should always be borne in mind in cases of nocturnal seizures. Because it is very rare in comparison with sleep epilepsy it is easy to miss: the diagnosis may be excluded by three early morning fasting blood sugars together with insulin levels.

The causes and diagnosis of vertigo create many problems. Vertigo can be so unpleasant and precipitous that a secondary vasovagal reaction is triggered with resulting loss of consciousness. Unfortunately, the converse also applies and on rare occasions vertigo may be experienced as an aura of an impending epileptic attack. It may be impossible to distinguish between the two but, in practice, a very careful history will usually suffice.

Syncope is the condition most commonly confused with epilepsy and may be defined as loss of consciousness due to a sudden decrease in cerebral blood flow. If an attack occurs in a situation where the patient is unable to get the head down so that blood can return, e.g. sitting in a chair or standing supported in a crowded train, a brief convulsion, sometimes associated with incontinence, can occur.

The commonest form is so-called reflex or vasovagal syncope. There is often an obvious precipitant like pain, the sight of blood, standing for a long period ('guardsman's faints'), micturition, coughing, sneezing, or lifting heavy weights. The onset usually consists of a feeling of dizziness, associated with tremor, a cold sweat, and fading of sounds and vision, following which consciousness is lost for a brief period. Pallor is almost invariable, and the pulse is often slow and faint. Recovery is relatively prompt. Typically attacks occur in adolescence and young adults, although they may occur in later years in the context of vertebrobasilar insufficiency or autonomic neuropathy, e.g. in diabetics.

Cardiac syncope (a sudden drop in cerebral perfusion due to cardiac causes) produces the same symptoms, although the prodrome is often more brief, and frequently associated with palpitations or extrasystoles of which the patient is aware.

Syncope on standing (orthostatic syncope) occurs in those with impairment of autonomic reflexes, orthostatic hypotension. The common causes are drugs and autonomic neuropathies as in diabetes.

Investigations

There is no known investigation that will prove or disprove a putative diagnosis of epilepsy. Investigation is designed to establish the type of seizure with a view to devising a rationale for treatment and, where it is suspected, to try to uncover an underlying cause.

In children and teenagers, overwhelmingly the most common cause for epileptic attacks is primary generalized epilepsy. If there is a family history, a history of morning myoclonus, or if an absence attack can be induced by hyperventilation, the need for further investigation is dubious. The incidence of underlying structural lesions as a cause for epilepsy increases with age and the need for investigation therefore becomes correspondingly greater, although elderly patients whose epilepsy often occurs in the context of cerebrovascular or degenerative cerebral disease seldom require extensive investigations.

An EEG in children and teenagers is valuable to confirm if possible the type of epilepsy suspected, to satisfy the patient and his family that he is having 'tests', and to buy some time to see whether further attacks occur when off treatment. Unless there are specific clinical indications on the history or examination often no more is necessary. An isolated attack in this age group requires no investigation at all unless there are strong political or social reasons to do so.

In adults start with an EEG; if this shows generalized paroxysmal activity and the history is compatible with the diagnosis of generalized epilepsy extensive further tests are not indicated. If the EEG shows focal slowing, the history indicates a focal site of onset, or there are abnormal neurological signs, a computerized tomographic (CT) brain scan is indicated. In the aged, modify the above approach to take into account previous cerebrovascular, cardiac or degenerative disease, and the practicality of doing anything if, e.g. an underlying tumour were shown.

Some doctors regard CT scanning as mandatory. This is an expensive investigation, the facilities for which are limited in the UK at present. A CT scan should therefore only be performed if there is a likelihood of its showing something which would significantly affect patient management. The tumour yield on CT scanning in children with fits is 0.02 per cent. In adults with their first fit starting after the age of 45 it is 10–15 per cent. In patients with no focal features on examination or on EEG, the CT scan can be predicted as normal in 94 per cent of cases, whereas if the EEG is focally abnormal or there are focal features on the history or examination, the CT scan will be abnormal in more than 50 per cent.

Management

General principles

'Epilepsy' as a diagnosis implies a continuing tendency to have seizures. One seizure does not constitute adequate grounds for a diagnosis of epilepsy. An abnormal EEG, a positive family history, or a continuing structural cause for the seizure must increase the risks of further fits, but none of these will make further seizure activity inevitable. Moreover, epileptic attacks may occur in the context of a self-limiting illness or an illness which can be terminated by medical intervention, e.g. encephalitis, meningitis or alcohol withdrawal. A continuing tendency to have attacks following a termination of the illness should not be presumed.

When to start treatment

All too often long-term treatment is started by general practitioners or casualty officers in response to what appears to be a crisis situation, a single seizure or series of seizures which has understandably provoked considerable alarm in the patient and his family. In general, most neurologists would agree that a single seizure should not be treated *unless* there is clinical or historical evidence to suggest that it has occurred in the context of a continuing illness.

At present, authorities differ in their advice about when to start treatment, which drug to use, and how long treatment should be continued. The available data are conflicting and inadequate, but studies in progress and projected should go some way to provide answers to these difficult questions.

Because of the inadequacy of the data, the decision to start drug treatment should not be undertaken lightly, and consideration should be given first to the need for treatment, and to other possible methods of controlling attacks. The need to treat simple partial seizures or morning myoclonus is questionable, particularly when they occur as part of a self-limiting syndrome like the benign focal epilepsies of childhood and adolescence.

Epileptic attacks which occur in response to a specific stimulus can sometimes be controlled by removal or modification of the stimulus. Attacks produced by flicker can be stopped on occasions by buying a smaller television, sitting 3–3.7 m (10–12 feet) away from the screen, using a remote controller to change channels, and turning the set off when it is not being watched. More elaborate manoeuvres using a Polaroid sheet in front of the screen, and wearing Polaroid spectacles are also possible. Flicker induced attacks seldom occur when the stimulus is below five cycles per second, and are far less common when the stimulus is coloured. Thus they are unlikely to occur in discotheques.

Other forms of seizure are more likely to occur with irregular hours or lack of sleep. These are usually those that occur in the mornings within an hour or two of waking. A change of life pattern, e.g. moving one's job nearer home, or a change from shift work to regular hours can often produce a dramatic reduction in the frequency of attacks. Certain patients have a prodrome of an impending attack which may last for one to 2 days. This often consists of a vague feeling of unease, ill-defined headache, irritability or stomach upset. These patients may be able to modify their lifestyle over the at-risk days so that they are not in a position of danger when the attack occurs. Other patients with simple partial seizures claim they can abort an attack by manoeuvres like grabbing the jerking limb with the unaffected hand, or thinking hard of something else, e.g. doing mental arithmetic when the aura occurs.

Often patients have more seizures when they are inactive e.g. after a hard day's work. Patients with epilepsy should be kept as active as possible, within the limits of their safety and that of others. The problem of the patient who has lost his job because of an epileptic attack, and cannot get another because the enforced idleness has increased the frequency of his attacks must be well known to most neurologists.

Anticonvulsants

Hard data on whether early treatment or delay in starting treatment affects prognosis do not exist at present. Similarly, little useful information is available on whether stopping treatment after a fit-free interval of (as yet) undetermined length affects prognosis as far as recurrence rate of seizures is concerned. The most difficult decision therefore is when to start treatment. In general, most neurologists tend to start anticonvulsants after the second seizure unless: (1) there is good clinical evidence or historical evidence after the first seizure to suggest that further seizures are very likely; (2) there is evidence to suggest that seizures will remit spontaneously, and there is no current danger to the patient of having them; (3) the patient himself is reluctant to start medication and there is no compelling reason, e.g. danger, to do so; (4) there are other possible ways of modifying the tendency to attacks which have not been tried.

The most important factor affecting the success of treatment is *compliance*. Full discussion with the patient and family must take place at an early stage, pointing out the possible effects of no treatment, the way treatment may modify these, the possible side-effects of treatment and how these can be countered, and the likely duration of treatment assuming that the response is as predicted. Nowadays, 85–90 per cent of patients with generalized seizures can be maintained almost attack free on *one anticonvulsant alone* providing the dose is adequate: the response of those with partial seizures and in particular complex partial seizures is less predictable and often frankly disheartening.

Current evidence suggests that all the major anticonvulsants available at present are equally effective: these are phenobarbitone, phenytoin, carbamazepine, and sodium valproate.

The choice of anticonvulsant for a particular individual must depend on two factors, convenience, and the incidence and severity of side-effects. Unfortunately these two factors often conflict: the incidence and severity of side-effects is frequently worse with phenobarbitone and phenytoin, but these drugs can be taken once daily because of their long half-lives, whereas carbamazepine and sodium valproate have fewer side-effects but have to be taken at least twice a day.

Phenobarbitone, phenytoin, and carbamazepine are not effective in simple absence seizures and the response of myoclonic seizures is unpredictable. The drugs of choice for these conditions are ethosuximide or sodium valproate. When absence seizures and tonic-clonic seizures occur in conjunction, sodium valproate is the drug of choice because it is effective against both types. The fashion at present is to use carbamazepine in many younger patients with generalized and complex partial seizures, and sodium valproate also in generalized seizures because the side-effects appear less. Myoclonus has been described in Chapters 2 and 9.

A discussion of the putative modes of action of the various anticonvulsants is beyond the scope of this chapter. A fuller description of the pharmacokinetics and possible side-effects of anticonvulsants is given in Table 11.4.

Phenytoin is effective against most forms of seizure except absence seizures. Its major advantage is that it can be taken once daily. Its major disadvantage is that side-effects like gum hypertrophy, coarsening of the skin and hirsutism are relatively common. For these reasons it is used less in children and adolescents. Another major disadvantage is that the 'window' between therapeutic and toxic levels is relatively narrow so that if the dose needs to be increased it should be done by small increments if symptoms of toxicity are not to occur: these include diplopia, slurred speech, unsteadiness, frank ataxia, and then drowsiness.

Phenobarbitone is very effective against most forms of seizure except absence seizures. Its major advantages are that it can be given once daily as it has a very long half-life and it is cheap. Its major disadvantage is that sedation is common, and because of the long half-life cannot be minimized by taking the dose at night. In addition, in children and adolescents, the mentally handicapped and the aged, paradoxical effects on behaviour like hyperactivity, irritability, aggressiveness and depression are quite frequent. Toxic effects are similar to those of phenytoin.

Carbamazepine is also very effective against most forms of seizure except absences. After chronic administration it has a relatively short half-life so that a twice daily dosage regimen is probably best. In patients not previously exposed to carbamazepine the plasma half-life is considerably longer so that the dose needs to be increased gradually. The drug is usually well tolerated, although the occurrence of skin rashes is more frequent than with phenobarbitone and phenytoin. Toxic effects are the same as for these two drugs.

Sodium valproate is effective against all forms of seizure, including absence and myoclonic seizures. It is therefore the drug of choice when more than one type of seizure coexists in the same individual. In comparison with other anticonvulsants it has a very short half-life and large variations in plasma levels between those taken before a dose and those taken 2 h after are common. It should therefore be taken two or three times a day and the usefulness of measuring plasma levels is dubious. Side-effects are uncommon but, on occasions, patients do complain of hair loss and tremor which can usually be eliminated by reducing the dose. Sedation is infrequent. In children a few fatal cases of hepatic failure due to sodium valproate have been reported, and in children and adults thrombocytopenia may occur, although it is very rare. Monitoring liver function and platelet counts early on in treatment is advised.

Ethosuximide is very effective against absence seizures. The half-life is long so that once daily medication can be given. Side-effects such as nausea, drowsiness and headache are not infrequent.

Clonazepam is at present a second line drug in the management of refractory absence and myoclonic seizures. Response to it can on occasions be dramatic. Unfortunately unacceptable sedation is quite common, and tolerance develops fairly rapidly so that a progressive increase in dosage is necessary. To minimize the risk of sedation the drug should be introduced very gradually.

Primidone has little or no advantage over any of the above anticonvulsants. Some 15–20 per cent of the ingested dose is converted to phenobarbitone, but there is some evidence that the other metabolite, phenylethylmalonamide, exerts a weak anticonvulsant effect as well. Sedation is extremely common and often severe, so that the starting dose must be low and increases in dosage small.

The cardinal principle of good anticonvulsant treatment is that it must be as simple as possible to minimize the possibility of drug interactions and to ensure good compliance. If fits continue after an anticonvulsant has been prescribed there are several possibilities: compliance is poor, the dose is wrong, the type of medication is inappropriate, or the patient has a form of seizure which is likely to respond poorly to whatever medication is prescribed. This last possibility should be known from the clinical history and the results of investigation, and in this case therapeutic idealism should be tempered with realism. The first two possibilities can be explored by measuring the serum anticonvulsant levels. If the level is low, the dose can be adjusted. If it is within the therapeutic range, it may be necessary to substitute another drug. There is seldom justification for adding another drug as current evidence suggests that seizures are no more

Table 11.4   Drug management of epilepsy

Drug	Daily average dose	Half-life (h)	Peak levels (h)
Ethosuximide	1–2 g (adult maintenance)	30	3–7
Carbamazepine	400–800 mg	Initially 20–40. With chronic administration 12–24	4–18
Clonazepam	2–6 mg	20–40 (adults) 15–30 (children)	1–4
Phenobarbitone	60–120 mg	2–5 (days)	4–12
Phenytoin	200–400 mg	Dose dependent. For average doses 20. For overdose may be 100	—
Primidone	500–1000 mg	5–12 (15–30 for phenylethylmalonamide (PEMA))	2–4
Sodium valproate	800–1500 mg	6–12	1–4

Therapeutic level (mg/l)	Drug interactions	Side-effects
40–100	Minimal	Headache, nausea, sedation, abdominal pain (common). Ataxia, psychosis, abnormal movements, rashes, blood, dyscrasias, hepatic and renal toxicity, lupus-like syndrome
5–10	Common, particularly with phenytoin, anticoagulants	Sedation, nausea, skin rashes, water retention, syndrome resembling porphyria. Leukopaenia
20–80 ng/ml	—	Sedation. Tolerance, leading to increased dose requirement
15–30	Common with phenytoin, valproate, anticoagulants	Sedation, macrocytic anaemia, rashes, paradoxical behavioural effects, osteomalacia (rare)
10–20	Common	Macrocytosis. Sedation. Gum hypertrophy, coarsening of features, lupus-like syndrome, blood dyscrasias, lymphadenopathy, splenomegaly, neuropathy, osteomalacia
Measured as phenobarbitone (15–30) and primidone (5–12)	As for phenobarbitone	In general as for phenobarbitone
Marked fluctuations over 24 hours. Therefore difficult to assess or interpret. Probably 50–100, if blood taken within 2 h of dose	Uncommon, except with phenobarbitone	Tremor, hair loss, nausea, alteration in weight (common). Thrombocytopaenia, abnormal liver function, hepatic failure (rare)

likely to come under control with two drugs than with one and as more drugs are introduced the possibility of side-effects and drug interactions increases.

When to stop treatment

In recent years it has become clear that chronic administration of antiepileptic drugs may produce subtle changes in cognitive function, mood and memory. A strong case can therefore be made for stopping treatment as soon as possible. Unfortunately, when a patient has been fit free on anticonvulsants for 2–3 years, it is not clear whether this remission represents a 'cure' or whether it merely represents 'control' which is dependent on continued antiepileptic therapy. Most clinicians agree that a trial of drug withdrawal in children or adolescents after a fit-free period of 2–3 years should be attempted unless there are compelling reasons against it, e.g. evidence of brain damage. A relapse rate of about 20 per cent can be expected in this group. In adults, however, the situation is rather more complex as the relapse rate is probably much higher (about 40 per cent), and other factors like driving, employment, reproductive need and so on, supervene. Most relapses occur within 6 months of reduction of anti-convulsant dosage.

A decision to withdraw anticonvulsants in adults should be taken by the patient himself on the advice of the clinician, after weighing up the risks of continued anticonvulsants against the risks of further seizures after drug withdrawal and the effect these might have on employment, driving prospects, leisure pursuits and so on (Table 11.5). Various factors will inevitably increase the risk of relapse, e.g. an underlying structural cause for attacks, the occurrence of partial as opposed to generalized seizures, or attacks which proved very difficult to control at the onset of treatment. In women the interaction of anticonvulsants with oral contraceptives necessitating a higher dose oestrogen preparation, and the faint possibility of teratogenicity, may be for them a potent argument in favour of drug withdrawal. In practice, it is extremely difficult to advise patients after taking all these factors into account: many prefer to remain on medication.

Table 11.5   Factors to be considered in stopping anticonvulsant therapy

Absolute requirements	Factors for	Factors against
(a) Fit-free interval of 2–3 years	(a) Childhood epilepsy	(a) Late onset epilepsy
(b) Patient's informed agreement	(b) Primary generalized epilepsy	(b) Partial seizures
	(c) Fits easy to control initially	(c) Underlying structural pathology
	(d) No underlying structural cause	(d) Continuing abnormal EEG
	(e) Normal EEG	(e) Epilepsy difficult to control initially
	(f) Non-driver	(f) Driver
	(g) Employment likely to be unaffected if further fits	(g) Employment likely to be affected if seizures recur
	(h) A woman of child-bearing age	

If a decision is taken to withdraw treatment, it must be carried out *slowly* over a matter of weeks, or even months in the case of phenobarbitone, to minimize the risk of withdrawal fits which may then be mistaken for a recurrence of the primary condition.

Epilepsy and pregnancy

Phenytoin, carbamazepine, phenobarbitone and primidone may all cause 'failure' of the contraceptive pill. This is probably caused by induction of hepatic microsomal enzymes thus accelerating the metabolism of sex hormones. Breakthrough bleeding is a warning of inadequate contraception and justifies changing to a higher dose oestrogen pill or to a different method of contraception. Sodium valproate does not have this effect, but its use in women of child-bearing age who may wish to become pregnant must be considered carefully because of possible teratogenicity.

Specific problems related to pregnancy are:

1. *Genetic aspects.* Apart from the rare metabolic and neurological diseases which are inherited and in which epilepsy is a prominent feature, there is no doubt that inheritance plays a prominent part in the genesis of primary generalized seizures. However, it appears that it is the EEG pattern of 3–6 Hz spike wave activity that is inherited and not the epilepsy; i.e. the threshold for having seizures is lowered but this factor has to interact with a number of other different and variable factors for seizures to occur. In general, there is a less than 10 per cent chance of a child 'inheriting' epilepsy if one first degree relative is affected: if two first degree relatives are affected, there is a 15 per cent chance.
2. *Possible teratogenicity.* The risks of epileptic mothers having an abnormal fetus is approximately double the rate in the population at large, regardless of drug therapy. Furthermore, the risk of serious fetal anoxia and/or abortion as a consequence of a prolonged generalized seizure during pregnancy must be taken into account. It is difficult to sort out specific abnormalities attributable to drugs alone from the above two factors, and considerable controversy exists on the matter. It appears that the safest drugs in pregnancy are carbamazepine, ethosuximide and phenobarbitone. Phenytoin has been implicated with hare-lip, various cardiac abnormalities, and the so-called fetal hydantoin syndrome. There have been suggestions that sodium valproate can rarely cause neural tube defects.

Teratogenicity, if it occurs, usually does so within the first 3 months of pregnancy. It is useless therefore to stop a drug once pregnancy has occurred. Pregnancy should be planned and the various pros and cons of continuing and stopping treatment weighed up beforehand.

In general, if the seizures are of a type that are no threat to the mother or fetus it is sometimes wisest to stop medication. Most neurologists agree that the risk to the mother and the fetus from major generalized seizures during pregnancy is greater than the risk from drugs, taking into account that 35–40 per cent of pregnant epileptic patients experience an increase in fit frequency.

Epilepsy and driving

A driving licence contains a statement saying that if there is a change in the holder's health which is likely to impair his ability to drive, and if it is likely to last more than 3 months, then *he* is statutory bound to inform the licensing authority. In law, all forms of epilepsy are regarded as coming under this provision.

A single fit does not constitute epilepsy: the current recommendations are that after such an occurrence a patient should not drive for a year. Where two or more fits have occurred the patient must inform the DVLC and the doctor must tell him to do this. From a medico-legal point of view, it is also advisable to enter in the notes that this has been done, and wherever possible to tell the patient in front of a witness. *All* forms of epilepsy are covered by the provision, and the doctor is allowed no clinical leeway. It may seem unreasonable to ban a person from driving if he has simple seizures confined to (say) one side of the face, but the law is the law.

Patients with epilepsy may drive once they have been fit free on or off treatment for 2 years. Alternatively, if seizures are confined to sleep, they must continue confined to sleep for a period of 3 years before a licence will be issued. The vexed question of stopping treatment in a patient who already holds a licence has been discussed.

Any seizure after the age of 5 years bars a person from holding an HGV or PSV licence, as does any unexplained attack of loss of consciousness in which all investigations are normal.

Medical management of a single seizure

Turn the patient on to his side into the recovery position. Remove objects likely to cause injury if encountered during the fit and loosen the collar. If the convulsive phase lasts for longer than 5–10 min, diazepam 10 mg or clonazepam 1 mg should be given intravenously over a period of about 2 min. If this is not possible, then paraldehyde 10 ml by deep intramuscular injection is an alternative. A glass syringe will need to be used for this.

Status epilepticus

Status epilepticus may be defined as recurrent seizures without recovery of consciousness in between. Because of different types of seizures it may be further classified into absence status and convulsive status. Absence status usually occurs in children: only the management of convulsive status will be discussed here.

Convulsive status epilepticus is a medical emergency, and carries with it a mortality of 5–20 per cent. In the majority of cases it occurs in the context of established epilepsy (60 per cent), or as the initial (15 per cent) or only (25 per cent) manifestation of epilepsy. If it occurs in the absence of a previous history of seizures, an underlying cause, e.g. glioma or encephalitis, should be considered.

Convulsive status, if not controlled, can produce serious long-term neurological deficit. Animal experiments have shown that during convulsions the cerebral oxygen demand goes up dramatically and that the blood supply can seldom match it so neuronal oxygen insufficiency soon occurs. Once this happens cell death follows, the region most at risk being the hippocampus. These changes occur regardless of whether the animal is paralysed and ventilated, although not as fast, so that anoxia and/or hyperthermia which are seen in status cannot be the only causes of neuronal damage. In humans, it appears that continuous convulsions lasting for longer than 2 h are frequently associated with permanent neurological damage so that allowing for a safety margin the doctor has about an hour to control status from the onset.

The management of status is summarized in Table 11.6.

Table 11.6 Status epilepticus

Causes (in order of frequency)	*Complications* Of status	Of treatment
Idiopathic epilepsy	(1) Hypoxia	(1) Respiratory depression
Tumour	(2) Pulmonary oedema	and apnoea (all drugs)
Miscellaneous	(3) Cardiovascular collapse	(2) Thrombophlebitis
(metabolic, toxic)	(4) Orthopaedic injury	(diazepam
Trauma	(5) Hypo/hypertension	chlormethiazole)
Encephalitis	(6) Chest infection	(3) Hypotension (all drugs)
Vascular	(aspiration)	(4) Cardiac arrhythmias
	(7) Hyperthermia	(phenytoin)
	(8) Dehydration	(5) Pulmonary oedema
	(9) Hypo/hyperglycaemia	(paraldehyde)
	(10) Renal and electrolyte	(6) Sterile abscess
	disturbances	(paraldehyde)

Management
1. Diazepam 10 mg i.v. over 2 min: can be repeated to a maximum of 50 mg in 6 h or diazepam infusion, 50 mg in 500 ml normal saline, to a maximum of 3 mg/kg over 24 h
2. Clonazepam 1 mg i.v. slowly, can be repeated to 3 mg over 6 h or clonazepam infusion 3 mg in 250 ml saline, usually 1–3 mg over 6 h is effective
3. Phenytoin i.v. slowly, less than 50 mg/min to a total of 15 mg/kg (best over 30–45 min) monitor heart rate, rhythm and blood pressure
   Phenytoin can be given orally or by nasogastric tube in a loading dose
4. If these measures fail, intubate, thiopentone infusion 1–2 mg/min i.v. (usually 1.0 g in 12 h) accompanied often by 'paralysing' drugs and ventilation
5. Other drugs sometimes used include chlormethiazole infusion and paraldehyde (i.m. or rectal)

1. Initial management

Oxygen is necessary in all cases. Diazepam 10 mg intravenously or clonazepam 1 mg intravenously should be given over 2 min, and an intravenous line with normal saline set up. Blood should be taken for electrolytes, urea, sugar, calcium, liver function, full blood count, and anticonvulsant levels if the patient is a known epileptic to establish whether poor compliance can be responsible for the status. If diabetes or alcohol withdrawal seem likely, 50 ml of intravenous glucose 50 per cent solution, and 100 mg of intravenous thiamine should be given. Blood gases should be measured. If there is clinical or biochemical evidence of hypoxia the patient should be intubated. All patients should be managed on an intensive therapy unit and pulse, blood pressure, ECG, rectal temperature and respirations should be monitored.

If at all possible get a brief history from relatives, ambulance staff or other witnesses. Is the patient a known epileptic? Does he take his medication regularly? If not a known sufferer with seizures, has there been a change in behaviour or function over the previous weeks or months which might suggest an underlying tumour: or very recent malaise and headache which might suggest developing encephalitis. If the former is true a CT scan should be performed *after* the fits are controlled. If encephalitis is suspected, the CSF should be examined immediately and a CT scan performed after the fits are adequately controlled. Note that a raised white cell count of 20 000 or more in the blood is quite common in status and should not be taken as an indication of underlying infection without corroborative evidence.

2. Further drug therapy

If the fits continue after the initial intravenous dose of diazepam or clonazepam, repeat intravenous bolus injections can be given every 10 min or more to a maximum of 50 mg of diazepam or 3 mg of clonazepam over 6 h. These benzodiazepines can also be given by infusion. If these measures fail to control the seizures, phenytoin to a total dose of 15 mg/kg can be given intravenously at a rate of not more than 50 mg/min, preferably over 30–40 min using an infusion pump. Watch the ECG for arrhythmias and monitor the blood pressure. Peak brain levels can be expected about 10 min after stopping the infusion. Phenytoin 100 mg can then be given as a bolus over 2–3 min 6-hourly and the dose adjusted by monitoring serum levels.

If the above measures fail, or if the patient shows signs of developing malignant hyperpyrexia as a consequence of the muscle activity, he must be paralysed and ventilated. At this stage a thiopentone infusion at a rate of 1–2 mg/min should be considered. If this stage has been reached, it becomes impossible to detect further seizure activity clinically since the patient is paralysed, so that EEG monitoring becomes necessary.

Other drugs which may be used to control seizures in status are:

1. Chlormethiazole 0.8 per cent given as an intravenous infusion. Usually a starting dose of 100 ml given over 5–10 min is used, and then the infusion continued at rates of about 0.5 g/h depending on the response. Peak levels are reached about 15 min after the bolus. Though effective in controlling seizures, the usefulness of this drug appears to be limited by the tendency for fits to recur as the infusion is stopped.
2. Paraldehyde is extremely effective but its use is limited by its propensity to cause sterile abscesses at the site of intramuscular injections and by the fact that it decomposes plastic bags and tubing; 10 ml of paraldehyde intramuscularly is the normal adult dose, or alternatively a rectal dose of 10 ml diluted in two volumes of arachis oil can be given. Apart from paraldehyde,

intramuscular injection of drugs has no place in the management of status epilepticus.

Metabolic and other medical complications which can occur as a direct result of the condition or its drug management are listed in Table 11.6.

3. Stopping intravenous therapy and converting to oral therapy

If status has come under control easily e.g. by repeated doses of intravenous diazepam, the patient should be maintained seizure free for at least 6–8 h before withdrawing intravenous therapy. If the course of status has been prolonged and difficult to control, a seizure free period of 24–48 h should be considered. Therapy should always be withdrawn slowly over 24–48 h. This gives the doctor the opportunity of converting to oral therapy via a nasogastric tube. Phenytoin is probably the drug of choice because there is a better match between therapeutic efficacy and blood levels than with most of the other anticonvulsants. Start with 100 mg orally 6 hourly, and adjust the dose in the light of serum levels. Carbamazepine, phenobarbitone, or sodium valproate can be added as required.

Sleep disorders

Sleep disorders may be classified into: too much sleep (hypersomnia or disorders of excessive sleep, DOES), too little sleep (insomnia or disorders in initiating or maintaining sleep, DIMS); dysfunctions or paroxysmal disorders associated with sleep (parasomnias). Into the last category come nightmares, sleep walking, sleep paralysis and sleep related epileptic seizures. Because of the disturbance to sleep that they cause they sometimes present as excessive daytime somnolence.

Disorders of excessive daytime somnolence (DOES)

The commonest disorders are narcolepsy, sleep apnoea and idiopathic hypersomnia.

Narcolepsy

This is characterized by disturbed nocturnal sleep and a tendency to be overcome during the day by uncontrollable attacks of somnolence at completely inappropriate times. Patients may drop off while eating and wake with their faces in the plates: or when driving or talking. Resisting the urge to sleep causes an increase in microsleep episodes and if these occur in salvo automatisms can happen.

Apart from excessive daytime drowsiness and a disturbed nocturnal sleep pattern, three other features are associated with the narcoleptic syndrome, hypnagogic hallucinations, sleep paralysis, and cataplexy. Hypnagogic hallucinations usually occur just as the patient is dropping off to sleep. They can involve any of the five senses and be extremely complex, and often very terrifying, particularly if they are associated with sleep paralysis. This again occurs just as the patient is dropping off to sleep when he becomes aware that he is unable to move a muscle: attempts to call out for help produce no sound. Attacks do not last for long but appear to last an eternity to the patient. Cataplexy is a precipitous drop in muscle tone, usually produced by emotion, fatigue, excitement, rage or sexual intercourse. Attacks may be generalized causing the patient to crumple to the floor, or they may affect a limited area of musculature, e.g. the head, when the jaw drops and the head will fall onto the chest.

The impression that the narcoleptic syndrome may be inherited has been confirmed by the recent finding of a strong association between it and the HLA antigen DR2.

Treatment is difficult and not entirely satisfactory. The patient should be advised to keep regular hours, and if disturbed nocturnal sleep is a prominent feature, a short-acting hypnotic like chloral hydrate is sometimes helpful. A regular postprandial nap sometimes helps to control episodes of microsleep. The most commonly used drugs are the amphetamines, pemoline and methyl phenidate, although this latter drug is no longer available in the UK except on a named patient basis. Each causes side-effects and tolerance may develop. Cataplexy, sleep paralysis, and hypnagogic hallucinations are more readily controllable with clomipramine or protriptyline.

Obstructive sleep apnoea

This is an important condition to recognize because in severe cases it may lead to cardiac failure and cor pulmonale. Not uncommonly it presents as daytime drowsiness as a consequence of disturbed night-time sleep. Characteristically it occurs in middle-aged men and post-menopausal women who are overweight and drink too much, although in younger people it can occur in relation to anatomical disorders of the nasopharynx, jaw and tongue, e.g. in Down's syndrome or in people with enlarged tonsils. Systemic hypertension is frequently noted. Common presenting complaints are excessive daytime drowsiness, fatigue, morning headaches and depression. Further questioning reveals a history of heavy snoring, restless sleep, confusion and disorientation at night. If available, a witness gives a story of sleep interrupted by snores which reach a crescendo following which breathing will cease for a variable period. If the cessation of respiration is prolonged, the patient usually wakes and appears confused for some minutes prior to dropping off to sleep again. Diagnosis is made on the very characteristic history and confirmed on polysomnography with monitoring of EEG, ECG, respiration, and oxygen saturation using an ear oximeter. Treatment often requires little more than weight reduction, abstention from alcohol, and the removal of factors likely to impair airway flow like smoking and allergens. Medications like medroxyprogesterone, protriptyline, and L-tryptophan are useful in specific cases. Nocturnal positive pressure inspiratory assistance may be of benefit. On rare occasions, surgical procedures to the palate or pharynx, lower mandible readjustment, or even tracheostomy have to be performed.

Table 11.7 Sleep disorders

Hypersomnia: disorders of excessive sleep (DOES)
(1) Psychological
(2) Psychiatric disorders, e.g. depression
(3) Abuse of drugs or alcohol
(4) Associated with obstructive sleep apnoea
(5) Associated with causes of parasomnia
(6) Narcoleptic syndrome
(7) Neurological disorders, e.g. hypothalamic lesions
(8) Idiopathic hypersomnia
Insomnia: disorders of initiating or maintaining sleep (DIMS)
(1) Psychological
(2) Psychiatric conditions, e.g. anxiety, hypomania
(3) Abuse of drugs or alcohol
(4) Associated with obstructive sleep apnoea
(5) Other medical or environmental conditions, e.g. thyrotoxicosis, allergy
Parasomnia
(1) Sleep walking
(2) Sleep terrors
(3) Sleep related bruxism
(4) Sleep epilepsy
(5) Restless legs syndrome
(6) Sleep paralysis
(7) Sleep-related head banging
(8) Sleep-related asthma
(9) Sleep myoclonus

Hypersomnia

Hypersomnia or excessive daytime drowsiness may occur as a consequence of disturbed nocturnal sleep, e.g. in obstructive sleep apnoea; or it may occur in the context of neurological disorders, particularly lesions affecting the hypothalamic area (e.g. Kleine-Levin syndrome); alternatively medical disorders like myxoedema sometimes may present with excessive daytime somnolence. Only after these possibilities have been explored can excessive daytime somnolence be said to be idiopathic hypersomnia.

Disorders of initiating or maintaining sleep (DIMS)

Insomnia must be one of the most frequent complaints in the population at large. It may be associated with a multitude of disorder such as thyrotoxicosis, psychiatric conditions, the abuse of stimulant drugs, nocturnal pain as in migrainous neuralgia, or conditions like the restless legs syndrome or nocturnal myoclonus. By far the commonest cause, however, must be the impression on the part of the patient that he is somehow 'missing out' on his sleep ration in comparison with others.

Parasomnias

Paroxysmal disorders associated with sleep include a number of ill-understood conditions like sleep walking, teeth grinding, nightmares, sleep-related head banging, sleep paralysis, sleep related myoclonus and sleep epilepsy.

12

Migraine

In Chapter 2 the symptoms of headache of acute onset are discussed. It is essential to emphasize that acute onset of headache may reflect an infection, e.g. meningitis, or haemorrhage, e.g. subarachnoid bleed. In both these situations there will be associated meningeal irritation with a stiff neck and positive Kernig's sign. These life-threatening conditions must not be missed.

The other common cause of headache with an acute onset is *migraine*. The diagnosis of the first attack may be difficult. Many definitions have been proposed which include recurrent episodic headache usually lasting hours, from 2 to 72. The headaches may be associated with visual upset (45 per cent), photophobia (82 per cent), nausea (87 per cent), vomiting (60 per cent) and prostration. Between attacks patients are normal. There may be a positive family history and an association with motion sickness. Many patients at the onset describe an aura or warning, most commonly with visual symptoms (45 per cent), but sometimes with more alarming focal sensory symptoms (33 per cent) or dizziness (72 per cent). Migraine is the commonest cause of headache and figures varying between 5 and 20 per cent have been suggested for the prevalence in the population. Women are affected more often than men, the peak incidence lying between the ages of 20 and 30, but it may arise in childhood, where there may be an association with cyclical vomiting and recurrent bilious attacks. The onset of migraine *de novo* in older patients (more than 55) is less common. In any series of chronic headache sufferers, migraine is one of the commonest causes.

Classical migraine

This describes episodes of acute headache, either generalized or lateralized to one side—hemicrania, preceded by a clear aura. The aura is most often a visual disturbance with complaints of spots, flashing lights, zig-zags, kaleidoscope effects, whorls or even fortification spectra (teichopsia). There may be visual loss, patchy scotomas or fragmentation, like a jig-saw puzzle with pieces missing, which may spread to a hemianopia or more complete field loss which can affect both eyes. On rare occasions distortion of size or shape may occur (like in 'Alice in Wonderland') or even formed visual hallucinations. Such visual auras may occur alone or be followed by sensory symptoms which may include tingling, paraesthesiae or numbness most commonly starting in one hand and spreading centrally, or involving the face or lips where the sensory upset may spread in a circumoral distribution to involve the lips, tongue, and nose in a 'snout' area. There may be accompanying slurring of speech and dizziness. Such auras usually last 10–20 min, sometimes longer (up to an hour or so), and as the symptoms abate there is the build up of an increasingly severe throbbing headache associated with nausea, photophobia, prostration and often vomiting. The headache may occur on the same side as the focal symptoms. Affected patients usually want to lie in a dark room. Exertion, activity, bending, coughing, light or noise will aggravate the headache. Many patients feel that the headache may ease after vomiting or a sleep. The pain is usually relieved within one to 2 days but may leave the patient weak and 'drained'. With increasing age the episodes become less severe: vomiting often ceases and the headache may be milder.

Common migraine

By contrast, in common migraine patients experience recurrent episodes of severe headache which is either generalized or lateralized but which have no preceding aura. The headache may be more frontal, or occipital, and may be described as throbbing, severe and accompanied by nausea, photophobia and prostration. Vomiting may occur. Again such headaches may last hours or a day or two. To compound the problem there is also evidence that many migraine sufferers also suffer with muscle contraction (tension) headache which may appear in the occipitofrontalis, masseter, temporalis and periorbital muscles. This may be the explanation why in some migraine attacks the headache may persist as a dull ache for days or even longer.

Frequency

This varies greatly but many patients experience recurring attacks of headache every 4–6 weeks often in 'groups' followed by long periods of freedom so they may suffer only two to four episodes yearly. Very frequent attacks can occur so that there is little or no clear symptom-free interval between: this may be termed status migrainosus.

Precipitants

Most patients recognize some triggers which precipitate an attack. These include anxiety or worry (70 per cent), light or glare (30 per cent), menstruation (39 per cent), certain food substances (13 per cent), alcohol (10 per cent), fatigue or missed sleep (43 per cent), relaxation (45 per cent), and hunger (7 per cent). Of the dietary triggers chocolate, cheese, citrus fruits, and onions are the most common offenders. In severe childhood migraine exclusion diets may be worth a trial in preventive treatment. Increasing interest has been shown in the possibility of food allergies causing migraine.

Many adolescent girls and young women describe an increased frequency of attacks just before or at the onset of their menstrual period. Conversely some women are free of migraine during pregnancy suggesting that hormone triggers play a role. Perhaps of equal importance is that in some women taking the oral contraceptive pill, migraine attacks may either appear for the first time, be aggravated or change their pattern. In the last instance focal neurological symptoms may appear in the aura. Such features are a contraindication to continuing the 'pill' as they may be the herald of a thrombotic cerebrovascular complication producing a stroke with a permanent deficit.

Physical triggers are also important. Light or reflected glare from water or working with a VDU may provoke attacks. Missed sleep and travel may also be incriminated. Certain exertional activities may provoke migraine: prolonged running or strenuous football. In the last, heading the ball or a clash of heads may be the mechanism. It is also possible to see migraine provoked or exacerbated by a head injury. There is also a group of patients who describe their headaches starting at weekends (Saturday morning headache) or on the first day of their holidays, perhaps due to a release from some stress.

Attention to potential precipitants is important. These can be recognized in two-thirds of patients and their avoidance, where possible, is part of treatment.

Migraine variants

In a small number of migraine attacks persisting neurological deficits may appear in association with the attack. Such migraine variants include:

1. Ophthalmoplegic.
2. Hemiplegic.
3. Retinal.
4. Basilar.

All these are uncommon but deserve mention as their recognition will aid diagnosis and often prevent unnecessary investigation. Again in the first attack it is necessary to exclude a number of potentially serious conditions. Computerized tomographic (CT) scans in some patients may show the presence of low density areas, suggesting that infarction can sometimes occur. Episodes that leave a permanent deficit are labelled *complicated migraine*.

Ophthalmoplegic migraine

Here an external ophthalmoplegia appears with complaints of diplopia most often from an oculomotor palsy, or less commonly an abducens palsy. The cranial nerve lesion is accompanied or preceded by headache and persists for days, sometimes weeks, long after the headache has receded. In the differential diagnosis of an acute painful ophthalmoplegia it is always important to exclude aneurysmal compression of the oculomotor nerve. This may require angiography in the first acute attack.

Hemiplegic migraine

Such patients develop an acute hemiparesis or hemiplegia followed or accompanied by severe headache. Again the weakness commonly lasts days or weeks, much longer than the headache. There is often a familial trend and patients may suffer recurring or alternating attacks. In the acute attack it is important to exclude an acute thromboembolic infarct, and in the young, unusual vasculitic conditions e.g. polyarteritis nodosa (PAN), meningovascular syphilis or moyamoya disease.

Retinal migraine

This may cause acute persisting visual loss in one eye, often with an altitudinal or scotomatous defect following a severe headache. In some patients an ischaemic papillitis has been described. Occasionally the visual loss may persist permanently.

Basilar migraine

If giddiness, circumoral sensory upsets or bilateral visual disturbances (suggesting occipital ischaemia) are included as symptoms of basilar migraine, then these are relatively common. Often more alarming transient brainstem neurological symptoms arise in basilar migraine. These include dysarthria, unsteadiness, double vision, tinnitus, confusional states or amnesia. A further rare complication is loss of consciousness, usually lasting 20–30 min, followed by severe headache. Such patients are often adolescent girls or young women and there is commonly sufficient warning so that they may go and lie down. The unconscious state appears to resemble sleep but the patient cannot be roused: there is full and complete recovery within 60 min, although the headache may last longer.

Migraine equivalents

These are rare transient episodes of disturbed neurological function which may be unaccompanied by headache or only by a very trivial mild discomfort. Here the differential diagnosis is focused on causes of transient cerebral ischaemia, particularly in older patients arising on an embolic basis or relating to paroxysmal changes of heart rate or rhythm. Such symptoms may include dysarthria or dysphasia, unsteadiness, confusion, amnesia or dreamy states and seldom last more than 60 min.

Childhood migraine

At least 5 per cent of schoolchildren suffer with migraine and although in many the episodic headache and accompanying symptoms are similar to those experienced by adults, there are some differences which deserve discussion. In particular a number of recurrent episodic disorders (periodic syndromes) arise. These include:

1. Cyclical vomiting.
2. Abdominal migraine.
3. Classical migraine } similar to those experienced in adults
4. Complicated migraine.

In abdominal migraine children complain of recurrent central periumbilical pain (an aching lasting minutes to hours), associated with anorexia, nausea and commonly vomiting. The child appears pale and unwell. In many children there is also headache and, if questioned, they may admit to a visual or sensory aura. Focal symptoms may sometimes be most easily described by a child with the help of drawings for many children will clearly depict their aura. Most of these children have a positive family history and many are also travel sick. A few describe symptoms compatible with benign paroxysmal vertigo of childhood.

In many children with migraine, the nausea, vomiting and sometimes the focal neurological symptoms may seem much more pronounced than the headache. There is always parental concern in children with recurrent headache. Very often this reflects fears of a cerebral tumour. It can be emphasized that in studies of children with headaches due to brain tumours, abnormal neurological or ocular signs were present on examination in 94 per cent within 2 months of the onset of symptoms. In any child with headache of uncertain cause, follow-up is important to see if any signs have appeared. Plain skull X-rays may prove helpful as 50 per cent of children with tumours will show abnormalities. In others where there is a strong clinical suspicion or the presence of abnormal signs, CT scanning will be undertaken. Children with migraine show no abnormal neurological signs and have normal neurological investigations.

Facial migraine and 'lower-half headache'

Recurrent episodes of migraine may sometimes cause pain in the face. Some of these attacks appear clearly defined as in migrainous neuralgia, chronic paroxysmal hemicrania and lower-half headache. Others are less specific and include a number of forms of episodic facial pain. In lower-half headache there are recurrent attacks of pain in the lower half of the face on one side, usually in the cheek spreading into the palate, ear, neck, and even downwards to the shoulder or upwards to the orbit. The pain is commonly severe and throbbing, accompanied by nausea and sometimes vomiting and may last one to 3 days.

Migrainous neuralgia, cluster headache, periodic migrainous neuralgia

This has many synonyms and is a very specific entity largely affecting middle-aged men. Patients describe recurrent episodes of very severe pain affecting one eye or the periorbital region on one side: usually one or two episodes recur every 24 hours. The attacks may awaken the patient from sleep and recur over several weeks in a 'cluster'. The pain is very intense, boring or throbbing, so that the patient will get up, walk about, or place a cold flannel over the eye. The pain usually last 45–120 min. Commonly there are associated vasomotor symptoms, conjunctival suffusion, ptosis, miosis, tearing and a blocked stuffy nose on the affected side (Fig. 12.1). There may be complaints that the cheek on the affected side or the periorbital region feels bruised and swollen. Alcohol may precipitate an attack. Between attacks patients appear normal although in the episode they may show oculosympathetic signs – ptosis, a small pupil and red eye. In many

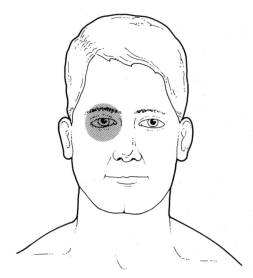

Fig. 12.1.   Migrainous neuralgia. Severe pain in or around one eye, often repeated nocturnal attacks, associated ptosis, miosis, tears, conjunctival suffusion, blocked nose, all ipsilateral to the pain

patients there are infrequent clusters separated by years, but in a few increasingly frequent attacks occur.

Chronic paroxysmal hemicrania

This describes acute brief episodes of severe pain rather like a migrainous neuralgia lasting 10–30 min affecting one side of the face and head usually in the temporo-orbital region. Patients may suffer 10–20 attacks daily over many years. The episodes are associated with vasomotor symptoms and largely affect young women. They can be triggered by neck movements, or pressure and show a specific response to indomethacin.

Causes of migraine

The main theories of the pathogenesis of migraine suggest that these episodes arise either on a vasomotor basis linked with various humoral factors, or from neural changes associated with a wave of electrical excitation or depression moving across the cortex. The true answer is unknown and probably involves features from both.

   The vasomotor theory proposes that the auras of classical migraine may be caused by vasoconstriction of cerebral arteries while the pain arises from vasodilatation of branches of the external carotid arteries. A fall in plasma 5-hydroxytryptamine occurs during a migraine attack, and its excretion product 5-hydroxyindole acetic acid (5HIAA) may be found in increased amounts in the urine. Serotonin is found in the platelets and it has been suggested that in the acute attack platelets may aggregate releasing serotonin. Certainly vaso-constrictor substances such as ergotamine may relieve or prevent the headache in an acute attack of migraine. Carbon dioxide inhalation, a potent cerebral vasodilator, may relieve the prodromal focal symptoms in classical migraine. Serotonin antagonists such as methysergide or pizotifen may prevent migraine.

Recent cerebral blood flow studies in classical migraine have shown an area of reduced perfusion over the hemisphere on the side opposite to focal neurological symptoms. However, this reduced perfusion lasted some 4–6 h and was not followed by increased perfusion. Furthermore, no such changes in blood flow were elicited in common migraine.

The neural theory proposes the auras arise from a wave of electrical depres-sion moving across the cortex. This was calculated by observations on the rate of spread of visual auras at about 3 mm/min, and this figure has been supported by animal experiments. Interestingly the recent cerebral blood flow studies have shown that the wave of reduced cerebral perfusion in classical migraine which starts in the occipital lobes, travels at about 2 mm/min. This suggests some link between the vascular and electrical theories although the full mechanism remains unknown.

Examination

Between migraine attacks patients should show no abnormal signs. During an acute attack patients may appear distressed, often pale, and nauseated. Occasionally they may show signs relating to their aura. In some of the compli-cated forms of migraine persistent neurological signs may remain for a time after the headache has eased. In a few rare instances migraine may be *sympto-matic* of some underlying cerebral arteriovenous malformation or vascular tumour. In such instances the patient may show persistent abnormal neurolo-gical signs, the presence of audible bruits over the skull or even a vascular birth mark. Many of these patients give a history of clearly lateralized vascular pattern headaches always occurring on the same side.

Investigations

In migraine, particularly in the first attack, and in migrainous variants some investigations may be undertaken. Tests may include those aimed at the general health of the adult patient, e.g. full blood count, erythrocyte sedimentation rate (ESR), blood glucose, urine analysis and chest X-ray, and those with a specific emphasis on the head, e.g. X-rays of the skull or sinuses. A good quality lateral skull film will show pathological calcification, or any signs of raised intracranial pressure (changes in the dorsum sellae, or in the sutures in children). It will also show if the pineal is calcified and, if so, further films can be taken to see if there is any displacement. CT brain scans may sometimes be indicated, particularly where there are clear focal features with persistent signs or the question of raised intracranial pressure is considered. In a few patients in a very acute first attack, hospital admission may prove necessary with a view to CSF examination to exclude a meningitis or subarachnoid haemorrhage. Again angiography may be indicated in patients with a persistent painful oculomotor palsy.

Treatment

In the acute attack explanation, reassurance and rest are all important. In the first attack many patients and their families are very frightened by this severe headache and even more so by any auras with focal neurological symptoms.

An appropriate dose of a simple analgesic (paracetamol, or soluble aspirin) is beneficial in the acute attack to control pain. This is made more effective if it is accompanied by a dose of metoclopramide 10 mg which will aid gastric emptying and prevent nausea. Prochlorperazine can also be used as an antiemetic. A number of studies have shown that oral preparations of analgesics are poorly absorbed in the acute phase of migraine because of gastric stasis, or are rejected by vomiting. In the adult, paracetamol 1.0 g or soluble aspirin 600–900 mg are the usual doses which can be repeated in 4 h. If these prove ineffective, mefenamic acid 250–500 mg, or naproxen 250–500 mg, may afford relief. The efficacy of these preparations can be enhanced by the prior administration of metoclopramide. In a few patients, about 1 per cent (particularly adolescent girls), metoclopramide and phenothiazines may produce an acute dystonic reaction.

There are many proprietary antimigraine preparations marketed. Many contain combinations of simple analgesics and metoclopramide, e.g. Paramax, Migravess, or simple analgesics, antihistamines and aperients, e.g. Migraleve.

Ergot derivatives, particularly ergotamine tartrate, have been used in the treatment of acute attacks for many years. Ergotamine is a potent vasoconstrictor and has proved effective in relieving attacks in about 50 per cent of patients. Oral preparations include Cafergot, Migril and Lingraine: some of these combine caffeine and an antiemetic. Ergot given by mouth is often poorly absorbed and in a proportion of patients may actually induce nausea and vomiting. To try to overcome this, ergot may be given by suppository, Cafergot, or by an aerosol inhaler, Medihaler. The other problem with protracted use of ergot is that it may produce habituation with headache appearing if the next dose is omitted. Ergot in excess may provoke vascular ischaemia in limbs and aggravate angina.

Prevention of migraine

Patients experiencing frequent attacks causing loss of time from work, school or running the home may need measures to prevent attacks of headache. It is always worth checking that there are no triggers that can be avoided with benefit, e.g. dietary, or the use of the contraceptive pill.

In a number of patients interval treatment may prove necessary. Here a preparation is taken regularly each day over a number of weeks, ideally about 12–16, to prevent the development of an attack. A variety of preparations have been used. These prove effective in about two-thirds of patients and the best include:

1. Serotonin antagonists, e.g. pizotifen, methysergide.
2. Beta-blockers, e.g. propranolol, atenolol, timolol.
3. Tricyclic antidepressants, e.g. amitriptyline, dothiepin.

Pizotifen

This can be given in a single dose at bedtime, 0.5–1.5 mg. It can also be used in children. It can be given twice daily building the dose up to 1.5 mg b.d. The main side-effects are drowsiness and weight gain.

Methysergide

This is a very potent antiserotonin agent but has the potential to produce a serious complication with prolonged usage in a small number of patients, namely retroperitoneal fibrosis. For this reason the smallest effective dose is used in a course lasting not more than 12 weeks with a break of at least 4 weeks. The starting dose is 1 mg b.d. which can be increased slowly to 2 mg t.i.d. It should be avoided in patients with any history of heart disease, renal disease or connective tissue disorders.

Propranolol

A less selective beta-blocker is highly effective in preventing migraine but needs to be given in a dose to produce blockade. In adults this is usually 80–160 mg daily. Side-effects include postural hypotension, nausea, weakness and cold extremities. It is contraindicated in patients with any history of asthma or heart failure.

Tricyclic antidepressants

These may be helpful particularly where there are emotional triggers or the patient has become depressed by the frequency of the headaches. They can be given in a single dose at bedtime e.g. amitriptyline 25–100 mg or dothiepin 25–75 mg. Lofepramine 70 mg b.d. or t.i.d. is claimed to have less anticholinergic side-effects and to be less sedating. Tricyclics may produce a dry mouth and drowsiness, and have the potential to aggravate glaucoma or urinary retention.

Clonidine in a dose of 25 μg b.d. increasing to 50–75 μg b.d. has also been used. Its action may be that of a noradrenaline agonist. It may cause a dry mouth, drowsiness or aggravate depression.

It is best to know one or two preparations well, their dose ranges, side-effects and likely duration of action.

Migrainous neuralgia

This may respond to the regular use of ergotamine. A Cafergot suppository inserted at bedtime for five successive nights can be used to prevent nocturnal attacks. The preparation is omitted on the sixth night to see if the cluster has stopped. If it has not, the five night cycle can be repeated. This will help some 70 per cent of patients. If this fails, methysergide in the lowest effective dose can be tried, but not for more than 12 weeks, or alternatively low dose lithium, 250 mg b.d. Lithium can produce tremor, gastrointestinal upset, weight gain, drowsiness and unsteadiness, although these are more common with higher doses.

Short courses of steroids have also been used in refractory cases. Nerve or ganglion injection or surgical section are measures that often prove disappointing in migrainous neuralgia.

Chronic paroxysmal hemicrania

Indomethacin is the specific treatment usually in doses of 25 mg b.d. or t.i.d. The main side-effects are gastrointestinal with indigestion, occasional dizziness, light-headed sensations and headache.

13

Head injury

Head injury is a common cause for admission to hospital with between 200 and 300/100 000 of the population being admitted each year in the UK. The young are affected more and men more than women. Most patients stay in hospital for less than 48 h. In the UK the majority of these patients will be seen and treated at the hospital where they were first admitted with only 3–4 per cent of head-injured patients being admitted into neurosurgical units. One half of all admitted head-injured patients will have sustained the injury in a road traffic accident and 50 per cent of all unconscious head-injured patients will have major additional injuries, particularly those involved in car accidents. The care of the head-injured patient is therefore linked inextricably with the management of multiple injuries, so that in considering the pathophysiology of head injury many systemic processes influence the management of these patients.

Local effects of head injury

There is the local effect of injury to the head, causing bruising or a laceration of the scalp, possibly producing a fracture of the skull which may be linear, basal or depressed. The dura may be torn and the brain contused and/or lacerated with associated haemorrhage. The initial impact produces a rise in intracranial pressure. The effect of this may be mild, producing temporary loss of consciousness, mild elevation of arterial pressure, suppression of the EEG and a few moments of apnoea. This relatively mild injury produces no visible brain damage, although the patient may be concussed. Concussion is a word commonly applied to a minor head injury, it is difficult to explain and probably is mainly due to brainstem dysfunction. Importantly, it is followed by a complete recovery.

More severe injuries will produce prolonged unconsciousness, severe elevation of blood pressure, persistence of apnoea with death occurring unless artificial ventilation is undertaken. These brains show evidence of subarachnoid haemorrhage and petechial haemorrhages in the brainstem.

Yet more severe injury will produce unconsciousness, pupillary dilatation, a massive rise in intracranial pressure, hypotension and rapid death. The pathology of the brains shows subarachnoid haemorrhage, blood in the basal cisterns and extensive brainstem haemorrhage.

Injury to the brain

The mechanical factors affecting the brain in injury are a mixture of flexion, extension and sideways motion with or without rotation. Basically three types of injury occur: diffuse axonal injury, polar injury and the shearing of bridging veins.

Diffuse axonal injury with the division of axons in the white matter of the cerebral hemispheres leads to unconsciousness, bilateral decerebrate posturing with a possibility of a permanent vegetative state. The distorting forces may affect the intracerebral vessels leading to the occurrence of small petechial haemorrhages.

Polar injuries affect the tips of the temporal lobes and undersurface of the frontal lobes and are a result of a mixture of a vertical and rotational movement. These areas may be contused or lacerated and, although obvious, do not affect neurological function initially. Later they may be associated with swelling which, because of space occupation, may lead to a rise in intracranial pressure.

These distortional forces may damage the bridging veins particularly those from the cerebral hemispheres to the sagittal and transverse sinuses leading to haemorrhages and haematoma formation.

Intracranial haematomas can be an early sequelae of head injuries and occur in some 3 per cent of all admitted head-injured patients. They are seen in 40 per cent of all unconscious head-injured patients.

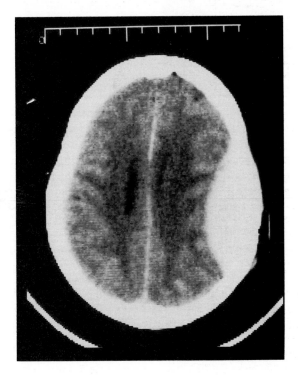

Fig. 13.1.   CT scan to show extradural haematoma

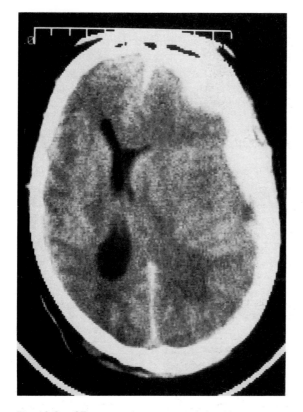

Fig. 13.2. CT scan to show acute subdural haematoma. Note the extensive shift

Extradural haematoma (Fig. 13.1) is a clot occurring between the skull and the dura as a result of a mild injury. It is a rare complication with only 0.5 per cent of head-injured patients admitted to hospital developing the condition. Commonly, because the injury is mild, early surgical removal of the haematoma should result in a neurologically intact patient.

Acute subdural haematomas (Fig. 13.2) are twice as common as extradural haematomas but carry a mortality rate that is twice as high. The reason for this is the association of acute subdural haematoma with severe underlying brain damage and rapid brain compression. A violent impact may produce such severe damage and haemorrhage that the patient is unconscious from the outset, rapidly developing the signs of brainstem compression and dying within 12 h. Occasionally the pattern of compression develops more slowly, although even with surgical intervention the mortality in this group remains between 70–75 per cent. A good recovery is rare and occurs mostly in young patients.

Chronic subdural haematoma (Fig. 13.3) is seen in the older age group and as the cause is usually a relatively minor injury and the progress of the complication slow, with treatment, the prognosis is good.

Intracerebral haematomas (Fig. 13.4) may result from penetrating injuries or be

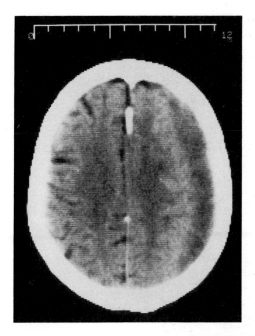

Fig. 13.3.   CT scan to show a chronic subdural haematoma. There is an absence of cortical sulci on the affected side, and a low density 'rim'

related to cerebral contusions. Successive CT scans show that after 48–72 h these haematomas are usually surrounded by an area of oedema. This is probably due to post-traumatic ischaemic brain damage. Intracerebral haematomas are associated with increased intracranial pressure, focal neurological deficit and an increased incidence of severely disabled patients.

Intracranial pressure and head injury

The normal range of intracranial pressure (ICP) is between 0 and 10 mmHg and raised intracranial pressure is regarded as being a measurement of more than 20 mmHg for longer than one minute. Raised ICP in the head-injured patient is associated with increased mortality. Patients whose ICP remains between 0–20 mmHg have a mortality rate of 23 per cent, while those whose pressure rises above 60 mmHg have 100 per cent mortality. A rising ICP is invariably accompanied by a decreasing level of consciousness and increasing neurological signs.

Continuing high ICP 24–72 h post-injury signifies the occurrence of brain oedema. The oedema is due to accumulation of water and is vasogenic, largely affecting the white matter. The endothelial cells of the cerebral vessels are responsible for the blood–brain barrier which normally prevents the passage of large molecules from the vascular compartment to the extracellular space. With brain trauma the tight junctions between the cells are affected and large molecules such as proteins along with electrolytes and fluid pass into the extracellular

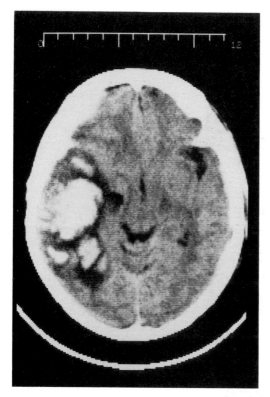

Fig. 13.4.   CT scan to show an extensive intracerebral haematoma. The blood shows as high density

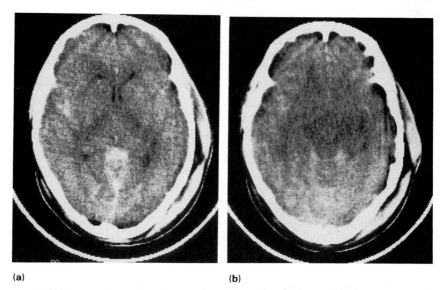

(a)   (b)

Fig. 13.5.   CT scan to show acute brain swelling. Note in **(a)** the small ventricles, and in **(b)** the obliteration of the basal cisterns

space. After head injury, oedema is usually found focally with contusions and haematomas, although, occasionally, it may spread throughout one or both hemispheres (Fig. 13.5). The oedema can produce a rise in ICP either locally or generally which then reduces cerebral blood flow.

Expanding lesions in head-injured patients produce a well established sequence of events. The ventricle on the side of the expanding lesion becomes

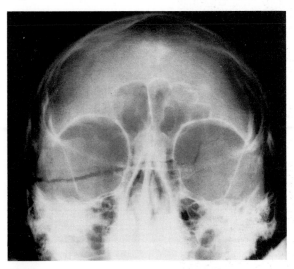

(a)

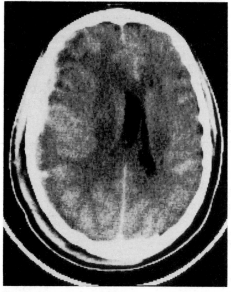

(b)

Fig. 13.6. (a) Skull X-ray showing an extensive fracture of the occipital bone seen through the orbit. (b) CT scan in the same patient showing contusion and swelling with ventricular shift

smaller. CT scans show a disappearance of the subarachnoid space in the supratentorial compartment and crowding of the brainstem in the tentorial hiatus occurs (Fig. 13.6). Central areas of the brain are pushed in a downward axial direction towards the foramen magnum. A mass in the temporal area causes displacement of the temporal lobe medially stretching and distorting the third nerve so producing a dilated pupil on the side of the lesion. Compression of the midbrain produces ischaemia of central areas leading to loss of consciousness and increasing neurological signs.

Cerebral blood flow and head injury

The brain receives about 15 per cent of the cardiac output. This produces a flow of around 800 ml/min of blood through the brain. There is a close relationship between cerebral metabolism and cerebral blood flow (CBF) while variations in regional CBF are due to the different functions of various parts of the brain. CBF is affected by arterial PO_2; an arterial PO_2 of below 50 mmHg produces an increase in CBF.

Variations in arterial P_aCO_2 can cause marked changes in CBF because CO_2 is a very potent vasodilator. If the P_aCO_2 is increased above 40 mmHg, CBF increases while it falls if the P_aCO_2 drops below 30 mmHg. The maintenance of CBF in response to various changes has been termed autoregulation and this may be impaired in ischaemia, hypoxia and brain trauma. Thus with trauma, an increase in intracranial pressure may cause the cerebral perfusion to fall.

Hypoxia is the most common early systemic disturbance. Immediately after an injury producing unconsciousness, the patient is pale, pulseless and apnoeic. With the return of spontaneous ventilation there is always patchy atelectasis of the lungs because of the failure of the alveoli to expand. The normal reflexes guarding the airway are impaired. If the trauma involves the brainstem then there will be abnormalities in rate, rhythm and adequacy of ventilation. Commonly, hyperventilation occurs with a fall in the P_aCO_2 and an associated respiratory alkalosis. In more than 75 per cent of unconscious head-injured patients the alveolar arterial gradients of O_2 tension are higher than normal so that the low arterial PO_2 is not simply due to diminished ventilation but also to abnormal ventilation – perfusion relations in the lung. The P_aCO_2 may sometimes rise producing an increase in intracranial pressure.

Arterial hypotension is usually due to hypovolaemia, so a fall in blood pressure suggests blood loss, perhaps from other injuries. In the unconscious head-injured patient a fall in blood pressure is invariably due to blood loss and will result in a fall of cardiac output and central venous pressure. Extremities are usually cold and clammy and the patient requires immediate transfusion.

Acute assessment and management

1. First aid.
2. Level of response.
3. History.
4. Clinical examination.

5. Investigation.
6. Care on the ward.

While immediate measures such as clearing an airway, stopping haemorrhage and dealing with surgical shock may be necessary in some cases, in many the condition of the patient will be good enough for a full examination to be completed on arrival in the Accident and Emergency Department. Priorities will vary from one patient to another and may alter in the individual patient depending upon the pace and change in the pathology.

1. First aid

A clear airway

A clear airway is essential at all times in the ambulance, in the emergency room, diagnostic department, intensive care unit and ward. The airway must be protected at all times in an unconscious patient. Initially this can best be done by attention to posture. The unconscious patient should be placed on his side with the head lower than the trunk allowing secretions to drain from the mouth. Twisting of the neck is to be avoided. The mouth and pharynx should be cleared of debris (using a finger if necessary). A pharyngeal airway should be inserted and the pharynx cleared by suction. If the cough and swallowing reflexes have been depressed or lost, provided that the procedure can be performed efficiently, a cuffed endotracheal tube should be inserted so that the trachea can be cleared by suction. Intubating head-injured patients can be difficult and should only be undertaken by experienced doctors. Following intubation, the chest must be auscultated to ensure equal air entry on both sides and the patients should have a chest X-ray to determine the level of the lower end of the endotracheal tube. Emergency tracheostomy has very little part to play in the management at this stage. A tracheostomy may be required later in the patient needing intubation for more than 14 days and in unconscious patients whose fractured jaws need splinting.

Haemorrhage

Any severe external haemorrhage should now be controlled: a pad and a firm bandage will usually stop a bleeding scalp wound. Branches of the supraorbital, temporal and occipital arteries may be clamped temporarily with a haemostat but, by far the best method is to suture the wound immediately. Penetrating wounds may cause severe haemorrhage if the sagittal or lateral venous sinuses are torn and this will be shown by the position of the wound and the colour of the blood. Elevating the patient's head and using a pad and bandage is usually sufficient to obtain control. A picture of pallor, low blood pressure and rapid pulse implying blood loss should never be attributed to the head injury. The restoration of the blood pressure takes precedence over the head injury and in these patients the abdomen, chest, pelvis and legs should be carefully examined. The observation of intra-abdominal haemorrhage is difficult in an unconscious patient because of the absence of rigidity or guarding. Signs such as superficial abdominal bruising, evidence of free fluid, absence of bowel sounds and increasing girth are useful, but in some cases intra-abdominal diagnostic peritoneal lavage may be necessary. Immediate and vigorous treatment of major thoracic or abdominal injuries requiring resuscitation and surgical action is the rule here, irrespective of the patient's state of consciousness. The emphasis must be on the restoration of adequate ventilation of the lungs and restoration of adequate circulation. In these circumstances the head injury has a lower priority but certain key points need to be remembered. First, the head injury should be assessed immediately before and after the anaesthetic. Second, premedication with drugs that depress consciousness or affect pupillary reaction should be avoided. Third, the anaesthetic should be as light and as short as possible and finally there should be no straining and no period of anoxia.

2. Level of response

The most important observation is the accurate assessment and recording of the level of consciousness. This must be simple, rapid, effective and understood by medical and nursing staff. Many problems arise from the use of vague terms such as semiconscious, stuporosed or comatosed, which fail to convey the exact clinical state of the patient. Unfortunately many hospitals have a variety of charts which fail to give a picture of the patient's progress. A clear and effective way of determining patients level of response is *the Glasgow coma scale* (*see* Table 3.6). Three features are independently observed: eye opening, verbal performance and motor response.

Using such a system an accurate base line of the patient's condition can be recorded so that subsequent observations will show the patient's progress.

3. History

Valuable information can be obtained by questioning anyone who arrives with the patient. Time, place and type of injury are essential pieces of information. Was the patient unconscious from the time of injury? Has the patient's level of consciousness changed since the injury? Has the patient had a convulsion? Was he found some distance from the vehicle? (those who have been thrown from cars or motor cycles or into the air often have neck injuries). All this information should be clearly and concisely recorded, thus providing valuable evidence of the clinical state as soon as possible after the injury. Any subsequent change in the patient's condition can be noted and assessed rapidly if there is adequate information on admission.

4. Clinical examination

Full examination of the patient often has to be delayed until the immediate threats to life have been countered and until the patient is fit for a possibly lengthy and disturbing undressing process in preparation for a thorough and complete examination.

Level of response

This should now be reassessed.

Pupils

The vital sign that an ipsilateral dilating pupil indicates rising intracranial pressure from a compressing supratentorial lesion, is well known: the important initial observation of equal reacting pupils before such dilatation, tends to be forgotten. Unilateral dilatation may be caused by direct injury to the eye, optic nerve damage or oculomotor nerve compression. If a head-injured patient is admitted with equal, reacting pupils and then develops dilatation of a pupil (provided there is also evidence of a deterioration in the level of response), a compressing extracerebral haematoma may be incriminated. Direct injury to the third nerve is the usual cause of a unilateral dilated pupil immediately following head injury. In these circumstances the pupil is likely to be dilated and unreacting to a bright torch from the moment of injury. If a dilated pupil does not react, either directly or consensually, then oculomotor nerve damage is the cause; if the pupil reacts consensually there is an optic nerve lesion. Ideally, the eyes should be examined before the lids swell; nevertheless, with due care and some assistance, the pupils can still be seen adequately, even in a restless patient with swollen eyelids. On no account must atropine be used to dilate the pupils to look for papilloedema.

Motor function

The examination of the limbs should be simple, rapid and should concentrate on movement of the limbs, either spontaneous or in response to stimulation. Tendon reflexes and plantar responses are of little value in the initial assessment of a head injury.

Weakness may be demonstrated relatively easily in an unconscious patient. A restless patient will show a discrepancy in the movements between the two sides, and painful stimuli may further emphasize this.

Severe weakness of one upper limb, with no involvement at all of the lower limb on that side, may indicate a brachial plexus lesion. Absence of movement, either spontaneous or on painful stimulation of either lower limb, while there is movement in both upper limbs, strongly suggests a spinal lesion.

Hemiparesis is usually attributable to direct injury to the cerebral hemispheres. If it is accompanied by a deteriorating level of response, with or without a dilating pupil, such hemiparesis may be caused by a compressing extracerebral haematoma. However, in such a case, the hemiparesis may be a false lateralizing sign following displacement of the cerebral hemisphere and midbrain, which are compressed against the free edge of the tentorium on the side opposite that of the compressing supratentorial haematoma. This will produce hemiparesis on the same side as the haematoma.

Other vital functions

The pulse, blood pressure, the rate and character of the breathing, and the temperature must all be noted. Progressive slowing of the pulse, a rising blood pressure and slowing of the respiratory rate are classic indicators of rising intracranial pressure. It is important to realize that these signs occur long after a deterioration in the level of consciousness and, when present with a compressing extracerebral haematoma, are signs of impending death. Slowing of the pulse is the first of these three signs, while respiratory slowing comes towards the end. The pulse rate in the head-injured patient is variable; the blood pressure may be normal or high; but the essential point is to note any change in these characteristics. Low blood pressure is usually due to surgical shock, although it may occur in terminal medullary failure. The one other exception is in an infant, where an extracerebral haematoma may produce a relative decrease in the circulating blood volume, leading to the signs of surgical shock. The temperature may be high, either because of blood in the subarachnoid space or following a hypothalamic disturbance; hyperpyrexia may occur very occasionally. In surgical shock the temperature may be low.

The head and face

First note any areas of bruising, laceration and swelling as these may help to lateralize and localize an ensuing extracerebral haematoma. Unless haemorrhage required attention earlier, wounds should be dealt with after a full examination and skull radiography. Epistaxis may indicate a fracture of the anterior cranial fossa floor and there may be associated subconjunctival haemorrhage, while bleeding from the ear is usually indicative of a fractured petrous bone. In these circumstances the use of an auroscope is unhelpful and may introduce infection. A bruise may become apparent, 24–48 h later, over the mastoid process. This is Battle's sign, which is confirmation of a fracture involving the petrous bone. Leakage of CSF, with rhinorrhoea and/or otorrhoea, suggests not only a fracture of the base of the skull but also a tear of the overlying dura. Meningitis is a possible consequence of this injury.

Head injury and maxillofacial injuries often occur together. Fractures of the mandible may be obvious because of swelling over the lower jaw, defects of occlusion, and malalignment. Although definitive care of facial and lower-jaw fractures can usually be delayed, particular attention must be paid to the airway.

Spinal injury

In the conscious patient, pain and stiffness of the neck should arouse suspicion: in the unconscious patient, unless there is a gross neurological deficit, a spinal cord injury will be difficult to detect. The danger of aggravating a spinal injury can be reduced by avoiding flexion of the patient: all parts of the body should be moved in a line. By turning the patient on to one side (log rolling), the contour of the spine can be inspected and each spinous process can be palpated. Detection of a cervical fracture-dislocation is extremely difficult. However, in the thoracic region, the presence of kyphos or a step-like configuration of the spinous processes is a clear indication of underlying damage. Certain other features may give a lead. If the spinal cord lesion is complete, there may be an absence of sweating up to that level and there may be a palpable bladder suggesting retention of urine, an unusual event after a head injury. However, it must be emphasized that even careful clinical examination of the fully conscious patient may give no clinical hint of fractures of the spine. It is, therefore, essential to radiograph at least the cervical spine in all severely head-injured patients.

Fractured limbs

In many cases of major head injury, provided that there is no real threat to life or limb, it is reasonable to delay treatment of limb fractures for hours or, in some cases, for days, while the condition of the patient is observed. A compound limb fracture will need early attention. However, provided that the patient's condition has been fully assessed and an anaesthetic is given carefully, there should be no detrimental effect to the head injury.

Alcohol

Alcohol and head injury are a common combination. The complexity of assessing and managing head injuries is increased when the patient has recently been drinking alcohol. The important guiding principle is never to assume that the level of consciousness, or a deterioration in the level of response, is caused by alcohol intoxication. Ignore the alcohol and treat the case in the usual way. Alcoholics tend to develop subdural haematomas; remember this when assessing a known alcoholic who has sustained a head injury.

5. Investigations

Blood samples are necessary for haemoglobin, blood gases, grouping and cross-matching. Urine should be analysed to exclude diabetes mellitus and also to assess haematuria. X-rays of the skull should be of good quality but unfortunately many such patients are restless, making this difficult. Lateral, antero-posterior and Towne's views should be taken but not basal views as the latter could damage the cervical cord if there was an unsuspected unstable cervical fracture. In severe injuries, X-rays of the cervical spine should be included.

Computerized tomography (CT) scanning has made a difference to the management of the head-injured patient as it will clearly show an intracranial haematoma, as seen in the illustrations. Unfortunately in the UK there are few scanners and in most district hospitals observations and plain X-rays are all that are available, so there has to be careful selection of patients for transfer to specialized centres.

6. The care on the ward

Before considering certain specific sequelae of head injury two essentials of the care of these patients should be emphasized. The most essential treatment of the severely head-injured patient is the detection, prevention and cure of life-threatening airway obstruction and haemorrhage. The second essential is to assess and observe the patient continuously, remembering that while surgery is rarely needed, the indications for such intervention are clear and concise.

It is important to realize that a straightforward diagnosis is not possible with a head-injured patient. Doctors and nurses have to cope with a developing process that is continuous from the moment of admission. The majority of patients are managed conservatively with detailed observations and scrupulous nursing care. Very few patients require surgery. In the UK a neurosurgical consultative system is readily available for discussion of difficult problems. Clinicians need to decide whether observations should continue, whether the patient should be transferred to a neurosurgical unit or whether, because of the patient's rapid downhill course, an operation should be performed immediately and locally. While the surgical techniques are not difficult and can be acquired by any competent surgeon, the problem lies in the correct interpretation of the clinical picture and the exact positioning of the burr holes. The CT scanner does solve this difficulty but, unfortunately, it is not available in many Accident and Emergency Departments.

Continuous observation with regular charting of the patient's clinical state, level of response, pupil size and reaction, pulse, blood pressure and temperature is mandatory. An unconscious patient requires particular care of the airway, physiotherapy, regular turning, care of the skin, bladder and bowels, meticulous fluid balance charts and adequate calorie intake. Careful observation and charting should enable the medical and nursing staff to decide whether a patient's condition is improving, static or deteriorating. An accurately completed, clear, simple chart is desirable but, unless deterioration can be recognized and appropriate action taken, obsessive recording of vital signs is valueless.

A deteriorating clinical state may be caused by several well-recognized complications. The most significant sign of deterioration is depression of the level of consciousness; when this occurs, the medical team must seek the cause.

Respiratory obstruction

This is the commonest cause of deterioration. The position of the patient needs to be checked. Blood gas analysis and the chest X-ray may help to determine the type of treatment necessary (physiotherapy, bronchoscopy) and the effectiveness of that treatment.

Epilepsy

This occurs in about 5 per cent of head-injured patients, more commonly in children, and at any stage after a head injury. The cardinal feature is a sudden deterioration in the level of consciousness, with or without convulsions, for convulsions may often go unobserved. Some recovery in the level of consciousness usually occurs shortly after the episode; however, a fit may be caused by an extracerebral haematoma, in which case the patient's condition will continue to deteriorate. If recovery is not rapid, it is therefore safer to assume that a compressing haematoma is present.

Patient's at risk – severely injured patients and those with depressed fractures, penetrating injuries and intracranial haematomas – should be given prophylactic anticonvulsive therapy, such as phenobarbitone (30 mg 8-hourly) or phenytoin (50–100 mg, 8-hourly).

Meningitis

Pyogenic meningitis usually develops within the first week after a head injury, most commonly following a fracture of the base of the skull with an associated dural tear. The symptoms of headache, stiff neck and pyrexia herald this complication. Meningitis will cause a deterioration in the clinical state of the patient, and must be recognized and treated immediately. The diagnosis should be confirmed by lumbar puncture and appropriate antibiotic therapy started.

Fat embolism

This relatively rare complication occurs within 72 h of injury. Major limb or pelvic fractures are usually present and the condition often follows corrective manipulation. The level of consciousness may deteriorate before the appearance of the characteristic petechial haemorrhages in the axillae, around the shoulders, thorax and abdomen. The classic signs of tachypnoea, tachycardia and fever suggest the diagnosis. If hypoxia occurs, the patient must be ventilated.

Intracranial haemorrhage – extradural haematoma

This most feared and rare complication typically occurs after a mild injury. More than one-half of the patients with this complication are under the age of 20, and it is a rare condition over the age of 40. It is also rare before the age of 2, when trauma tends to indent the pliable skull and dura together so damage tends to occur to the brain, and haematomas are subdural. In an adult the blow causes the dura to become separated from the skull immediately below the point of impact and this is where the clot forms. The bleeding may be arterial or venous, and not necessarily from the middle meningeal artery. It should be considered if there is a deterioration in the level of consciousness which is not attributable to the common causes mentioned previously. Again, the single most important indication is a deterioration in the level of consciousness. To wait for the classic textbook description of unilateral dilated pupil, hemiparesis, slowing of the pulse and a rising blood pressure is to accept a morbidity and mortality of 50 per cent. Restlessness is usually due to a full bladder but increasing restlessness is often an additional sign of an evolving haematoma.

While the observation that extradural haematomas 'should be dealt with at the hospital where the condition is diagnosed and as soon as it is diagnosed' is the ideal solution, certain questions must be answered. On which side of the head should the burr holes be made? Where should the burr holes be made? Recently, it has been reported that, for a successful outcome, the haematoma must be removed within 2 h of the first sign of deterioration, an event which will vary from one patient to another. Nevertheless, in the UK there should be time for neurosurgical consultation.

If the pupil is not dilated, a fracture shown on X-ray (Fig. 13.7) or bruising

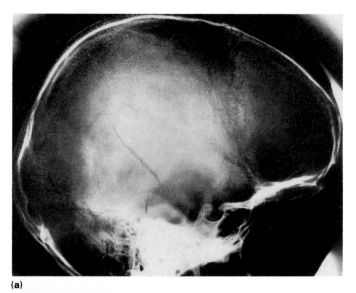

(a)

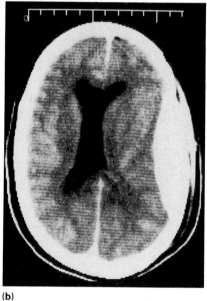

(b)

Fig. 13.7. (a) Lateral skull X-ray showing a fracture of the temporal bone. (b) CT scan in the same patient showing an extradural haematoma

and oedema of the scalp, will indicate the side to place the burr hole. Bruising is often apparent only after the scalp has been shaved. The burr hole should be placed over the midpoint of the fracture, or in the centre of the area of bruising and swelling if no fracture is present. If there is neither fracture nor evidence of scalp trauma, then the burr hole should be made in the 'standard' position. This is midway between the external canthus and the external auditory meatus and immediately above the zygomatic arch. If this burr hole is negative, a second may be placed above the ear in the posteroparietal region. It is not within the scope of this chapter to describe the surgical techniques involved.

If the exploratory burr holes do not reveal an extradural haematoma, then it is probably wiser for the general or orthopaedic surgeon not to open the dura. If the dura is blue and bulging, indicating a subdural haematoma, the best course of action would be to consult a neurosurgeon again and to transfer the patient to a neurosurgical unit.

Acute subdural haematomas are relatively common, ocurring at any age following high speed and severe impact injuries, tend to be sited low in the frontotemporal region and carry a poor prognosis.

Chronic subdural haematoma

Only 50 per cent of adults with chronic subdural haematoma give a history of trauma and the injury has usually been a mild one. In patients without a history of preceding trauma there may be an identifiable cause such as a vascular lesion, haemorrhagic disease or the patient may have been on anticoagulants. Factors such as cerebral atrophy, alcoholism and epilepsy predispose to the formation of subdural haematoma. Chronic subdural haematoma tends to occur in older people over the age of 50 with a greater number of males being affected. Most

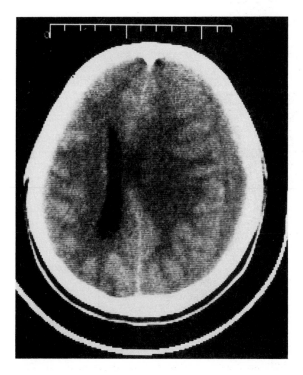

Fig. 13.8. CT scan to show an isodense subdural haematoma

haematomas are in the parietal area and the vast majority are unilateral. Headache is the most frequent and non-specific symptom with personality disorder, paresis and impairment of consciousness occurring frequently. While it is emphasized that major fluctuations in consciousness and neurological signs are characteristic features in chronic subdural haematomas, these only occur in one-third of the cases.

When there is a history of preceding injury there is generally a delay of 1–2 months between injury and symptom and often the injury is so trivial that the patient or their relatives fail to remember it. It is a difficult diagnosis to make on clinical grounds as the presenting features can mimic a variety of other conditions such as psychiatric illness, brain tumour and cerebrovascular disease.

A skull X-ray may show a displaced calcified pineal gland and an isotope brain scan in the majority of cases will show an abnormality localized to the site of the haematoma. Increased uptake is usually easy to detect when the haematoma is unilateral. The CT scan demonstrates the subdural haematoma as an area of low density on the outside of the brain and gives information about the site and size of the haematoma as well as the amount of midline shift. However, there are subdural collections that are isodense with the brain (Fig. 13.8) and this can produce diagnostic difficulties if the subdural is bilateral.

The haematomas usually drain through one or two burr holes, although in a few cases, if the haematoma is clotted or multilocular, a craniotomy may be required.

Special complications

Cerebrospinal (CSF) rhinorrhoea and otorrhoea

Cerebrospinal rhinorrhoea is the more frequent of these two complications; neither usually persists for longer than a week. Cerebrospinal fluid is differentiated from nasal secretion by the presence of sugar and the absence of eosinophils.

Conscious patients should be nursed with the head raised, thus reducing the CSF pressure and they should be warned not to blow their nose because of the possibility of introducing infection. Prophylactic antibiotics should be given until the leak stops. Sulphadimidine (0.5 g, 6-hourly) is the drug of choice as it readily crosses the blood–CSF barrier.

Occasionally, cerebrospinal rhinorrhoea is associated with fractures of the middle third of the face: correction of these fractures frequently stops the flow of CSF.

Indications for the transfer of patients for possible neurosurgical intervention are persistent (for over one week) or recurrent CSF leak, and the occurrence of meningitis.

Traumatic aerocele

Air very occasionally enters the cranial cavity after fractures of the base of the skull, and may be associated with rhinorrhoea. The air will be visible on skull radiographs, particularly in brow-up lateral views, which is one of the important reasons for taking a horizontal ray lateral radiograph. The air may be subarachnoid, subdural, in ventricles or as an aerocele in the brain itself. Patients with large amounts of air in the ventricles or frontally should be referred to a neurosurgical department for a dural repair when they are sufficiently recovered, as the situation is not urgent. Very occasionally a frontal aerocele may cause gradual clinical deterioration by increasing intracranial pressure and surgery will be required urgently.

Post-concussional syndrome

After a head injury many patients complain of a variety of symptoms often over a longer period of time. Headache and dizziness are the most common, but other symptoms such as lack of concentration, impairment of memory, fatigue, irritability and depression are also frequent. A number of factors may produce this syndrome and there is no single aetiological mechanism. In most patients the post-concussional symptoms have both organic and psychological causes. Headache and dizziness tend to decline in incidence over a period of time although both may still be present up to 2 years following a relatively minor injury. Impairment of concentration and memory, irritability and fatigue tend to fluctuate over the months following a head injury and very often become more prominent as time progresses. Depression is a symptom which is psychological in origin, occurring when there is no suggestion of structural damage to skull or brain. Indeed, many of the symptoms which are grouped together under the general heading of post-concussional syndrome can be ascribed to a true reactive depression.

Some of these symptoms have been ascribed to malingering. While true conscious malingering for financial or other personal gain does occur, it is a rare phenomenon. It is important that, when faced with a patient who has had a head injury and is complaining of post-concussional symptoms, each symptom should be assessed and carefully analysed with particular reference to the time of its onset in relation to the injury. A sympathetic and understanding approach may help the patient to cope with what can be a most distressing sequel of head injury.

Post-traumatic epilepsy

Post-traumatic epilepsy may be early, occurring in the first week after a head injury and this happens in 5 per cent of closed head injuries. Later epilepsy occurring after the first week following injury also occurs in about 5 per cent of all head-injured patients admitted to hospital after non-missile injuries. Early fits are more commonly focal, although temporal lobe attacks in the first week after injury are uncommon. Patients who have early epilepsy, those who have been unconscious for more than 24 hours, patients with acute intracranial haematomas and those with depressed fractures, all have an increased risk of late epilepsy. Risk of late epilepsy after a depressed fracture is not dependent on the site of the fracture nor whether or not the fracture is elevated if the dura is torn. If focal neurological signs are present, if loss of consciousness exceeds 24 h, or if there has been early epilepsy then the risk of late epilepsy is increased.

Electroencephalographic (EEG) abnormalities are likely to be present in those patients who have suffered severe brain damage and these patients are more prone to epilepsy. The EEG changes become less apparent with time, but this change is not a particularly useful prognostic indicator. It should also be noted that around 20 per cent of patients who subsequently develop late epilepsy have a normal EEG in the early stages after injury.

Children are different when compared with adults with regard to the occurrence of post-traumatic epilepsy. Early fits are more common in children and occur with milder injuries, particularly when the child is under the age of 5. Children under the age of 16 are less liable to develop late epilepsy after depressed fractures than are adults. In addition, it has been suggested that late epilepsy may develop after a longer interval in children than in adults.

Anticonvulsant therapy is to be recommended in patients with a high risk of late epilepsy. It is felt that the benefit of anticonvulsant therapy may be due to the prevention of the development of an epileptic focus rather than the suppression of epileptic activity. The treatment should therefore be started as soon after the injury as possible, ensuring that adequate blood levels of the anticonvulsant are obtained within the first 24 hours. Oral dosage should then be substituted as soon as possible and an attempt made to maintain this for one year. While it should be recognized that such treatment may reduce the incidence of early epilepsy it can never be completely successful; many of the fits occur in the first hour or so after injury. The implications of post-traumatic epilepsy do not differ from those of epilepsy in general; the most serious, of course, being the socioeconomic consequences.

Admission to hospital

Which head-injured patient should be admitted to hospital? This difficult question, of course, applies only to those with mild head injuries. Recent guidelines have been produced. Briefly, many mildly head-injured patients can go home provided they are accompanied by a responsible person. Detailed instructions to the responsible person on the timing of observations, the changes to be looked for, and with clear directions on what to do if changes occur are mandatory. The following should stay in hospital.

1. Patients who cannot remember the incident and those who have a skull fracture.
2. Patients with residual symptoms (headache, drowsiness, vomiting) and those with neurological signs.
3. Children, particularly if the parents are worried, for they are much more difficult to assess than adults.

14

Raised intracranial pressure

Because the skull is not compressible, except in young children, raised intra-cranial pressure (ICP) produces a somewhat unusual and unique pathophysio-logical process. When assessing what may occur to a patient when such a process takes place it is necessary to consider two broad aspects: (1) the symptoms and signs, and (2) the various shifts and herniations that may occur within the cranium (*see* p. 293).

Symptoms and signs

1. Headaches

The cardinal symptom is headache: this may have an explosive onset, as in the case of an intracranial haemorrhage, or if there is a sudden rise in ICP, e.g. due to acute hydrocephalus. Alternatively, a slowly progressive but, nevertheless, inexorable increasing headache may occur, e.g. from the growth of a tumour. The headaches of raised ICP usually take the pattern of being worse in the morning and gradually regressing as the day goes on; inevitably, as the ICP rises, this diurnal pattern may disappear and the headaches will be more or less constant. The headaches may worsen on coughing, straining or when there is a sudden change in posture; the sudden increase of the symptoms may sometimes make the patient scream with the pain. Occasionally these very acute crescendo headaches may be associated with visual symptoms including transient loss of vision referred to as visual obscurations or amblyopic attacks. Although not common, there are occasions when the headaches may localize the site of the lesion: they may be unilateral with a supratentorial tumour or occur in the occipital and upper cervical regions in the presence of a posterior fossa tumour.

2. Vomiting

Nausea and vomiting are commonly associated with headache. Sometimes vomiting may occur in the absence of nausea: it then is often effortless and may even be projectile, and may be present with little, if any, headache. If vomiting is the dominant symptom it may arise from a lesion in the floor of the fourth ventricle. Vomiting, when associated with headache, may be particularly distressing for the patient since the act of vomiting will increase the ICP and worsen the headache.

3. Impairment of consciousness

This implies a serious rise in ICP and so tends to occur as the stage of decompensation is reached. Deep coma may occur early in the presence of an intracranial haematoma. Acute hydrocephalus may produce a sudden crescendo headache which may lead to loss of consciousness: this on occasions may be associated with acute loss of lower limb function. The mechanism of impaired conscious level relates to the degree of transtentorial herniation with consequent pressure on the midbrain. The introduction of the Glasgow coma scale (*see* p. 93) helps to assess the conscious level.

4. Visual disturbances

Impaired acuity and visual obscurations have already been mentioned. The well-known sign of papilloedema as a manifestation of raised ICP should not need to be stressed. However, what does need to be emphasized is the fact that papilloedema may be absent in the presence of a large intracranial mass: indeed less than 50 per cent of adults with intracranial tumours have any papilloedema, although the incidence in children is higher. The specific reason why some patients develop disc swelling while others do not is unclear. The crucial message for the clinician is to realize that raised ICP must not be discarded as a diagnosis simply because the discs are flat. If papilloedema is allowed to worsen there will eventually be a progressive decline in visual acuity and even blindness. Because the pupillary responses are so important as part of the assessment of patients with raised ICP, the pupils should not be dilated in order to inspect the fundi. Rarely the visual acuity may decline with hydrocephalus in the absence of papilloedema, and here the dilated third ventricle may directly exert pressure on the optic nerves and chiasm.

Diplopia usually results from an abducens nerve palsy producing paresis of the lateral rectus muscle. This sign is a false localizing one in that it is rarely related to a specific anatomical lesion within the cranium. In contrast, an oculomotor nerve palsy is frequently localizing in that it almost always occurs on the same side as the supratentorial mass producing the raised ICP, and indeed this is one of the characteristic features of transtentorial (uncal) herniation.

5. Other focal signs

There are some focal neurological signs which relate to the mass lesion that has produced the raised ICP. A homonymous hemianopia points to a lesion occupying the posterior half of the hemisphere; the classical superior quadrantic homonymous hemianopia suggests a temporal lobe lesion and the inferior quadrantic homonymous hemianopia a parietal lobe lesion (*see* Fig. 3.1). It is unusual for extracerebral lesions to produce such a field defect, although this does occasionally occur. A hemiparesis or hemiplegia may frequently arise from masses in the supratentorial compartment, especially in the posterior frontal or frontoparietal regions. Hemisensory signs will tend to be produced with lesions arising in the parietal area. Although a hemiparesis or hemiplegia will usually be opposite to the side of a mass lesion, there are occasions when the signs will be on the same side as the lesion that has produced them. This neurological contradiction usually relates to a particular displacement of the midbrain and is explained in the next section.

Shifts and herniations

The intracerebral compartments are separated by dural sheets and the tentorium separates the cerebral hemispheres from the cerebellar hemispheres laterally and the medulla and pons in the midline. The midbrain straddles the tentorial hiatus. The part of the hemisphere that is adjacent to the tentorial edge is the medial part of the temporal lobe, the uncus anteriorly and the hippocampus posteriorly. The blood supply to these medial temporal structures comes from the posterior cerebral arteries. There are three main patterns of shifts or herniations: subfalcine, transtentorial (uncal), and foramen magnum (tonsillar).

1. Subfalcine herniation or cone

Part of one hemisphere is shifted under the falx towards the opposite side (Fig. 14.1). This usually results in an altered conscious level and this merges with transtentorial herniation which commonly follows. Focal signs may be absent.

2. Transtentorial (uncal) herniation or cone

This is the commonest form of coning. The medial temporal structures that pass through the tentorial hiatus will inevitably press upon the oculomotor nerve, as this runs along the free edge of the tentorium, and the midbrain. Thus the cardinal features of transtentorial herniation are an alteration in pupillary size and a decreasing level of consciousness (*see* p. 95). As the downward movement increases, the pupil size will increase and the conscious level will decline further: ultimately the contralateral pupil will enlarge and the patient lapses into an irreversible coma from which recovery is unlikely. As part of the shift, small perforating blood vessels passing into the brainstem may tear causing small haemorrhages. Finally, the more caudal part of the brainstem will pass down to, and then through, the foramen magnum, thus producing the foramen magnum (tonsillar) cone.

Kernohan's notch effect describes the displacement of the midbrain laterally as well as downward causing the cerebral peduncle opposite to the supratentorial mass, and opposite to the initial direction of the displacement, to impinge against the sharp tentorial edge. An indentation into the cerebral peduncle will thus be produced and those pyramidal fibres in the peduncle are compromised. Since these pyramidal fibres are destined to cross at a more caudal medullary level, the resulting clinical picture is one of a hemiparesis that is not only obviously contralateral to that cerebral peduncle that has been indented but is

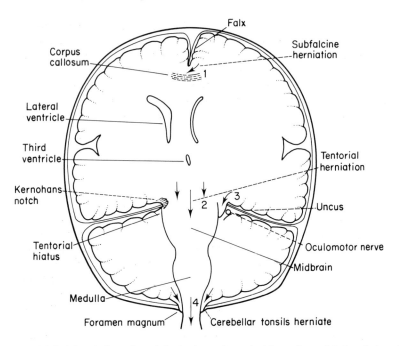

Fig. 14.1. Coronal section of the brain to show the sites of possible herniation. Note: the oculomotor (III) nerve lies by the free edge of the tentorium cerebelli. 1. Subfalcine herniation; 2. transtentorial herniation; 3. uncal herniation; 4. tonsillar herniation (foramen magnum)

ipsilateral to the offending supratentorial mass (Fig. 14.1). This is one of the explanations of a neurological situation where a hemiparesis may be very misleading if used to lateralize the offending intracranial mass, and indeed this could be classified as a form of false localizing sign.

3. Foramen magnum (tonsillar) herniation or cone

The commonest predisposing factor to this form of shift is a neglected and advanced transtentorial herniation. Here, there is downward movement of the medial cerebellar structures and lower brainstem leading ultimately to 'jamming' of these structures through the foramen magnum where the cerebellar tonsils will compress the medulla. If a posterior fossa mass is present, herniation through the foramen magnum may occur without any transtentorial shift. The clinical features may include severe occipital and cervical pain with, at times, neck stiffness and even head retraction. These last two features together with the patient's complaints of severe headache may lead to a fatal conclusion by the clinician that such a patient may have a meningitis. The disastrous consequences of completing the cone by performing a lumbar puncture may be avoided if the clinician carefully analyses the way the history has evolved in conjunction with the physical signs.

Another important feature of this variety of coning is respiratory irregularity.

Cardiovascular abnormalities may also occur, although the classical brady-cardia and elevated blood pressure tend to be late events, and may not always occur. The absence of these signs must never be used to exclude the presence of an impending cone since the end stage is the cessation of respiration from which the patient will very rarely recover. It should also be remembered that very occasionally a large posterior fossa mass will promote an upward movement through the tentorial hiatus, producing the so-called upward cone (*see* Chapter 3).

Hydrocephalus

Anatomy

Cerebrospinal fluid (CSF) is produced by the choroid plexus in the lateral, third and fourth ventricles. It is also possible that some may be produced by the epen-dymal lining of the ventricles. CSF leaves the ventricular system through the single midline fourth ventricle foramen of Magendie and the paired fourth ven-tricle lateral recesses, the foramina of Luschka. The fluid then circulates in the subarachnoid spaces (cisterns) around the brainstem and passes through the tentorial hiatus and over the cerebral hemispheres where it is eventually absorbed through the arachnoid granulations into the intracranial venous sinuses, the main one of which is the superior sagittal sinus. For hydrocephalus to develop there will have to be either overproduction in the presence of normal circulation and absorption, or conversely there will have to be impairment of the latter in the presence of normal production. Such impairment amounts to an obstruction and if this occurs within the ventricular system, or at the exit fora-mina of the fourth ventricle, it is referred to as an obstructive or non-communicating hydrocephalus. If it occurs within the basal cisterns or at the surfaces of the cerebral hemispheres it is referred to as a communicating hydro-cephalus. Thus a tumour that would narrow part of the ventricular system or block the aqueduct will produce a non-communicating (old terminology internal) hydrocephalus, while scarring of the basal cisterns and arachnoid granulations in relation to previous haemorrhage or infection would produce a communicating (old terminology external) hydrocephalus.

Symptoms and signs

The features of raised ICP predominate and therefore headaches and vomiting are common and such symptoms frequently progress. A decline in general mental function may also take place and ultimately the level of consciousness may fall, although this is a late feature. The signs may include papilloedema and cranial nerve palsies, especially the abducens, and in the terminal stages there may be pupillary irregularities. Two other signs that may be present are those of lower limb weakness with ataxia, and a defect of upward gaze. The former is usually ascribed to the fact that the fibres for lower limb function are closer to the ventricles than the fibres for the more rostral parts of the body. The defect of upward gaze is usually related to the disturbance of the back of the midbrain (tectum) which may be distorted by pressure from the dilated temporal horns thus causing pressure in the region of the tentorial hiatus.

Childhood hydrocephalus

Various congenital obstructions to the CSF pathways may arise (*see* p. 371). Congenital aqueduct stenosis producing hydrocephalus may occur in some children with spinal dysraphism (e.g. meningoceles, meningomyeloceles) and also be associated with maldevelopment of the basal cisterns. Unlike the adult, the skull of a baby or young child may enlarge, increasing the skull circumference. Often young patients appear very irritable with frequent crying, the latter sometimes high pitched and termed the 'cerebral cry'. The anterior fontanelle widens and becomes tense, although if there is a slower rise in ICP the fontanelle may simply be delayed in closing. It should be stressed that any cause of raised ICP may produce a similar clinical picture and sometimes the investigation of a child suspected of a congenital hydrocephalus may reveal either an intracranial tumour or a chronic subdural effusion.

Normal pressure hydrocephalus (NPH)

This is an adult disorder that usually occurs from middle age onwards and its pathogenesis is somewhat obscure; indeed, its title is probably inaccurate. The first reports described adults who proved to have hydrocephalus (or more specifically a degree of ventricular dilatation) but who were found to have normal or low CSF pressure when measured at lumbar puncture. It is now known, however, that if such patients are subjected to 24 hour intracranial pressure monitoring, the pressure waves do rise and thus it is misleading to use the term normal or low pressure hydrocephalus. Some patients may have a past history of an intracranial haemorrhage or meningitis but, in these situations, it may prove difficult to distinguish this form of hydrocephalus from the more conventional form of communicating hydrocephalus. Patients usually present with the triad of dementia, lower limb weakness with ataxia, and urinary incontinence. It is not necessary for all three to be present. The symptoms may improve if a correct diagnosis is made and treatment instituted by the insertion of a shunt.

It is sometimes difficult to differentiate NPH with ventricular dilatation from degenerative disorders, e.g. Alzheimer's disease, where there is widespread cortical atrophy (*see* p. 233).

Diagnosis of hydrocephalus

At all ages the diagnosis can easily be confirmed by a CT scan (*see* Fig. 18.2). More information about the surrounding brain may sometimes be obtained with a magnetic resonance imaging (MRI) scan. Plain skull X-rays in children may show suture splaying and in adults a demineralized pituitary fossa. In addition, there may be changes related to the cause of the hydrocephalus, e.g. calcification in a suprasellar craniopharyngioma, or what appears to be a small posterior fossa in long-standing aqueduct stenosis. Isotopic-labelled albumin, radio-iodinated human serum albumin (RIHSA), can be injected by lumbar puncture into the CSF and used to evaluate the distribution and absorption of CSF by scanning the patient at various intervals. This may prove useful in patients suspected of having normal pressure hydrocephalus.

Treatment

Treatment may fall into two approaches: (1) dealing with the lesion causing the hydrocephalus, and (2) the insertion of a shunt system to relieve the ventricular obstruction and allow drainage of the CSF. Sometimes the two may be combined and a preoperative shunt may make the course of the subsequent major operation easier. The principle of shunting is to insert a catheter into the ventricle and link this to a subcutaneous tube that will drain the CSF either into the peritoneal cavity or into the right atrium of the heart (ventriculoperitoneal and ventriculoatrial shunt respectively). Part of the system may contain a valve mechanism that may be complex or simple but is constructed to ensure that the correct flow of the CSF is to drain downwards in a caudal direction. For aqueduct stenosis the insertion of a shunt is commonly used, but a ventriculocisternostomy (bypass tube) may still be employed (Torkildsen's operation). This will drain from the lateral ventricle to the cisterna magna.

Complications may arise from shunts. These include blockage, infection, or the development of a subdural effusion.

Benign intracranial hypertension

A number of mechanisms may be responsible for this curious disorder which most often occurs in young women. The presentation is usually with the symptoms and signs of raised ICP. The precise aetiology is still controversial. In some adolescent girls and young women there appears to be an endocrine link and the patient is often very obese. It may also follow an infection or head injury, particularly in young children. A relationship to certain drugs now seems well established and these include the contraceptive pill, certain antibiotics, e.g. tetracycline, and withdrawal from steroid treatment.

Symptoms and signs

The patient usually gives a relatively short history of some weeks' duration with symptoms of headache and vomiting. Cranial nerve palsies, especially the abducens, may also occur but the most florid sign is that of significant bilateral papilloedema. This may be so severe that ultimately in some patients it may affect the visual acuity with progressive visual loss and the appearance of consecutive optic atrophy. The patient may appear well in other respects and this is often paralleled by the absence of any impairment of conscious level or any alteration of intellectual function. These latter features may contrast with those found in patients with raised ICP from a tumour. Although the condition may be drug-induced, it is important, particularly in women who are taking the contraceptive pill, to consider the possibility that the underlying aetiology may be due to a superior sagittal sinus thrombosis. It is quite possible that a condition that has been described in the older neurological texts as otitic hydrocephalus (raised ICP in relation to a chronic ear infection) might have been a form of benign intracranial hypertension in association with a lateral sinus thrombosis.

Investigations

The diagnosis is made by exclusion of other causes of raised ICP. The condition may be suspected on clinical grounds, although many doctors have made the mistake of suspecting the disorder in a young, somewhat obese, fertile woman only to discover that the CT scan has shown an intracranial tumour. The definitive investigation is a CT scan which usually reveals small, sometimes slit-like ventricles with no evidence of any shift or mass lesion. Clearly such CT scan appearances may also occur with bilateral isodense subdural haematomas and this diagnosis should always be considered. Lumbar puncture will confirm the presence of raised pressure with a normal CSF in benign intracranial hypertension.

Treatment

Drug therapy has been suggested but no single drug has been shown to be totally satisfactory. Diuretics are often effective and acetazolamide has also been used on the grounds that it has some inhibitory effect on CSF production. Steroids have also been tried, but it is questionable whether they should be used since they may even cause the disorder. Other treatments have included regular lumbar punctures although this only temporarily lowers the pressure. In many instances it is likely that the disease is self-limiting, but if the vision is threatened, decompression of the optic nerves may be necessary. Patients require regular follow-up with measurements made of their visual acuity and fields, including the size of the blind spots.

Intracranial tumours

Gliomas

These are the most common primary brain tumours and the term implies a glial origin. The glia is a form of cerebral connective tissue and the commonest cell type is the astrocyte; hence the astrocytoma is the commonest primary brain tumour. Oligodendroglia is a less prevalent element of the cerebral connective tissue and similarly the oligodendroglioma is a much less common tumour. The two other neoplasms that are frequently classified in the group of glial neoplasms are the ependymoma and the medulloblastoma; in fact the last tumour is not universally regarded as being necessarily a glial origin tumour.

The astrocytoma and oligodendroglioma may be classified into one of four grades (1–4) depending upon the degree of malignancy as revealed by the histological appearances of anaplasia, frequency of mitoses, presence of necrosis, and giant cells, etc. The most common primary malignant brain tumour is the astrocytoma grade 3–4. A very malignant variety of this tumour is sometimes known as the gliobastoma multiforme. Such tumours rapidly grow, giving a short history which may be only weeks to a few months, but occasionally may be only a few days. In general, the symptoms relate to the raised ICP due to the mass effect of the tumour, and the focal disturbance related to the tumour site (Fig. 14.2). Symptoms may also include focal and major epileptic seizures.

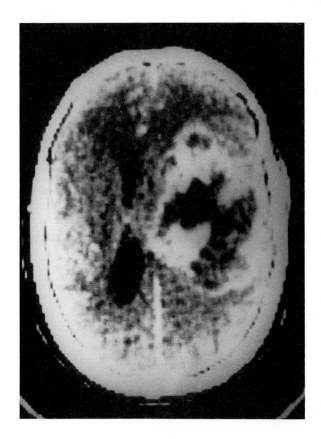

Fig. 14.2. Extensive right frontal glioma causing shift across the midline. Note peripheral enhancement and necrotic centre

Focal weakness and sensory loss may arise. Dominant hemisphere symptoms may include speech dysfunction and complex sensory problems may appear with parietal lobe lesions. The more slowly growing tumours (grade 1–2) are quite rare and usually present with a much longer history which may sometimes be years: in this respect epilepsy may be a very common symptom.

Treatment

The treatment of the malignant astrocytoma remains largely unsatisfactory because cure is so very rare, even with radical surgery. Nevertheless, the free interval (i.e. that between surgery and recurrence) is very much better than it used to be especially with the combination of radiotherapy (DXT) and some-times chemotherapy. DXT remains the best adjuvant treatment although it is not possible to predict which patients will benefit from the treatment. Indeed, the mean increase in the free interval may only amount to months. The place of chemotherapy is more controversial, although in those studies where there have been a few long-term survivors, such patients have usually been those who have had additional chemotherapy.

For patients with deep-seated tumours or those in poor neurological condition a biopsy may be all that is required. This may be the conventional burr hole biopsy or the more modern stereotactic biopsy and the indications are to exclude any unexpected benign pathology (such as an abscess) and to confirm the histological diagnosis. The last may aid management and help with the prognosis. The stereotactic biopsy carries a lower risk to the patient than the conventional burr hole biopsy since the latter may sometimes produce acute oedema and haemorrhage, both of which may cause clinical deterioration and even death.

Swelling around a tumour may often dramatically be relieved for a time by the use of steroids. Dexamethasone 4 mg t.i.d. is a dose commonly given to adults to start treatment. The dose can be lowered, depending on the patient's response and state. In some patients steroids may be maintained for some time with considerable symptomatic benefit. With prolonged steroid treatment it may be wise to add some ranitidine or cimetidine to reduce the risks of gastric irritation.

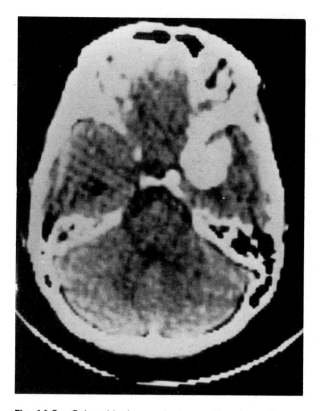

Fig. 14.3. Sphenoid wing meningioma with enhanced mass on the right side

Meningiomas

These tumours, almost all of which are histologically benign, arise from the brain coverings (i.e. the meninges) in the region of the arachnoid granulations. The tumour is much rarer than the glioma and the common sites include parasagittal (30 per cent), convexity (30 per cent), sphenoid wing (15 per cent) (Fig. 14.3), and subfrontal (15 per cent) (Fig. 14.4). Other less common sites include intraventricular, torcula (confluence of the sinuses) and posterior fossa. As with gliomas, the symptoms and signs depend upon the space-occupying effect which causes raised ICP, and the site of the brain from which the tumour arises. Thus a parasagittal tumour may produce epilepsy, often focal, which may involve the legs but can spread to the arms. Later, appropriate weakness and sensory loss in the limbs on the side opposite to the tumour may appear. A dominant hemisphere pterional meningioma may produce dysphasia as well as a contralateral brachiofacial weakness, and a subfrontal meningioma may produce dementia and, if elicitable, anosmia. The natural history of the meningioma will clearly be a good deal longer than that of a glioma although occasionally it may be relatively short.

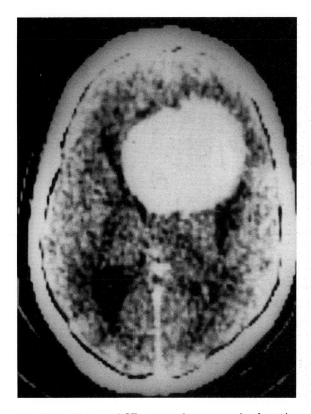

Fig. 14.4. Enhanced CT scan to show a massive frontal meningioma

Treatment

Although histologically benign these tumours may prove difficult to remove and those related to the parasagittal area present a hazardous prospect because of the involvement of the superior sagittal sinus. Convexity tumours are totally removable both in terms of their bulk and their origin, and these tumours carry the best prognosis. The basal and sphenoid wing tumours may prove difficult to remove completely and thus may recur. The tumour may be radioresistant, although radiotherapy may be used to try to halt the rate of growth. At operation both arteries and veins may have become adherent to the tumour capsule and obviously every effort must be made to avoid damage to these. Postoperative oedema leading to neurological deterioration may sometimes occur and this may be reduced by steroids. In general, the prognosis is far better than that for a patient with a glioma. Nevertheless, recurrence may occur, especially with parasagittal, basal and sphenoid wing tumours: in such situations a further operation may prove necessary.

Pituitary tumours and craniopharyngiomas

These two lesions are grouped together because the clinical features may be similar. The main components of the problems that are produced are neurological, visual and endocrine. These often include symptoms of optic nerve and chiasmal compression, and the features of hydrocephalus due to a large tumour that has expanded upwards to obstruct the foramen of Monro. If there is lateral expansion this may involve the cavernous sinus or the temporal lobe producing corresponding cranial nerve palsies (III, IV, VI and V a and b) and temporal

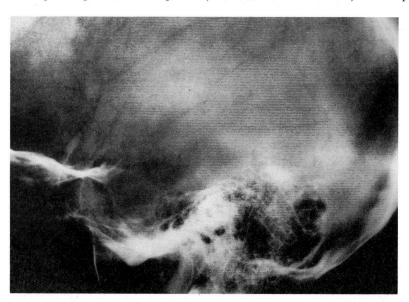

Fig. 14.5. Lateral skull film to show an enlarged pituitary fossa with loss of the dorsum sellae

lobe epilepsy respectively. The *visual disturbances* are common, usually the classical bitemporal hemianopia (*see* Fig. 3.1) but a frequent symptom is failing vision in one eye. Some patients may only notice the decline in visual acuity at a late stage. Examination may sometimes, in a situation where one eye is considerably worse than the other, surprise the patient who was unaware that the so-called good eye was also affected. A very marked asymmetry of acuity with very poor vision in one eye, and relatively good if not normal vision in the other, would perhaps be more in favour of a suprasellar meningioma than a craniopharyngioma or pituitary tumour.

The *endocrine manifestations* relate to the type of tumour although it must be stressed that with modern endocrine assay techniques there is increasing evidence that many of the pituitary tumours are in reality mixed in terms of their cellular content and endocrine disturbances (*see* p. 414).

The most common tumour, the chromophobe adenoma, predominantly produces hypopituitarism as indeed does the craniopharyngioma. The syndrome of acromegaly, while by definition being a form of hyperpituitarism from excess growth hormone, may in fact have some features of hypopituitary dysfunction (e.g. reduced sexual function). With such tumours neurological complications do occur and these will include optic pathway dysfunction, but it is uncommon for these tumours to reach the very large size that may occur in chromophobe adenomas (Figs. 14.5 and 14.6). The tumour that produces Cushing's disease very rarely leads to neurological complications, although the well known endocrine disturbance will occur. Acromegaly and Cushing's disease may be produced by microadenomas. The most common microadenoma, however, is the prolactinoma which produces excess prolactin secretion which is now recognized as an important cause of infertility with amenorrhoea in females and occasionally sexual dysfunction in males.

Craniopharyngiomas probably arise from remnants of Rathke's pouch which form an expanding cyst in the suprasellar region. As this enlarges it may extend up into the third ventricle and down to involve the optic chiasm and pituitary gland. It may occur in children as well as adults and quite commonly may produce diabetes insipidus or features of hypothalamic upset.

Treatment

Relief of optic nerve or chiasmal compression is clearly mandatory. Unfortunately, if vision is severely compromised the results of surgery may be disappointing; nevertheless, it is surprising that in some patients with very poor acuity there may be very good return of vision. Complete removal of large pituitary tumours is rarely, if ever, attainable and certainly for chromophobe lesions the aim should be to achieve a satisfactory decompression of the optic nerves and chiasm and then to institute postoperative DXT since such treatment has been clearly shown to reduce the chances of recurrence. There is now an increasing vogue for pituitary surgery to be carried out trans-sphenoidally rather than through a frontal craniotomy, and experts may even be able to remove quite large tumours through the sphenoid sinus route. For the microadenomas the trans-sphenoidal route using the operating microscope is ideal because it avoids the need to expose the optic nerves or chiasm, and there is a better chance of

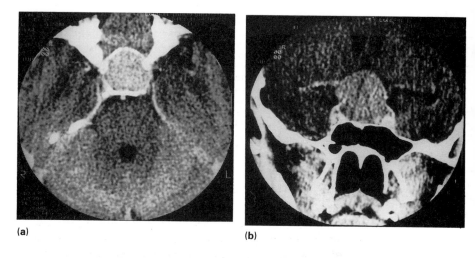

(a)   (b)

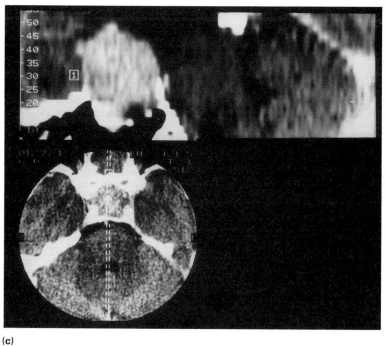

(c)

Fig. 14.6.   (a) Axial view of an enhanced CT brain scan to show a pituitary tumour. (b) Coronal section from the same patient to show the tumour rising well above the pituitary fossa. (c) Sagittal reconstruction from the same patient taken at the level indicated

preserving some normal pituitary tissue. However, bromocriptine can be used to shrink prolactinomas and may be the treatment of choice. Following surgery and irradiation for pituitary tumours, such patients will require careful endocrine assessment to see what hormonal replacement therapy is necessary and some patients will require cortisone and thyroxine.

Surgery for craniopharyngiomas may be formidable as such lesions may be very large and the attempt may be accompanied by the risks of damage to the hypothalamus or the floor of the third ventricle. Some lesions may be excised; in others the cyst drained and this followed by DXT. With incomplete removal recurrence is common.

The investigation of patients suspected of having supratentorial tumours

To some extent this is directed by the symptoms and signs found. For example the presence of a bitemporal hemianopia or features of hypopituitarism would indicate the need for careful assessment of endocrine function (*see* p. 414) and X-rays directed towards the pituitary fossa. Common measures are included in Table 14.1. In all adults suspected of an intracranial mass a chest X-ray should be taken to exclude a primary bronchogenic carcinoma or the presence of metastases.

A good quality lateral film of the skull should be taken. This may show the presence of pathological intracranial calcification, erosion of the dorsum sellae, or pituitary fossa enlargement (*see* Fig. 14.5). If the pineal gland is calcified other skull views may be taken to see if there is any shift from the midline. The

Table 14.1 Investigations in patients suspected of a cerebral tumour

Blood tests
Full blood count, ESR
Specific: as indicated e.g. Wasserman reaction or equivalent, acid phosphatase, serum proteins
Endocrine status: pituitary tumour
Plain X-rays
Skull
Pineal shift if calcified
Sella erosion or pituitary fossa enlargement
Abnormal calcification
Others: abnormal density, enlarged exit foramina
Chest
Primary tumour, metastases, cardiac contour
CT brain scan
Enhanced series
Evidence of shift, hydrocephalus
High or low density areas may enhance
MRI brain scan
Particularly useful in posterior fossa, basal lesions, craniocervical junction
Radionuclide scan
Screening test for meningiomas, metastases, abscesses, some gliomas
Angiography
Selected mass lesions to elucidate circulation, e.g. giant aneurysms, angiomas

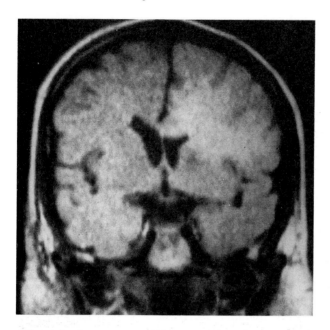

Fig. 14.7. Coronal section MRI scan to show displacement of the lateral ventricle from an infiltrating glioma

bones of the skull may occasionally show abnormalities of density, widening of the exit foramina or, in children, splaying of the sutures. Computed tomography (CT) brain scans with enhancement are the investigations of choice in patients suspected of mass lesions (*see* Figs. 14.2–14.6). Occasionally special views, e.g. coronal reconstructions, may aid definition. MRI scans may also prove useful in selected instances (Fig. 14.7).

Radionuclide scans may be very helpful where access to CT scanning is limited. They will show most meningiomas, metastases and abscesses but only a proportion of gliomas. Angiography may be necessary in selected patients where a knowledge of the blood supply to a tumour may help the surgeon, or when rarely a giant aneurysm may present as a tumour. Some examples are shown in Figs. 14.2–14.14.

Blood tests may be indicated in the assessment of endocrine status and in the screening of some primary tumours, e.g. acid phosphatase from prostatic carcinoma.

Metastases

Metastases are common in the supratentorial (hemisphere) or infratentorial (posterior fossa) compartments. There is no certain method on clinical grounds of identifying a metastatic lesion as opposed to a primary brain neoplasm, although a history of a known primary tumour elsewhere would heavily favour any neurological syndrome as being due to a metastatic lesion. Occasionally in

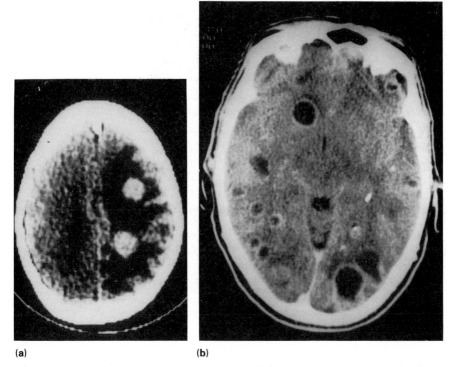

(a)   **(b)**

Fig. 14.8. (a) Enhanced CT brain scans to show two solid metastatic lesions with considerable surrounding oedema (low density). (b) Multiple cystic metastatic lesions with ring enhancement

such patients other pathology, e.g. meningiomas or subdural haematomas, may be found. Clearly if a patient has clinical evidence of more than one neurological lesion this may be due to metastatic disease (Fig. 14.8). The clinical features relate to the site of the lesion or lesions and any space-occupying effect.

The common primary sites are lung and breast; therefore examination of the breast and a chest X-ray are always important. The other primary sites that may metastasize to the brain are the kidney, gastrointestinal tract, melanomas of the skin, and lymphomas. *Almost never !*

Treatment

If clinical examination and investigations confirm dissemination then neurosurgical intervention is probably unjustified. A burr hole or stereotactic biopsy may occasionally be necessary to confirm the diagnosis. Sometimes removal of a single intracranial metastasis may be justified, particularly if the primary is in the breast. Other metastases from this site may be controlled with DXT and chemotherapy. These metastases may be shown by isotope bone or liver scans. Technically a solitary metastasis is often not difficult to remove as such a tumour may be firm and discrete, tending to shell out from the surrounding brain.

Clearly, any decision must take into account the patient's age, general medical condition, and particularly whether there is any evidence of metastases elsewhere. The prognosis for most patients with cerebral metastases is generally poor. In some patients cranial irradiation may improve survival and where appropriate hormonal therapy or other forms of chemotherapy may be indicated.

Primary cerebral lymphoma, microglioma

This tumour can arise in the hemispheres, cerebellum or brainstem. It usually causes diffuse infiltration of the white matter by large mononuclear lymphoma cells. Commonly there are frequent mitoses indicating the malignant nature of the tumour. There is a marked increased incidence in immunocompromised patients. The history is usually short and symptoms depend on the site, e.g. focal epileptic seizures or a progressive hemiparesis, although there may often be a rapid decline in alertness with later symptoms of headache and features of raised ICP. Tumour cells may be shed into the CSF where they can be identified, and there may also be a CSF pleocytosis. The CT brain scan may show diffuse low density in the white matter.

Steroids and radiotherapy may prolong life although the response may be variable.

Pineal region tumours

These rare tumours occur more commonly in males with a maximal incidence between the ages of 15 and 25. They have been mistakenly referred to in the past as pinealomas. This term, however, implies a tumour of pineal parenchymal tissue and such tumours (pineocytoma or the more malignant pineoblastoma) are very rare. The commonest pineal tumour is the germinoma, a tumour that is not only locally malignant but may seed through the CSF pathways. Another very rare tumour of embryonic yolk sac origin is a chorion carcinoma; again this is highly malignant and may disseminate along CSF pathways. These tumours, the pineal parenchymal tumours, and the rare dermoid and its varieties, constitute most of the pineal region tumours. Occasionally, a glioma arising in the region of the tectum may present as a pineal region tumour, and two other masses that may arise in the pineal region include the very rare carrefour meningioma and, in young children, the vein of Galen aneurysm.

The clinical features of tumours in the pineal region are those of raised ICP, usually due to obstruction of the upper aqueduct and posterior part of the third ventricle together with pressure on the midbrain. The latter is usually the tectal region and the signs are referable to the eyes. There may be a combination of large poorly reacting pupils with light-near dissociation, a defect of upward gaze and a defect of convergence, Parinaud's syndrome. Sometimes convergence nystagmus is present and rarely the entire globes seem to exhibit nystagmus when convergence is attempted (nystagmus retractorius). Papilloedema is common.

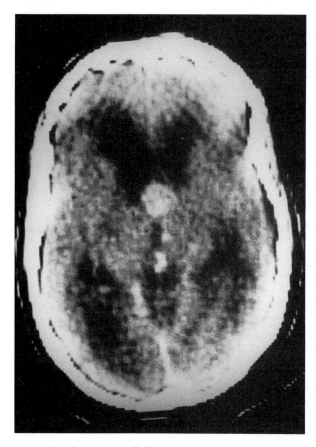

Fig. 14.9. Enhancing colloid cyst causing an obstructive hydrocephalus

Treatment

This is controversial although any hydrocephalus is usually alleviated by shunting. In some patients surgery combined with radiotherapy is undertaken; in others a biopsy for confirmation of the diagnosis. Certain tumour markers may be found in the blood and CSF and these include alpha-fetoprotein which may be raised in germinomatous tumours, and chorionic gonadotrophin which may be raised in yolk sac-chorionic carcinomatous tumours. DXT is useful in the radiosensitive germinomas, whereas the yolk sac tumours tend to be more chemosensitive. The rare dermoid may prove difficult to remove because of ramifications passing into the surrounding brain tissue.

Posterior fossa tumours

Medulloblastoma and ependymoma

The *medulloblastoma* is a highly malignant tumour and is the commonest child-hood tumour, although occasional examples do occur in adults. The tumour is rapidly growing and the origin is usually close to the fourth ventricle. The clinical presentation commonly relates to a disturbance of that area and especially to obstruction of the flow of CSF. Thus raised ICP due to hydrocephalus is common. However, because the tumour is often strategically close to the fourth ventricle floor, vomiting is very common and indeed may precede the other symptoms. Although the duration of history is usually short, frequently less than 3 months, rarely a child may persistently vomit for longer periods, and only be diagnosed when symptoms of raised ICP appear. Some children may appear wasted. The most common neurological signs are papilloedema and truncal ataxia, the latter because of frequent involvement of the vermis. Limb weakness and cranial nerve involvement (commonly the abducens, and rarely lower cranial nerves) may sometimes occur. Medulloblastomas may 'seed' along the neuraxis.

The *ependymoma* is also a tumour most often presenting in childhood although it is rarer than the medulloblastoma. It may also arise in adults. Unlike the medulloblastoma some ependymomas may be of low grade and therefore far less aggressive: others may be highly malignant. Ependymomas arise with almost equal frequency in the supra- and infratentorial compartments. On clinical grounds there is no certain method of distinguishing between a fourth ventricle medulloblastoma, an ependymoma or even an astrocytoma which may have spread into the fourth ventricle. Some ependymomas may show calcification.

Cerebellar astrocytoma

This tumour may be solid or cystic and when presenting in childhood it is frequently very slow growing and relatively benign. Occasional recurrence may sometimes follow many years after surgery. The duration of symptoms is often longer than with other childhood tumours of the posterior fossa. Sometimes the tumour may be very diffuse in terms of its cerebellar spread (Fig. 14.10) but still be of a low grade nature. The common cystic variety will consist of a large cavity containing clear yellow fluid, and in part of the wall the actual tumour nodule will be present. In contrast most astrocytomas that arise in adults in the cerebellum tend to be more aggressive. It is clear that the medulloblastoma and the astrocytoma frequently represent opposite ends of the spectrum in that the former is a highly malignant tumour of childhood but the astrocytoma is relatively benign. Many childhood cerebellar astrocytomas arise in one hemisphere causing ipsilateral clumsiness. Sometimes they may cause head tilt. Although symptoms and signs of raised ICP may appear with both of these tumours, there will usually be more truncal ataxia in the medulloblastoma patient, and more unilateral limb ataxia in the astrocytoma patient.

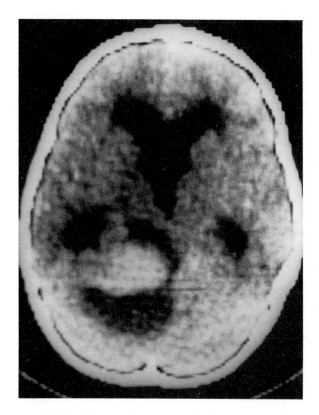

Fig. 14.10. CT scan showing a cerebellar astrocytoma causing a degree of hydrocephalus

Investigations

Plain X-rays of the skull in a child may show splaying of the sutures but changes in the vicinity of the pituitary fossa are less common with raised ICP. Very occasionally there may be calcification in a slow growing astrocytoma or an ependymoma. The definitive investigation is CT scanning and this will usually show hydrocephalus, sometimes gross, and the tumour (Fig. 14.10). The tendency for the medulloblastoma and sometimes the ependymoma to seed throughout the CSF pathways should always be considered. Extradural metastases, most often to bone, may rarely occur in patients with medulloblastomas following surgery.

Treatment

The various posterior fossa tumours under discussion may be partially or totally removed, but those involving the floor of the fourth ventricle may not be totally removable because damage here causes severe neurological deficits. With the cerebellar astrocytoma, provided the solid part of the tumour has been removed no more need be done and there is no need to attempt to remove the wall of the cyst. Most medulloblastomas and some ependymomas are very radiosensitive but, because these tumours may seed along the neuraxis, treatment must include the whole brain and spinal cord. Chemotherapy may be a useful adjuvant especially in the treatment of recurrent medulloblastomas. The prognosis for children with these tumours is very much better than it used to be and certainly cure with the cystic astrocytomas may be anticipated. With the medulloblastoma the outlook is far less good although there is 5-year survival in some two-thirds. The prognosis seems better for older patients.

Haemangioblastoma

The other common tumour of the cerebellar hemisphere is a haemangioblastoma. Like the astrocytoma this may be cystic or solid. The cystic tumour, which in reality is a cavity containing the same golden yellow fluid as the astrocytoma with a similar appearing tumour nodule in the wall, certainly cannot either on clinical grounds or CT scanning be distinguished from the astrocytoma apart from the age of the patient: a haemangioblastoma is a rare tumour of childhood whereas the cystic astrocytoma is a rare tumour of adults.

The clinical presentation of a patient with a haemangioblastoma is usually one of ataxia, this being more in the limbs than the trunk, although the latter can occur if the vermis is involved. The ataxia usually progresses over some months, but sometimes only weeks. Symptoms of raised ICP are common since hydrocephalus usually occurs before the diagnosis. Sometimes the tumour may arise in the lower vermis or the tonsil, and there may be severe occipital or suboccipital pain and even head retraction. When such a patient presents with a stiff neck, an erroneous diagnosis of meningitis may be made. Lumbar puncture should not be performed as it may be very hazardous.

The large solid haemangioblastoma may be associated with a family history of such tumours, and these may not only have been present in other members of the family within the cerebellum but anywhere along the neuraxis. There may be a link with von Hippel-Lindau disease where cerebellar haemangioblastomas may be associated with retinal angiomas and even other problems, e.g. renal carcinoma. In any patient with a haemangioblastoma polycythaemia may also be present.

CT scanning will commonly give the diagnosis (Fig. 14.11), although in selected patients vertebral angiography may prove helpful.

Treatment

Surgical removal is the treatment of choice and may be relatively simple if the tumour is small or cystic. This may cure the patient: the prognosis being good and recurrence rare. However, the large solid lesions may prove much more difficult to remove since heavy blood loss may ensue.

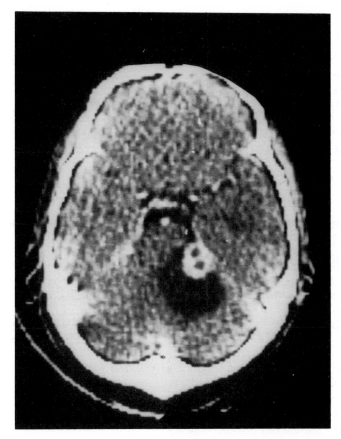

Fig. 14.11. CT scan showing an extensive low density area in the posterior fossa. Note the enhancing nodule on the side wall; this was a haemangioblastoma

Metastases

These are also common in the posterior fossa. Details have been given on p. 306.

Cerebellopontine angle tumours

Acoustic neuroma (Schwannoma)

The most common extrinsic posterior fossa tumour is the acoustic neuroma, a benign tumour arising from the eighth nerve. The common early symptoms include a progressive unilateral hearing impairment which eventually leads to complete deafness; sometimes there may be episodic vertigo but more commonly unsteadiness and usually facial sensory impairment. As the tumour enlarges medially it may compress the brainstem; this may cause quite severe ataxia and CSF obstruction, the latter producing hydrocephalus. The facial, abducens and bulbar cranial nerves may sometimes be involved. The headaches from raised ICP may be severe and additional lower limb ataxia may be accentuated by this as well as from brainstem distortion. Nystagmus is

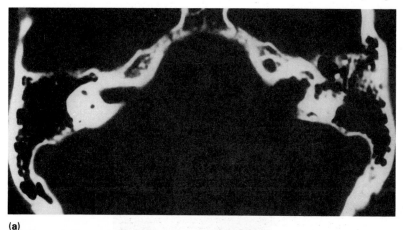

(a)

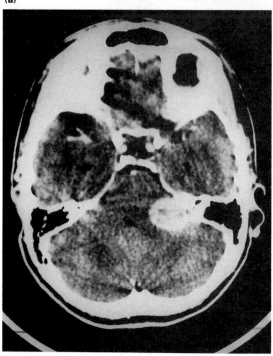

(b)

Fig. 14.12. CT brain scan with adjusted window width, (a) showing a very widened porus. (b) The enhanced view delineating the acoustic neuroma which is displacing the fourth ventricle

commonly present, initially fine and directed away from the side of the nerve deafness due to the peripheral vestibular disturbance; later coarse ipsilateral nystagmus may arise as the brainstem is compressed. The ipsilateral corneal reflex is commonly depressed or absent and this may appear relatively early. Papilloedema appears in about 25 per cent of patients and is not always associated with hydrocephalus. A proportion of patients present with large tumours and serious brainstem distortion and this makes a formidable surgical challenge with often a high morbidity, whereas removal of a small tumour is much easier with lower risks and often a good chance of sparing the facial nerve and even sometimes the eighth nerve, particularly if the tumour has largely arisen from the vestibular division.

Investigations

There is nerve deafness with absence of loudness recruitment, a canal paresis and abnormal auditory evoked potentials. The well recognized erosion of the porus (internal auditory meatus) is only evident when the tumour has reached a certain size, although is present in some 60 per cent of patients at the time of

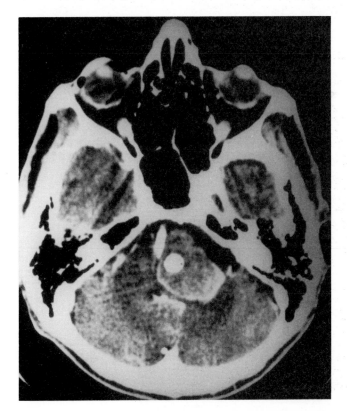

Fig. 14.13. Enhanced CT brain scan showing a very large aneurysm arising from the basilar artery. This was compressing the fourth ventricle and presented as a posterior fossa mass

presentation. Tomography of the internal auditory meatus may prove helpful, but CT scanning with enhancement will detect all but the very smallest lesions. With different bone window settings (Fig. 14.12) the porus can be well shown. MRI scanning may also prove helpful in doubtful cases. If the tumour is very small it may be necessary to inject some contrast intrathecally and carry out cisternography. Traditionally, the acoustic neuroma produces a high level of CSF protein although lumbar puncture should not be carried out in the presence of a large tumour. Bilateral acoustic neuromas may occur particularly in association with von Recklinghausen's disease (neurofibromatosis).

Treatment

A cure can be achieved by surgical removal but, with large tumours, there are significant risks, particularly of damage to the facial nerve and brainstem. The use of the operating microscope may reduce the risks but even when the facial nerve seems to be preserved it sometimes fails to function. In the elderly or frail with large tumours an intracapsular removal may be used, although further slow growth of the remnants occurs. Preoperative shunting in patients with

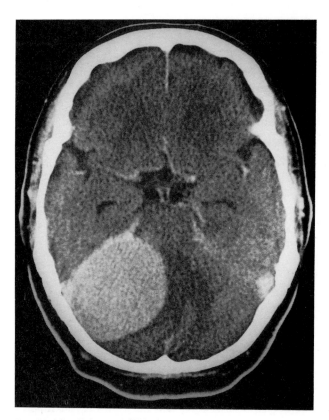

Fig. 14.14. Enhanced CT brain scan to show a large posterior fossa meningioma

significant hydrocephalus may prove very useful and reduce subsequent operative risks.

Other cerebellopontine angle tumours

These are rare and include aneurysms (Fig. 14.13), meningiomas (Fig. 14.14),
epidermoids and trigeminal neuromas. Most present with symptoms and signs
of raised ICP and later brainstem dysfunction. The epidermoid (cholesteatoma)
is a lesion that is more common in women and is of developmental origin. It is
the angle tumour most associated with a facial paresis. It should not be confused
with a chronic middle ear infection which is sometimes referred to as a cholesteatoma and is linked with suppuration and an accumulation of debris which
may erode bone and behave like an expanding mass. Because the epidermoid is
a developmental lesion it is rarely totally removable and sometimes the lesion
does spread up to, or even arise from, the floor of the middle fossa. The trigeminal neuroma is rare and usually presents with facial sensory symptoms,
including pain (but almost never true trigeminal neuralgia), visual symptoms
(which may include diplopia), and ataxia.

CT scans with enhancement or MRI scans will usually confirm the diagnosis.

Chordoma

This is a rare tumour arising from notochordal remnants and like the dermoid
may appear at the spinal or cranial end of the neuraxis. The former are virtually
restricted to the sacral and sacrococcygeal region and the latter to the region of
the basisphenoid and clivus. At the skull base the medial temporal structures
and cavernous sinus may be invaded, producing disturbance of the IIIrd to
VIth cranial nerves. The tumour is often slow growing and symptoms of raised
ICP tend to occur late. Rarely the tumour may arise in relation to the optic
nerves and a chiasmal syndrome may occur. Tumours arising from the clivus
usually produce brainstem dysfunction with or without cranial nerve palsies.

Plain X-rays will frequently reveal bony destruction. For intracranial lesions
CT scanning usually shows an avascular mass which may enhance.

Complete surgical removal is often not possible, although a degree of decompression may be achieved. For clival lesions a transoral transclival route may be
used which allows better access.

Intracranial abscess

For practical purposes the two main varieties are intracerebral abscess and subdural abscess (empyema). Extradural abscess is rare although it may occur
during the phase of development of an intracranial abscess from local sinus
infection (i.e. an osteomyelitis of part of the bone may develop) and it may also
follow a penetrating injury.

Pathogenesis

Depending on the site of the abscess, the source tends to vary: thus a temporal
lobe and cerebellar abscess usually results from chronic otitis media and a

frontal lobe abscess from local sinus disease. Abscesses of metastatic origin tend to occur in the parietal or occipital region but the source is not always found. An abscess may follow some local dental problem or result from chronic suppuration, e.g. bronchiectasis. An important but sometimes forgotten cause of metastatic abscess is subacute bacterial endocarditis (SBE) which arises from septic embolic infarction. Penetrating foreign bodies, including pencil tip injuries, have also been reported as causes. Subdural empyema usually follows a pansinusitis. The specific pathways by which infection spreads to the brain remain unclear. Direct spread, e.g. from chronic otitis media or retrograde septic thrombosis have all been suggested, and obviously metastatic arterial spread in SBE must clearly occur at some time in the evolution of a cerebral abscess.

The common organisms are streptococci, both aerobic and anaerobic, and bacteroides, but any organism is capable of producing a cerebral abscess. However, staphylococcal infection is relatively uncommon unless there is an adjoining osteomyelitis of the bone usually in relation to a previous injury. Although it is likely that a phase of cerebritis occurs prior to the formation of the abscess with encapsulation, it is also not clear why some patients are able to develop a well-formed encapsulated abscess with very little in the way of systemic upset, while others may be very ill, with typical features of infection, and have a diffuse cerebritis.

Symptoms and signs

A cerebral abscess acts as an intracranial space-occupying lesion like a tumour. Even in the cerebritic phase the intense inflammatory reaction produces an abnormal and swollen area of brain. However, of all the intracranial space-occupying lesions, an abscess tends to produce more elevation of ICP due to the intense inflammatory reaction and oedema. Although the symptoms and signs of raised ICP may be marked, there are two clinical traps. First, papilloedema may be absent and second, the raised ICP may produce neck stiffness which can lead to the erroneous diagnosis of meningitis. These two features may give the clinician a false sense of security regarding a lumbar puncture which may provoke a fatal cone.

Headaches of increasing severity leading subsequently to confusion and drowsiness frequently occur in patients with intracranial pus. The duration of symptoms may be variable but is, on the whole, days or at the most weeks. A pre-existing local infection such as sinus disease or chronic middle ear disease may be elicited and the presence of valvular heart disease should alert the doctor. In patients with known sinus infection, the development of rather intense and unremitting headaches which alter from being purely frontal to generalized is suspicious. If other features of raised ICP appear, such as vomiting, this is stronger support for the presence of an abscess.

Focal symptoms and signs will usually relate to the site involved, e.g. dysphasia in a dominant temporal lobe abscess, ataxia and nystagmus in a cerebellar abscess. With regard to a cerebellar abscess, hydrocephalus may develop and also add to the patient's headache. Most patients appear generally ill but in a few this is not apparent, perhaps because the abscess is well walled off. Pyrexia and changes in the white count and ESR do not always occur.

Patients with subdural empyema tend not only to be more ill than patients with an intracerebral abscess but also have more florid features of raised ICP, particularly very severe headaches. The patient will have pus that has spread extensively over the subdural space producing an underlying cerebral septic thrombophlebitis. Epilepsy often occurs. An unusual neurological syndrome of a cerebral paraplegia (i.e. lower limb weakness not due to a spinal lesion but due to an abnormality of the leg areas of the cortex) may arise from the collection of pus in the interhemispheric fissure.

Investigations

Blood should be taken for a full count, ESR and blood cultures. Plain X-rays of the skull may show opaque sinuses or abnormalities in the region of the mastoids suggesting a source of infection. The CT scan, with enhancement, is the definitive investigation (Fig. 14.15). Isotope scanning may be helpful and is often positive: it is useful where there is no ready access to a CT scanner. Lumbar puncture is mentioned to be condemned because of the dangers. Any

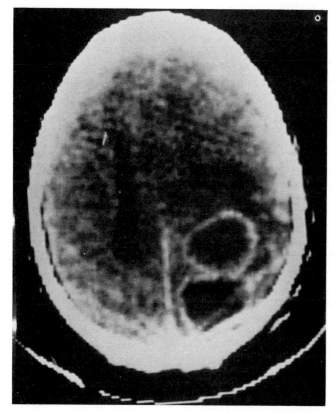

Fig. 14.15 Multiloculated occipital lobe abscess with surrounding oedema and ring enhancement

patient showing meningeal irritation and focal symptoms and signs should undergo a CT scan before embarking on CSF examination. In instances where the CSF has been examined it may be normal or show a pleocytosis, often with polymorphs and lymphocytes; the protein may be elevated. Rarely an abscess may rupture into the CSF pathways (either into the subarachnoid space or the ventricular system) producing an appearance of the CSF similar to that of a meningitis.

Treatment

Aspiration of the abscess through a burr hole, or multiple burr holes for sub-dural pus, tends to be the most favoured treatment, although controversy persists as to whether this is the best method or whether craniotomy should be carried out. Whatever is performed the important priorities are to institute the correct antibiotic therapy and reduce the ICP. Raised ICP is shown by a depressed conscious level and supported by the presence of much oedema around the abscess on the CT scan. It can be controlled by an intravenous infusion of mannitol followed by steroids for a short period. Antibiotics are given intravenously in large doses. Cultures and sensitivities of any organisms isolated from blood cultures or aspirated pus enables the selection of the best antibiotics, although such answers may not be available for 24–48 h. The organisms most commonly found are streptococci or bacteroides and these are usually sensitive to a combination of penicillin and metronidazole, the latter to cover any anaerobic organisms. Other antibiotics may also be added initially. Because epilepsy is a common complication of an intracranial abscess, anticonvulsants should also be started.

The abscess may need to be aspirated at fairly frequent intervals and CT scanning is most helpful in assessing progress. It should be stressed that metronidazole should not be stopped until the laboratory has confirmed beyond all doubt that no anaerobic organisms are present. Usually the intravenous antibiotic therapy is continued for a minimum of 3 weeks, and then if the patient's condition is satisfactory, and the abscess shows evidence of regression on the CT scan, an oral preparation of the drug may be given (if appropriate). If there is any doubt about the patient's condition or the shrinkage of the abscess cavity, then intravenous therapy should be continued.

Once the patient's condition has improved, and while still receiving antibiotics, the primary source of infection may be dealt with if this is known, e.g. a sinus infection or chronic otitis media. Patients with SBE are likely to require prolonged antibiotic treatment and should undergo a full cardiological assessment.

Parasitic cysts

Hydatid cysts

These arise from infection by *Echinococcus granulosus* and are found in sheep-raising areas. The ova are excreted in dog's faeces. Sheep and cattle may also be intermediate hosts. In a small number of infected patients, particularly children, a parasitic cyst appears in one cerebral hemisphere presenting like an expanding mass lesion. Cysts are more commonly found in the liver and lungs.

Treatment is by the careful surgical removal of the intact cyst avoiding puncture and spillage.

Cysticercosis

Larvae from the pork tapeworm, *Taenia solium*, may invade man producing multiple encysted lesions. These may occur extensively in muscles, often the thighs, and sometimes produce multiple cystic lesions in the brain. The cysts are irritant and may present with a meningoencephalitic picture, with features of multiple mass lesions, but most commonly with epileptic seizures. Sometimes the cysts may block the CSF pathways producing an obstructive hydrocephalus with symptoms of raised ICP. The larvae commonly calcify producing a typical appearance in infected limb muscles and multiple calcified intracranial lesions seen on a skull X-ray.

In a few patients there may be an eosinophilia. There may be signs of meningeal irritation with a CSF pleocytosis and elevated protein. A complement fixation test, best performed on the CSF, has also been used.

Treatment includes anticonvulsant drugs to control seizures, and now a course of praziquantel with steroid cover. Obstructive hydrocephalus may require a shunting procedure.

15

Infections of the central nervous system

The common syndromes of central nervous system infection are meningitis, when inflammation is largely confined to the meninges, and encephalitis, where the brunt of the inflammation is borne by the brain itself. Either syndrome is frequently accompanied by some features of the other but, for ease of discussion, they are usually considered as separate entities.

Meningitis

Acute meningitis is sometimes a medical emergency and one of the cornerstones of the management of meningitis is the speedy recognition of those cases that require the prompt initiation of appropriate antibiotic therapy. Most such cases are due to acute bacterial infections and characteristically the cellular response in the cerebrospinal fluid (CSF) is predominantly polymorphs, producing a purulent meningitis. The other traditional group of meningitis cases are those with a largely lymphocytic CSF pleocytosis. Although most of the latter group have a viral aetiology, there are a number of other treatable causes that always need to be considered.

Initial assessment of the patient

Meningeal inflammation from whatever cause is characterized by: (1) headache, often severe and described as bursting in nature; (2) photophobia; (3) spinal muscle spasm, detected by neck rigidity and positive Kernig's sign (pain from hamstring spasm provoked by attempting to extend the knee with the hip flexed); and (4) fever. In severe bacterial meningitis there may also be cerebral oedema and raised intracranial pressure leading to alterations in consciousness, vomiting and seizures. It is not difficult to recognize such classical features of meningitis but in some patients, notably neonates, young infants, immunocompromised patients and the very old, the signs are often much more subtle. In neonates apathy, irritability, lethargy and loss of appetite may be the only features and, in the elderly or immunocompromised patient, fever and confusion may develop without any specific evidence of meningeal irritation and be mistakenly ascribed to some concomitant illness or other infection.

Once the possibility of meningitis has been recognized then the next step

Table 15.1   The predominant infectious causes of meningitis

Common pathogens
  Neisseria meningitidis
  Streptococcus pneumoniae
  Haemophilus influenzae
  Enteroviruses
  Mumps virus
Rarer causes
  Mycobacterium tuberculosis
  Listeria monocytogenes
  Gram-negative bacilli
  Staphylococci
  Leptospira
  Borrelia burgdorferi (Lyme disease)
  Human immunodeficiency virus (HIV)
  Other viruses
  Cryptococcus neoformans
In the newborn
  Group B streptococci
  Escherichia coli
  Other Gram-negative bacilli
  Listeria monocytogenes
  Staphylococcus aureus

depends upon an assessment of the patient's condition and the speed of progression of the illness (Fig. 15.1). Most patients will not have any specific clinical findings and will have had symptoms for more than 24 h by the time they are first seen by a doctor. Any of the organisms listed in Table 15.1 may be responsible for the illness in this group and a decision regarding therapy depends upon the results of lumbar puncture (LP). In contrast, about 25 per cent of patients with bacterial meningitis will have a very acute and rapidly progressive illness. In these cases, in those who are semicomatose or comatose whatever the time course of their illness, in neonates, and if meningococcal infection is likely (patients with a typical rash), then providing an initial brief examination fails to reveal papilloedema or focal neurological signs, a LP and blood cultures should be obtained and empirical therapy directed at the likely pathogens started before the CSF result is available (*see* below). Papilloedema is unusual in meningitis and its presence should prompt an urgent search for an intracranial space-occupying lesion by CT scanning before LP can be contemplated.

The microscopical and biochemical examination of the CSF will usually give a clear indication of the type of organism causing the meningitis (Table 15.2), but there is a good deal of overlap between the findings in the various categories and a Gram's stain of the CSF is mandatory in all cases.

Acute bacterial meningitis

Almost any bacterium is capable of causing meningitis but, for many species, this is only as part of a generalized illness. There are, however, a few bacteria which consistently cause meningitis as a primary manifestation of disease (Table 15.1) and, in most instances, the likely aetiology of purulent meningitis

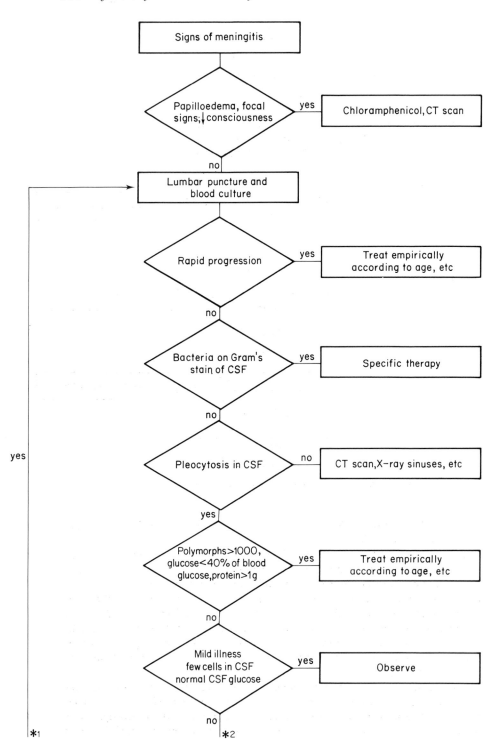

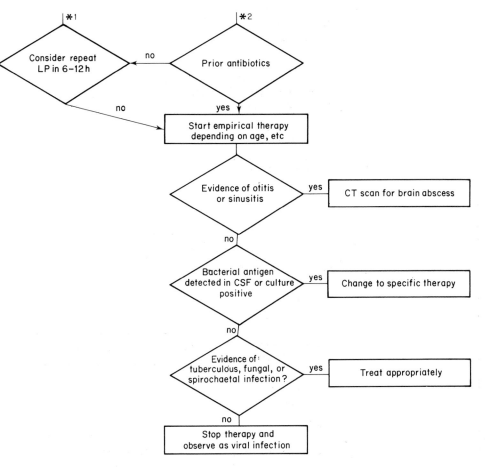

Fig. 15.1. Algorithm for the management of acute meningitis

can be further narrowed down by a consideration of the patient's age and previous health (Table 15.3).

The annual incidence of bacterial meningitis is between 3 and 5/100 000 overall population; the incidence is highest in the first month of life and nearly 75 per cent of sporadic cases occur in children under 15 years old.

In most cases of bacterial meningitis the immediate source of the pathogen is the nasopharynx; the bacteria colonize the mucosa and then spread via the bloodstream to the subarachnoid space. The factors that determine the likelihood of bloodstream invasion are largely speculative but the major factor that enables bacteria to cross the blood–brain barrier is the presence of capsular polysaccharide.

The purulent exudate that develops in the subarachnoid space during bacterial meningitis has profound effects. The normal flow of the CSF is obstructed and the reabsorption of CSF by the arachnoid villi is reduced. Hydrocephalus is produced and this causes interstitial oedema. Vascular permeability and

Table 15.2   Lumbar puncture findings in meningitis of different aetiologies

	Normal	Pyogenic bacteria	Viral meningitis	Tuberculous meningitis
Appearance	Clear	Turbid/purulent	Clear/opalescent	Clear/opalescent
Cells	0–5/mm³	5–2000/mm³	5–500/mm³	5–1000/mm³
Predominant cell type	Lymphocytes	Polymorphs	Lymphocytes	Lymphocytes
Glucose	2.2–3.3 mmol/l*	Very low	Normal†	Low
Protein	200–400 mg/l	Often > 900 mg/l	400–900 mg/l	Often > 1 g/l
Other tests		Bacteria on Gram stain: bacterial antigen detectable		Bacteria on Ziehl-Neelsen or fluorescent stain

* Approximately 60% of blood level
† May be low in mumps meningitis

Table 15.3   Causes of purulent meningitis under specific circumstances

Historical data	Organism
Age	
Neonate	*E. coli*, Group B streptococcus, *Listeria*
Child under 6 years old	*H. influenzae*, meningococcus, pneumococcus
Over 6 years old	Meningococcus, pneumococcus
Underlying disease	
Diabetes mellitus	Pneumococcus, Gram-negative bacilli, staphylococci
Alcoholism	Pneumococcus
Associated finding	
Petechial or purpuric rash	Meningococcus
URTI, otitis, sinusitis	Pneumococcus, *H. influenzae*, anaerobes
Pneumonia	Pneumococcus, meningococcus
Critical care patient	Gram-negative bacilli, *Staph. aureus*
Open skull fracture or craniotomy	Gram-negative bacilli, staphylococci
CSF rhinorrhoea	Pneumococcus, Gram-negative bacilli
Intracranial shunt or reservoir	*Staph. epidermidis*
Other factors	
Family cases	Meningococcus: *H. influenzae*
Recurrent	Pneumococcus

URTI: upper respiratory tract infection

cellular damage are induced by toxins released from bacteria and white blood cells and thus cerebral oedema worsens. Vasculitis and thrombosis of the superficial meningeal vessels cause major changes in cerebral perfusion and, ultimately infarction.

The diagnosis of bacterial meningitis is made by culturing the blood and by examination of the CSF (*see* Table 15.2).

The treatment of bacterial meningitis requires the administration of antibiotics that achieve high levels in the CSF. This usually involves parenteral administration. Furthermore, the penetration of most antibiotics is proportional to the degree of meningeal inflammation and therefore the dose should generally not be reduced as irritation diminishes and the patient improves. General supportive measures are also important and some patients will require fluid replacement, antiemetics, anticonvulsants and treatment of raised intracranial pressure. Fever usually settles within a few days and any recurrence of pyrexia during antibiotic therapy is likely to be due to drug fever, subdural effusion or empyema, thrombophlebitis (cerebral or leg vein), or an unrelated infection.

Particular forms of bacterial meningitis

Neisseria meningitidis (meningococcus)

This Gram-negative diplococcus is the most common cause of bacterial meningitis in the UK. It may occur at any age but is predominantly a disease of children and young adults. Occasionally small clusters of cases occur in

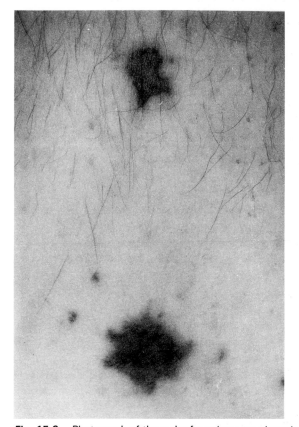

Fig. 15.2. Photograph of the rash of meningococcal septicaemia

susceptible populations and in parts of sub-Saharal Africa large epidemics are frequently seen. There are nine different serogroups of meningococci: group B is the most common serogroup seen in the UK, with smaller numbers of groups C, A, and W135.

The organism is usually carried asymptomatically in the nasopharynx and is transmitted by droplets. The incidence of carriage is high but only occasionally is acquisition followed by bacteraemia and meningitis. There is usually an abrupt onset of symptoms and there may be rapid progression to confusion and coma. The meningitis is always part of a bacteraemic process and two-thirds of patients have a petechial or purpuric rash (Fig. 15.2). Occasionally, acute fulminant meningococcaemia, often without meningeal involvement, is accompanied by widespread skin lesions, disseminated intravascular coagulation (DIC) and circulatory collapse. This is the Waterhouse-Friderichsen syndrome. Metastatic infection in the joints, myocardium, and lungs may also occur.

Neurological complications are infrequent in meningococcal meningitis and the prognosis in cases other than those with circulatory collapse is excellent. Immunologically-mediated complications, notably reactive arthritis, pericarditis and fever sometimes appear 10–14 days after the onset of the disease.

Diagnosis is made by finding *N. meningitidis* in the CSF or blood and treatment is with intravenous benzylpenicillin (20–30 mg/kg body weight 4-hourly) given for 5–7 days. Chloramphenicol (15–25 mg/kg body weight 6-hourly) should be used in penicillin-allergic patients. The widespread resistance of meningococci to sulphonamides precludes empirical use of these antibiotics. There is no evidence of any benefit from steroid or heparin therapy for severe cases, but plasmapheresis and leucopheresis are sometimes helpful.

Close contacts of the patient (family, room-mates, nursery school contacts) are at an increased risk of cross-infection. As penicillin will not eradicate meningococcal carriage, the patient and all such contacts should be given rifampicin (600 mg (or 10 mg/kg body weight) b.d. for 2 days) to eliminate the organism from the nasopharynx. Polysaccharide vaccines are available against meningococci of groups A, C, Y and W135 but not group B.

Streptococcus pneumoniae (pneumococcus)

This form of meningitis tends to occur at the two extremes of age. Predispositions to infection include splenic dysfunction (including sickle cell disease), alcoholism, abnormal humoral immunity (e.g. patients with multiple myeloma), and CSF leaks following skull fractures. Repeated attacks may occur. In half the cases the source of infection cannot be determined and meningitis is presumed to follow primary bacteraemia from the nasopharynx: in others it is associated with pneumonia or infection in the middle ear or paranasal sinuses.

Pneumococcal meningitis is often the most severe of the common forms of meningitis with coma and seizures frequently appearing early in its course.

Treatment is with benzylpenicillin (or chloramphenicol for the penicillin-allergic patient) for 10–14 days. Penicillin-resistant strains of pneumococci have appeared in South Africa, Spain and elsewhere, but fortunately such organisms have not yet become widespread. Cefuroxime or cefotaxime can be used to treat almost all such strains.

Neurological complications (venous sinus thrombosis, hemiplegia, ventriculitis, hydrocephalus) are frequent after pneumococcal meningitis and the mortality remains between 20 and 40 per cent.

Haemophilus influenzae

This is almost exclusively a disease of children between the ages of 4 months and 6 years and is caused primarily by capsulated, type b strains of the small, Gram-negative bacillus. Meningitis is often a complication of a primary respiratory or ear infection, which is frequently acquired from another family member with a similar illness, and begins insidiously with drowsiness or irritability. Inappropriate ADH secretion, deafness, cortical vein thrombosis and sterile subdural effusions are common complications. The latter can be detected by transillumination of the head and may require repeated aspiration or surgical drainage.

Chloramphenicol given for 7 days is the treatment of choice in the UK. Cefuroxime (50 mg/kg body weight 6-hourly) or a third-generation cephalosporin are suitable alternatives: ampicillin-resistance is becoming common among *H. influenzae* and ampicillin should only be used once the organism is known to be sensitive. The mortality is still 5–10 per cent.

Household contacts under the age of 4 years are at increased risk of secondary disease but the efficacy of rifampicin prophylaxis (600 mg (20 mg/kg body weight) daily for 4 days for *all* family members if there is such a young child in the house) is unproven. A vaccine against *H. influenzae* type b is given to infants in the USA.

Neonatal meningitis

Meningitis in the newborn is a serious problem with a high mortality and morbidity. In the UK its incidence is about 1/2500 live births and is particularly seen in low birthweight infants (below 2.5 kg). The organisms that are responsible are chiefly Group B streptococci (GBS) and *Escherichia coli*, particularly strains carrying the K1 capsular antigen. Other less common organisms include *Listeria monocytogenes*, *Pseudomonas aeruginosa* and *Staphylococcus aureus*. Although the majority of infecting bacteria arise from the mother's genital tract and colonize the infant during birth, others are introduced from environmental sites as a result of invasive procedures.

The classical features of meningitis are often absent in the newborn and the signs are usually non-specific. Fever, poor feeding, lethargy, apathy and irritability may predominate. Diarrhoea, apnoea, respiratory distress or jaundice may suggest disease of another system and brief tonic spasms may not be recognized as convulsions. Neck stiffness is rare and the diagnosis of neonatal meningitis requires a high index of suspicion.

Meningitis caused by GBS presents in two distinct ways, depending upon its time of onset after birth.

1. Early onset (first week of life). This is frequently associated with prematurity or obstetric complications and the organism is from the maternal birth canal. The infant has a fulminant illness with a high mortality. Septicaemia and

respiratory symptoms (often confused with respiratory distress syndrome) are prominent.

2. Late onset (after the first week of life). This is a more insidious illness with meningitis a prominent feature and a mortality of only about 15 per cent. Infection is often acquired from hospital personnel or equipment.

The diagnosis of neonatal meningitis depends upon the LP findings but it should be remembered that in the neonate normal CSF may have up to 30 cells/mm^3 (often neutrophils) and a protein concentration up to 1.5 g/litre. The treatment usually recommended for neonatal meningitis is immediate empirical administration of a combination of ampicillin and gentamicin. The penetration of aminoglycosides into the CSF is variable and levels should be measured. Intrathecal and intraventricular gentamicin have both been advocated but the efficacy and safety of these approaches remains controversial. An alternative is to use a third-generation cephalosporin such as ceftriaxone or cefotaxime which penetrate well into the CSF and are effective against most of the likely organisms. Treatment can be modified upon the basis of Gram's stain or culture of the CSF. The prognosis of neonatal meningitis remains poor with mortality up to 50 per cent in premature infants; neurological and psychological sequelae are found in one-third of the survivors.

Other types of purulent meningitis

Shunt-associated meningitis

About 25 per cent of patients with ventriculoatrial or ventriculoperitoneal shunts for hydrocephalus develop meningitis. Most cases are due to *Staphylococcus epidermidis*; many of the remainder are due to *Staph. aureus* or Gram-negative bacilli. The route of infection is usually direct inoculation at the time of shunt implantation and 70 per cent of infections occur in the 2 months after surgery. Systemic and intraventricular therapy with antibiotics (vancomycin seems best for staphylococci) often must be combined with removal of the shunt.

Gram-negative enteric bacilli

Other than during the neonatal period this is primarily seen in patients with head injuries, those who have had neurosurgery, alcoholics and elderly diabetics. Therapy should be with a third-generation cephalosporin (e.g. cefotaxime or ceftazidime) until the species and sensitivity of the responsible organism are known.

Listeria monocytogenes

This is chiefly a disease of neonates or pregnant, debilitated or immunocompromised adults (especially recipients of renal transplants). Either meningitis or a diffuse or focal meningoencephalitis may occur and, despite the name of the organism, polymorphs usually predominate in the CSF pleocytosis. Ampicillin, given for 3 weeks with or without gentamicin, is the best therapy. Co-trimoxazole should be used in the penicillin-allergic patient.

Bacterial meningitis of unknown cause

A difficult dilemma arises when the CSF examination suggests a bacterial cause (*see* Table 15.2) but no organism can be seen on Gram's stain. This often results from outpatient antibiotic therapy which has partially treated a bacterial meningitis; viral meningitis, however, is also frequently associated with polymorphs in the CSF during the first few hours of infection and occasionally it also produces a slightly low glucose level. Distinguishing between the two is not always easy. If the patient is relatively well then it is usually safe to observe him and repeat the LP 6–12 h later; by then, in viral infections, the CSF pleocytosis has often become lymphocytic. Special studies of the CSF may also help: bacterial antigens can be detected by counterimmunoelectrophoresis, latex agglutination or enzyme-linked immunosorbent assay (ELISA); high lactate levels suggest bacterial infection; and the limulus lysate test for endotoxin indicates a Gram-negative infection. These tests may enable a more specific diagnosis to be made earlier than the culture results. If the patient is obviously ill or the second LP has an increased polymorph percentage or falling glucose level then bacterial infection must be assumed and treatment directed at the organisms most likely to be involved must be started *without delay*.

Except in neonates and certain other special instances (*see* above and CNS infection in the immunocompromised patient *see* below), the vast majority of cases of bacterial meningitis are caused by pneumococci, meningococci and *H. influenzae* (the latter almost always in preschool children). Chloramphenicol, cefuroxime or a third-generation cephalosporin is suitable empirical therapy against these three pathogens. In patients over the age of 6 years, *H. influenzae* is very rarely a cause of meningitis and empirical penicillin alone is recommended. Chloramphenicol or cefuroxime can be given to the penicillin-allergic patient. Giving more than one antibiotic in these circumstances is of no additional benefit.

Lymphocytic meningitis

If examination of the CSF shows an excessive number of lymphocytes and a raised protein but no organisms are seen on Gram's stain then the likeliest cause is a viral infection. There are, however, other causes of this CSF picture and many of them require specific therapy. These other possibilities must, therefore, always be considered before assuming that the illness is viral in aetiology (*see* Fig. 15.1).

Tuberculous meningitis

Tuberculous meningitis can occur at any age. In children or adolescents it is usually a manifestation of primary tuberculosis but in adults it is frequently the result of rupture of a subependymal tubercle that has lain quiescent for many years.

The clinical presentation is very variable and depends upon a number of factors: the thick meningeal exudate; vasculitis; cerebral oedema; and the presence of tuberculomas. The illness often begins with a period of general ill-health and malaise which lasts for a week or two before meningeal symptoms appear. Changes in consciousness, seizures and focal neurological signs, particularly VIth-nerve palsies then develop.

Diagnosis can be confirmed by finding *Mycobacterium tuberculosis* in the CSF on Ziehl-Neelsen stains (a large quantity of CSF, up to 10 ml, should be sent for examination if tuberculosis is suspected), but treatment often has to be given on suspicion when the other CSF results, particularly the glucose level, are suggestive (*see* Table 15.2). In children the chest X-ray often shows evidence of pulmonary tuberculosis, but in adults the X-ray is generally normal. The Mantoux test is negative in 10–30 per cent of cases.

Therapy of tuberculous meningitis must take into consideration the ability of drugs to cross the blood–brain barrier. The two drugs that attain the best CSF levels, pyrazinamide and isoniazid, are usually given together with rifampicin and either intramuscular streptomycin or oral ethambutol for the first 2–3 months of therapy. Treatment is then usually continued with isoniazid and rifampicin for a further 7–10 months. Pyridoxine supplements should also be given to prevent isoniazid toxicity. Modern drug regimens have made intrathecal streptomycin unnecessary.

Steroids are probably beneficial in patients with high CSF protein levels and impending spinal block, significantly elevated intracranial pressure, or with focal or general neurological signs. Most patients will recover completely if therapy is started before consciousness is depressed but some develop hydrocephalus or spinal arachnoiditis. Therefore the patient needs close monitoring during the early stages of therapy with frequent CSF examinations and CT scanning to detect progressive changes. Even with early diagnosis the mortality is 10 per cent and another 10–30 per cent have residual neurological damage.

Cryptococcal meningitis

Meningitis due to the yeast, *Cryptococcus neoformans*, is usually seen in patients whose immunity is depressed by steroids, diabetes, lymphoproliferative disorders or AIDS. The organism is widely distributed in nature and infection is acquired by inhalation. Normal hosts are able to contain the infection in the lungs but in those with abnormal T-cell function dissemination to the meninges and other organs is frequent.

The symptoms of cryptococcal meningitis tend to be intermittent over several weeks and meningism is less common than fever, confusion, memory loss and depressed consciousness. Visual disturbances and cranial nerve palsies may be present. The organism may be seen in the CSF using either Gram's stain or an India ink preparation, but the most accurate diagnostic test is the detection of cryptococcal antigen in the CSF or blood using latex agglutination or ELISA.

Treatment is with intravenous amphotericin B. There is no additional therapeutic benefit from using a lower dose of amphotericin combined with 5-flucytosine but toxicity may be lessened. Treatment needs to be continued for at least 6 weeks during which time cryptococcal antigen levels in the CSF should decline.

Parameningeal suppuration

A suppurative process adjacent to the meninges may be associated with the CSF changes of an aseptic meningitis; a history of sinusitis or ear infection should suggest the possibility and indicate the need for a CT scan.

Spirochaetal infection

Leptospirosis

A lymphocytic meningitis, often in conjunction with conjunctivitis and abnormal liver function should raise the possibility of leptospirosis. It is contracted from mammals and is typically a disease of agricultural or abattoir workers. Penicillin therapy is usually recommended.

Lyme disease

This illness is due to *Borrelia burgdorferi*, a spirochaete transmitted by ticks. The first symptom is often a specific rash (erythema chronicum migrans) at the site of the bite but this can be followed several weeks or months later by arthritis, meningoencephalitis and carditis. Symptoms can be relapsing or chronic. Treatment is with high dose penicillin or tetracycline.

Syphilis

See p. 341.

Viral meningitis

A wide variety of different viruses has been implicated in meningitis but the majority of cases are caused by enteroviruses (coxsackie, ECHO and polioviruses, *see* p. 338) or mumps virus. The clinical features of meningitis are not specific, although clues to the aetiology may be obtained from the epidemiological history. Enterovirus infections are spread by the faecal–oral route and are more common in the late summer; small epidemics may occur. A macular rash (and occasionally other rashes) is not unusual. Parotitis would favour mumps; a shingles rash, varicella-zoster virus; genital herpes, herpes simplex type 2; and a history of exposure to small rodents, lymphocytic choriomeningitis (LCM) virus.

The responsible virus should be sought from cultures of the CSF, stools and throat swabs. Serological tests are rarely helpful for enteroviruses but a rising titre can be measured in mumps and other viral infections. Whatever the cause, the management of viral meningitis is purely symptomatic and recovery is usually rapid and complete within a few days.

Encephalitis

Most cases of meningitis are complicated by some degree of inflammation of the brain so that meningoencephalitis probably more correctly reflects the extent of the pathological process. There are, however, some forms of central nervous system infection in which widespread involvement of brain tissue regularly occurs so that disturbances of consciousness, personality, thought and motor function predominate. Some of these, e.g. herpes simplex encephalitis and rabies, are due to direct invasion of the brain cells but others are caused by a secondary immunological response to infection or immunization (parainfectious or postinfectious encephalitis, *see* p. 351). Clues to the aetiology can sometimes be found in the epidemiological history or clinical examination (Fig. 15.3).

Herpes simplex encephalitis

In the UK the most common form of sporadic encephalitis is that due to herpes simplex virus (HSV). It occurs at all ages and is not seasonal. In the neonate, HSV encephalitis is usually part of a disseminated infection contracted from maternal genital lesions. In other patients, the encephalitis is only rarely a primary HSV infection, although there is still debate as to whether it is usually caused by reactivation of latent HSV type 1 (from the trigeminal ganglion or the brain) or by reinfection with a different exogenous HSV strain.

The disease typically has an acute onset with fever, early deterioration in consciousness, seizures and rapid progression. The virus has a particular predilection for the temporal or frontal lobes and the necrosis and oedema often produce focal symptoms (anosmia, olfactory or auditory hallucinations, etc). Focal temporofrontal abnormalities are also commonly detectable clinically or on EEG, isotope scan or CT scan. The diagnosis can only be confirmed prospectively by detection of the virus in a brain biopsy since evidence for specific antibody production in the CSF is only available retrospectively.

The drug of choice for the treatment of HSV encephalitis is acyclovir which is clearly beneficial providing therapy is started before severe brain necrosis has occurred. Therapy (10 mg/kg body weight 8-hourly) should be given for 2 weeks. With such a safe, effective drug available the arguments for diagnostic brain biopsy are less convincing and acyclovir should be started whenever the clinical picture suggests HSV infection. Until the patient responds or serological proof of HSV infection is obtained, however, investigations aimed at other treatable causes of the symptoms should be continued.

Arbovirus encephalitis

In many parts of Asia and the Americas encephalitis is caused by various arboviruses (*arthropod-borne* viruses) transmitted by mosquito or tick bites. Cases are only very rarely seen as importations into the UK.

Rabies

This almost inevitably fatal encephalitis is transmitted in the saliva of infected mammals by bites (or licks onto mucous membranes). Dogs, wolves, cats and bats are the animals that most often transmit the virus to man. There are very

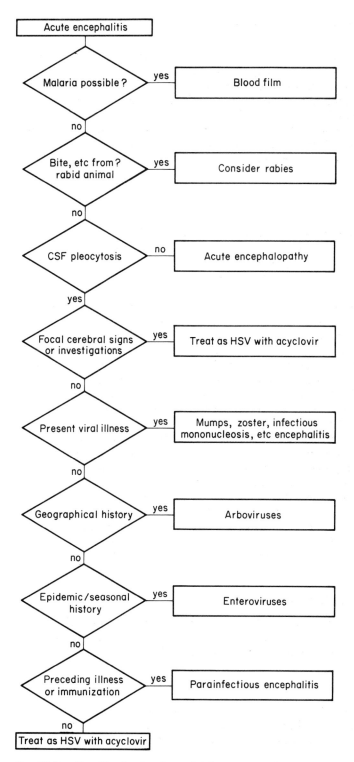

Fig. 15.3. Algorithm for the diagnosis of acute encephalitis

few areas of the world where rabies is not endemic (the British Isles is, at present, a notable exception).

The virus enters the peripheral nerves and spreads retrogradely along the axons to reach the central nervous system; the site of the inoculation largely determines the incubation period which can be many months following bites on the legs. The first symptoms are often non-specific but include paraesthesiae at the inoculation site (often long after the wound has healed). Excitability and spasms of the pharyngeal and laryngeal muscles induced by draughts of air or the sight of water (hydrophobia) are typical. The illness is rapidly progressive and, despite intensive care, paralysis, coma and death are the rule.

Prophylactic vaccines are available and should be given as soon as possible after exposure to the saliva of a potentially rabid animal. Specialist advice should be sought.

Cerebral malaria

Malaria should *always* be suspected as the cause of any neurological symptoms in a patient who has returned from an endemic area within the past 2 months. It is a medical emergency.

Although four species of *Plasmodium* infect man, only *P. falciparum* causes cerebral malaria. Falciparum (malignant tertian) malaria is endemic in much of the tropical and subtropical world. It is transmitted by the bite of an infected mosquito and after a short intrahepatic cycle the parasites invade red blood cells. Fever always occurs and often it is not periodic. Non-specific influenza-like symptoms are frequent. In severe disease vascular damage and sludging of the parasitized red cells lead to blockage of capillaries and hence ischaemia of vital organs. Cerebral malaria leads to lethargy, drowsiness, coma and almost any other CNS symptoms and signs: it can progress to death with frightening rapidity. Haemolysis and disseminated intravascular coagulation compound the severity of the illness.

The diagnostic test is examination of a peripheral blood smear. It can sometimes be difficult to differentiate between the species of *Plasmodia* but if over 1 per cent of the red cells are parasitized or ring forms are seen then falciparum infection should be assumed.

For cerebral malaria intravenous quinine therapy should be used and specialist advice obtained.

Chronic and progressive viral encephalitis

In addition to these acute infections there are several chronic and progressive neurological conditions due to viral infections. These chronic infections are exemplified by subacute sclerosing panencephalitis (SSPE), which is a very rare fatal infection due to a measles virus and which becomes manifest as a progressive neurological deterioration only several years after an apparently uncomplicated attack of measles, and progressive multifocal leucoencephalopathy (*see* below).

CNS infection in the immunocompromised patient

Infections of the CNS are not uncommon in patients with compromised host defences and are often caused by pathogens that do not usually infect the normal host. Abnormalities of immune function are normally classified under one of four headings: (1) defects in polymorph function; (2) defects in humoral immunity; (3) defects in cellular immunity; and (4) splenic dysfunction. Each of these categories is associated with a predisposition to infection of the central nervous system by certain opportunistic pathogens (Table 15.4).

Table 15.4 Major opportunistic pathogens causing syndromes of central nervous system infection in immunocompromised patients

Immune defect	Meningitis	Encephalitis	Brain abscess
Polymorph defect	Gram-negative bacilli Candida	Gram-negative bacilli Candida	Aspergillus
Antibody defect	Pneumococcus H. influenzae	Enteroviruses	
Cellular immune defect	Listeria Cryptococcus Tuberculosis	Listeria Cryptococcus Toxoplasma Varicella/zoster Papovaviruses	Nocardia Aspergillus Toxoplasma
Splenic dysfunction	Pneumococcus H. influenzae		

Patients with inadequate polymorph function, typically those with severe neutropenia, are prone to infection with Gram-negative aerobic bacteria (*Escherichia coli, Klebsiella, Pseudomonas aeruginosa*, etc) and certain fungi. Defects in the ability to mount an antibody response are accompanied by an increased risk of infection by encapsulated bacteria and by a rare chronic encephalitis caused by enteroviruses. Such defects are seen in patients with B-cell lymphoma or leukaemias and myeloma. Patients with defects in cell-mediated immunity (organ transplant recipients, patients with Hodgkin's disease and other lymphomas, those receiving steroid therapy and patients with AIDS) are highly susceptible to intracellular microorganisms.

Loss of splenic function, whether by disease or surgery, is associated with abnormal phagocytic function and lack of opsonizing antibodies and predisposes the individual to infection with encapsulated bacteria. It should be appreciated that, as a result of surgery or therapy with cytotoxic or immunosuppressive drugs or corticosteroids, many patients have abnormalities of their immune system that fall into several of these categories and are thus prone to a wide range of opportunistic pathogens.

The features of meningitis caused by *Listeria* and *Cryptococcus* have already been described (*see* p. 330, 332). Brief mention of some other opportunistic pathogens is given below but for all such infections specialist advice is recommended.

Candida

Meningitis due to *Candida* is usually part of disseminated disease in a patient with neutropenia or following parenteral hyperalimentation. It is a subacute or chronic infection similar to cryptococcosis.

Nocardia

This branching bacterium typically causes a single brain abscess as part of a disseminated infection.

Aspergillus

CNS infection with these fungi occurs in neutropenic patients and those with defects in cellular immunity. Single or multiple brain abscesses are found, often in conjunction with a CSF pleocytosis and signs of meningitis.

Toxoplasma gondii

Cerebral toxoplasmosis has become of major importance in patients with AIDS, in whom it is the most common opportunistic infection of the CNS. There are a variety of presentations ranging from confusion and headache to focal neurological signs: often fever is absent. Diagnosis is usually suspected by finding an enhancing lesion on CT scan, typically in the deep white matter. Serological tests can help in patients with lymphoma but are often unhelpful in those with AIDS. Biopsy of a suspicious lesion may be needed. Treatment is with pyrimethamine and sulphadiazine.

Varicella/zoster virus

Visceral dissemination of chickenpox or shingles is not uncommon in the immunocompromised patient and encephalitis may result, usually between one and 6 weeks after the rash. Acyclovir should be given.

Progressive multifocal leucoencephalopathy

This rare progressive demyelinating disease is caused by a papovavirus. It presents either as dementia or with focal signs and relentlessly progresses to death within a few weeks.

Poliomyelitis

The three strains of polioviruses are enteroviruses and, like others in this genus (*see* above), usually produce an asymptomatic or mild, non-specific infection. Aseptic meningitis also occurs and in a small minority of cases extensive neuronal necrosis, especially of the anterior horn cells in the spinal cord causes paralytic disease.

Poliomyelitis is now extremely rare in the UK but is still an important disease among children in less developed areas of the world. The viruses are spread by the alimentary route, either via faeces or oral secretions and where poor sanitation and overcrowding exist almost all persons over the age of five have antibodies to all three strains.

The vast majority (90–95 per cent) of infections are clinically inapparent. In the remainder, 2–5 days after exposure there is a 'minor illness': fever, headache, sore throat, vomiting and malaise are common complaints but resolve within a day or two. In a minority of cases (1–2 per cent overall) the 'major illness' follows several days later. This is an unremarkable viral meningitis and in some cases there is no further progression. In about 0.15 per cent of all poliovirus infections, however, muscle pains herald the development of frank paralysis a few days later.

The paralysis is of the lower motor neurone type with flaccidity and absent tendon reflexes. Characteristically it is asymmetrical, proximal more than distal, affects the legs more than the arms, and progresses over 24–48 h.

Bulbar polio

In a small number of cases the nuclei of the cranial nerves, particularly the IXth and Xth, are involved. Dysphagia, nasal speech and respiratory difficulties follow. Very rarely the respiratory and vasomotor centres in the medulla are involved.

In any form of neurological poliovirus infection the CSF findings are those of an aseptic meningitis (*see* above). The virus can be cultured from the stools or throat washings (but seldom from the CSF).

No form of treatment will affect the neurological outcome once paralysis has become established. Management consists of respiratory support if there is bulbar or respiratory muscle disturbance, prevention of contractures and rehabilitation.

Paralytic polio can be prevented by immunization with either inactivated (IPV) or live oral (OPV) vaccines. Both forms have been widely used. In the UK, OPV is given as part of the primary immunization course in infancy. Occasionally vaccine-associated paralysis has been reported and OPV should not be given to immunocompromised hosts or their household contacts.

Tetanus

The clinical manifestations of tetanus result from the effects of an exotoxin (tetanospasmin) produced by *Clostridium tetani*, a spore-forming, strictly anaerobic, Gram-positive rod. Disease results after a wound is contaminated by bacterial spores, which then vegetate and elaborate toxin.

Any age group may be affected but in the UK most cases are in the elderly, who are often unprotected by vaccination. Any trivial injury may be contaminated but severe trauma with extensive tissue necrosis is particularly liable to infection. Intravenous drug abuse and the traditional practice in some societies of using animal dung on the neonatal umbilicus are other particularly hazardous practices.

The incubation period is between 3 and 21 days (usually 5–10 days). Tetanospasmin has its major effect upon the spinal cord where it impairs inhibitory synapses. This produces muscle rigidity and spasm, and sympathetic overactivity. Most cases have masseter spasm and trismus as the presenting symptom. This produces the characteristic sardonic smile (risus sardonicus). Stiffness of the spinal and abdominal muscles also occurs and opisthotonos can result. As the disease progresses severe spasms of muscles occur and may result in apnoea and choking. Sweating, tachycardia and other signs of autonomic dysfunction may appear. The shorter the incubation period and the faster the progression of the disease, the more severe the illness is likely to be.

There are no specific diagnostic tests for tetanus and diagnosis is based only upon the overt clinical signs. The CSF is normal and often there is no evidence of the original wound.

Specific treatment should be given with a single dose of human hyperimmune immunoglobulin, 3000–6000 units i.m. and benzylpenicillin 4 million units/day in divided doses for 10 days. Surgical excision of the injured tissue should also be contemplated.

The mainstay of treatment of tetanus is expert nursing and medical care in an intensive care unit. The patient should be kept quiet to minimize the number of spasms and in the most mild cases this and sedation may be all that is needed. In more severe cases paralysis and intubation are necessary. Aggressive nutritional support, control of autonomic dysfunction and prevention of pneumonia and pulmonary emboli are all vitally important.

An attack of tetanus does not confer immunity to further attacks and all patients should be given a course of vaccination. Everyone should receive a complete basic course of toxoid given as part of the normal childhood immunizations with further routine boosters given every 10 years thereafter.

The use of tetanus toxoid and hyperimmune globulin should be considered in all patients with wounds and depends upon the immunization history and the type of wound (Table 15.5).

Table 15.5 Guidelines for tetanus prophylaxis

History of tetanus immunization	Clean minor wound[1]		All other wounds[1]	
	Td[2]	TIG[3]	Td[2]	TIG[3]
Within past 1 year	No	No	No	No
Within past 5 years	No	No	Yes	No
Within past 10 years	Yes	No	Yes	No
More than 10 years ago	Yes	No	Yes	Yes
Never fully immunized	Yes[4]	No	Yes[4]	Yes

[1]A clean minor wound is one less than 6 h old which is clean and non-penetrating. All other wounds are tetanus prone
[2]Td = Adult type of tetanus and diphtheria toxoids
[3]TIG = 250 units of human tetanus hyperimmune globulin given i.m.
[4]Proceed with a full course of basic immunization

Syphilis

Syphilis is due to infection with *Treponema pallidum*, a slender spirochaete between 5 and 15 μm in length. It cannot be cultured on artificial media and diagnosis therefore depends upon direct visualization or serological testing.

Transmission is almost always venereal although infection can occur *in utero* or as a result of blood transfusion. The true incidence in the UK is unknown but it is more common in urban areas and has increased recently among homosexual males.

The clinical features of syphilis reflect a complex interaction between the organism and the immune system.

Primary disease

One to 6 weeks after infection a painless papular lesion develops at the site of inoculation. This develops into a shallow, indurated ulcer (the chancre) accompanied by regional lymphadenopathy. Untreated it heals within 2–3 weeks.

Secondary disease

This occurs 6–8 weeks later, corresponding to the time of maximal antigenic load. There is an erythematous papular eruption, often involving the palms and soles, which may coalesce to form moist, highly infectious, condyloma lata around the genitalia. There is a bacteraemia and the nervous system becomes infected. CNS symptoms are rare but occasionally a lymphocytic meningitis may develop. Secondary disease spontaneously heals after 4–6 weeks but in one-quarter of patients relapses occur at some time over the next 4 years.

Latent syphilis

During this stage there are no clinical symptoms and the infection can only be detected by positive serological tests.

Tertiary disease

Approximately one-third of patients will develop clinical evidence of late disease as a result of continuing destructive inflammation. This may only become manifest several decades after infection. The cardiovascular system (aortitis), musculoskeletal structures and the nervous system (20–30 per cent of cases) are commonly involved. There are a number of varieties of neurosyphilis and more than one can occur in any individual.

Gumma

This is a nodule of granulomatous inflammatory tissue that may produce the neurological signs of a progressive space-occupying lesion.

Meningeal

This occurs 5–10 years after the primary infection and produces a subacute or chronic meningitis. There may also be focal signs as a result of endarteritis of the cerebral vessels. The CSF is abnormal with a mononuclear pleocytosis, raised protein and sometimes a reduced glucose concentration.

General paralysis of the insane (GPI)

Ten or more years after infection about 5 per cent of untreated syphilitics develop progressive dementia, speech and thought disorders, long tract signs and exaggerated tendon reflexes.

Tabes dorsalis

This syndrome may be delayed by 20–30 years and results from progressive demyelination of the posterior columns and dorsal nerve roots. It is characterized by ataxia, paraesthesiae, sensory loss and clusters of severe instantaneous pains in the legs or trunk (lightning pains). The loss of sensation leads to retention of urine and faeces, Charcot's joints and trophic ulceration. Optic atrophy and Argyll Robertson pupils (small, irregular pupils that react to accommodation but not to light) occur in tabes dorsalis and GPI.

The demonstration of *Treponema pallidum* by darkfield microscopy is the method of choice for a suspected syphilitic chancre or condyloma lata.

In the other forms of disease diagnosis is based upon serological tests, which fall into two groups: the non-specific (reaginic) antibody tests and those for specific treponemal antibodies. The rates of positive tests in untreated syphilis at various stages are summarized in Table 15.6. The reaginic antibody tests (particularly the VDRL) are useful as screening tests or for monitoring the response to treatment but false positive results are common and any positive result in the serum therefore needs further confirmation. A positive VDRL test from the CSF is diagnostic of neurosyphilis. The FTA-Abs is the standard specific antibody test. A positive result is diagnostic of present or past infection but once positive the FTA-Abs usually remains so for life, with or without treatment, and the test cannot therefore be used to document the adequacy of therapy.

Table 15.6   Rate of positive serological tests (%) in various stages of syphilis

Stage of disease	VDRL	FTA-Abs
Primary	75	85
Secondary	99	99
Latent	75	98
Tertiary	70	98

VDRL: venereal disease research laboratòry test; FTA-Abs: fluorescent treponemal antibody absorption test

Penicillin remains the treatment of choice for all stages of syphilis. The recommended regimens and follow-up are summarized in Table 15.7.

Table 15.7 Treatment and follow-up of syphilis

Stage	Treatment	Follow-up
Primary or secondary	Benzathine penicillin 2.4 million units i.m.	1, 3, 6, 12 months
Tertiary (cardiovascular)	Three, weekly doses of above	Above and then every 6 months for 2 years
Neurosyphilis or latent disease with abnormal CSF	Penicillin G, 12–24 million units (mU)/day i.v. for 10 days; or procaine penicillin, 2.4 mU/day i.m. plus probenecid for 10 days	As above for tertiary disease and CSF every year for 3 years
Penicillin-allergic patients		
Primary or secondary	Tetracycline or erythromycin 500 mg 4 times a day for 15 days	
Late	Tetracycline or erythromycin 500 mg 4 times a day for 30 days	

16

Demyelinating diseases of the central nervous system

Multiple sclerosis (MS)

This condition causes patches (plaques) of inflammatory damage largely affecting the white matter of the central nervous system. The plaques contain areas of myelin loss (demyelination) with variable degrees of secondary axonal degeneration. The hallmarks of multiple sclerosis are those of anatomical and temporal dissemination, i.e. the plaques occur at different sites on different occasions.

Epidemiology and aetiology

The cause is unknown although a number of theories have been proposed. These will be discussd briefly. The condition shows a curious geographical distribution with zones of high and low incidence in the world: high-risk zones include the northern temperate zone and low risk areas the equatorial regions. In high risk areas the prevalence lies between 50 and 200 per 100 000 while in low risk areas the value is less than 10 per 100 000. Migration studies suggest that it is where the first 15 years of life are spent that determines whether a person is subject to a high or low risk.

In most sufferers the condition starts in early adult life, women are more affected than men, and the peak age of incidence is about 30. Recently, genetic studies have tried to answer the question raised by the appearance of several affected people in the same family. However, in such affected members the increased frequency did not suggest a Mendelian trait (25 or 50 per cent frequency) and in monozygotic twins the prevalence of the unaffected twin developing the disease is only 30 per cent. Certain HLA tissue antigens (e.g. HLA DR2) have an increased incidence in patients with MS, although this appears to be polygenic.

It has been proposed that exposure to a possible virus with a very long latency may allow the condition to develop in certain people who have defective immunological defences. Such defects of the immune system may be genetically determined. However, despite extensive viral studies no such organisms have been isolated. Animal experiments have now produced a relapsing and remitting demyelinating disease by the injection of encephalitogenic protein (a sterile extract of nervous tissue) in Freund's adjuvant. This causes experimental allergic encephalomyelitis which is a cell-mediated disorder and microscopically appears similar to the plaques of MS. Furthermore, the presence of oligoclonal IgG in the CSF of MS patients supports the synthesis of immune proteins in the CNS.

Pathology

Demyelination will produce multiple plaques in the white matter of the brain, spinal cord and optic nerves. Most commonly such plaques are concentrated around the ventricles, the optic nerves and chiasm, in the brainstem, cerebellum, and posterior and lateral columns of the spinal cord. In the latter, the cervical and thoracic regions are most affected. In an acute lesion there is perivenous inflammation with infiltration of mononuclear cells and lymphocytes, oedema and destruction or thinning of myelin. The axons are relatively spared although with more severe damage there may be both neuronal and axonal loss. In more chronic lesions there will be loss of myelin, often axons, and prominent fibroglial proliferation causing scarring. The old term for such scarring was sclerosis. Over many years the CNS of affected patients may show multiple plaques and the brain atrophies. Many such plaques can now be demonstrated during life by magnetic resonance imaging (MRI) scans.

Symptoms and signs

The presentation is very varied. About half the patients may start with a single symptom, the other half with multiple. Common symptoms include:

1. Sudden visual loss or blurring from an acute optic neuritis (see p. 158). This may cause a drop in acuity with often a central scotoma and afferent pupillary defect. This occurs in about 25 per cent.
2. Sudden weakness, numbness or sensory symptoms in one or more limbs. This is the presentation in about 50 per cent. Such symptoms may reflect plaques in the posterior columns or dorsal root entry zones where they may produce tingling, paraesthesiae, numbness, a sensation of tight bands or even more bizarre sensory features like itching, tickling, or insects under the skin. Feelings of burning or coldness may reflect involvement of the spinothalamic pathways. These sensory symptoms may vary in extent and often progress over a few days. Severe sensory loss may lead to a de-afferented limb which appears clumsy and 'useless', which is particularly noticeable in the hand where there will be difficulty in performing fine manipulative tasks, and there is also sensory ataxia. Sensory upsets are often accompanied by Lhermitte's phenomenon (barber's chair sign) where neck flexion produces tingling or an electric-shock sensation down the back and sometimes into the legs. This suggests damage to the posterior columns in the cervical cord. Although this is found commonly in MS it may also occur with other pathology at that site.

   Motor symptoms may produce spastic weakness, most marked in the legs, where there may be complaints that the leg feels heavy, stiff and may drag.

There is often inability to run as an early feature. Commonly patients may complain of problems with one leg but in fact show signs of pyramidal tract involvement of both legs, with exaggerated reflexes, extensor plantar responses and often absent abdominal reflexes.

In the spinal cord the intermedio-lateral columns may be affected which will cause urinary symptoms with urgency, frequency and even retention with incontinence. Bowel symptoms include constipation and in the male there may be complaints of impotence.

3. Disturbances in the brainstem and cerebellum are the presenting features in about 15 per cent and may lead to:

(a) Visual upset with blurred or double vision, or oscillopsia (sensation of objects moving). These may arise from palsies of individual ocular muscles, most often from oculomotor or abducens nerve involvement, but also from an internuclear ophthalmoplegia. The latter arises from damage to the medial longitudinal fasciculus. Coarse nystagmus may lead to oscillopsia and varying patterns of nystagmus suggest central brainstem involvement, e.g. coarse horizontal, multidirectional, vertical, rotatory or combinations of these.

(b) Balance and coordination disturbances may arise from plaques in the cerebellum or its connections. These may be aggravated by sensory ataxia (from position sense loss). Charcot's triad describes nystagmus, a scanning dysarthria and intention tremor all pointing to a cerebellar lesion. Unsteadiness may point to a midline or a lateralized cerebellar fault. The intention tremor may be mild, or so gross that patients may be totally dependent, even unable to lift a cup to their lips.

(c) Facial sensory and motor symptoms may occur with pontine plaques. Symptoms include numbness in the face often remitting within a few weeks, or even the development of trigeminal neuralgia. Neuralgia starting in a young patient should alert the doctor to the possibility of MS presenting in this way, or to some other causes of symptomatic tic (*see* p. 165). Involuntary movements may also occur with facial myokymia, a fine ripple under the skin in the cheek from a 'continuous rhythmic fascicular contraction'. Myokymia may also arise from other pontine pathology. Hemifacial spasm may rarely arise in MS. A lower motor neurone facial palsy (of Bell's pattern) may also occur and sometimes this may be the clue to a previous episode.

(d) Acute vertigo lasting days and usually linked with vomiting, ataxia and prostration may occur. This is accompanied by nystagmus and is relatively common as a manifestation of a brainstem plaque. If this has been a retrospective episode, it has often been attributed to an infective labyrinthine disorder. The symptom of dizziness is common but needs careful evaluation (*see* p. 34). Hearing loss is uncommon in MS.

(e) Bulbar symptoms with slurring dysarthria and problems swallowing may reflect medullary plaques. Severe bulbar damage may lead to life-threatening respiratory complications necessitating urgent hospital admission.

(f) Paroxysmal brainstem disturbances may also be found lasting seconds or minutes and include dysarthria, pains, ataxia, tonic spasms and sensory upsets.

4. Cerebral disturbances may arise but are less common. Many patients with long-standing MS show clear evidence of a decline of cognitive function and sometimes this appears slowly progressive. A hemiplegia or hemianopia are uncommon features. Cerebral plaques lead to a greater incidence of epileptic seizures. Depression and sometimes euphoria may also arise. In a few patients there may be marked behavioural problems. Patients with brain-stem upset may show emotional lability.

Course and prognosis

Most commonly, the condition runs a relapsing and remitting course with a relapse rate of about 0.3/year. In early attacks there is often full recovery, but over many years patients often show persisting signs following incomplete recovery. Perhaps some 60 per cent of patients change from a relapsing-remitting course to a progressive pattern at some stage. Cumulative disability may lead to a progressive paraplegia, or even tetraplegia with, in some instances, a totally dependent paralysed patient with double incontinence. Such patients will show an increased mortality, a figure of 20 per cent has been suggested for patients with disease of 20 years' duration.

About 10 per cent of patients show a slow grumbling progression from the onset. This is most often found in middle-aged patients presenting with a spastic paraparesis. In a number of patients, perhaps as high as 20 per cent, the disease runs a benign course seeming to 'burn out' leaving little or no residual disability.

Many patients recognize that relapses may be precipitated by intercurrent infections, illness or even trauma, including surgery. Emotional shock may also be a trigger and sometimes immunization. Becoming over-tired also appears to make some patients more vulnerable to relapse. An increased temperature or a hot bath may often transiently aggravate the symptoms and sometimes the signs of MS patients. Pregnancy *per se* probably does not increase the relapse rate, but there appears to be a greater risk in the immediate months postpartum and affected patients should be encouraged to have small families.

In patients with chronic and progressive disease a number of problems arise. These include:

1. Increasing spasticity usually arising in patients whose leg weakness has con-fined them to a bed or wheel-chair. Such patients may sometimes develop extensor, or more commonly flexor spasms with the legs drawing up. Such spasms are often painful, may disturb sleep or prevent the maintenance of a comfortable position.
2. Bladder disturbance with incontinence is common. The combination of an immobile incontinent patient with impaired saddle sensation lying in a wet bed predisposes the development of bed-sores. Persistent incontinence in the male can usually be managed by the use of a condom drainage appliance but in the female such appliances are unsatisfactory and here incontinence may be managed by (a) pads, (b) catheters, indwelling or intermittent (even self-inserted), or (c) urinary diversion usually to an ileal conduit draining to an ileostomy bag. Long-term catheterization poses problems from blocked

catheters, recurrent and resistant urinary infections and these may show retrograde spread to the kidneys.

Constipation is more easy to manage with attention given to appropriate diets, aperients and even enemas. In some patients manual removal may prove necessary.

Impotence in the male is a real problem although there are a few specialist centres which try to help patients with such difficulties.

3. Skin ulceration with the development of pressure sores. These have already been mentioned and linked with incontinence. The important point here is prevention with the avoidance of any prolonged pressure on an immobile area. Such ulcers may become very deep and indolent causing systemic upset, anaemia, and even osteomyelitis in underlying bone. Often secondary anaerobic infection occurs in such wounds. Severe ulceration may require hospital admission with a view to debridement and even plastic surgery with rotation of skin flaps to cover extensive areas.

4. Decline in mental function with additional depression, apathy and increasing dependence in the chronic patient. These may impose enormous burdens on devoted families so that facilities for respite care, adequate holiday breaks or even long-term institutional care may require provision.

Variable figures are given for survival. Many patients live for more than 30 years. In one survey about one-third were working and two-thirds able to walk after 25 years. However, another survey suggested some 20–25 per cent of patients had died within 20 years of the onset of their illness.

Investigations

Despite numerous claims there is no single laboratory test that is pathognomonic for MS. The diagnosis is clinical and rests on the establishment of multiple lesions disseminated anatomically and temporally which have not been shown due to other pathology.

There may be laboratory support for MS in changes in the CSF. About one-third of patients may show a mild lymphocytic pleocytosis, usually less than 50 cells/mm^3. The CSF sugar is normal and cultures are sterile. The total CSF protein will be elevated in 30–40 per cent, usually a mild rise of less than 1 g/litre. However, if this protein rise is differentiated, it occurs in the globulins and the gamma globulin fraction is increased above 13 per cent of the total protein in some 60–70 per cent of patients. CSF protein electrophoresis will show the presence of discrete oligoclonal bands in 90–95 per cent of patients. Such bands may also arise in other uncommon inflammatory CNS disorders (e.g. syphilis, subacute sclerosing panencephalitis) so these changes are not completely specific.

Evoked potential studies have been used with increasing frequency to demonstrate the presence of multiple lesions. Again, such studies are not pathognomonic for MS but the demonstration of an optic nerve lesion in a patient with a spastic paraparesis would be strong support for demyelination. The most used evoked potentials are visual, auditory brainstem and somatosensory. The presence of significant delay in central conduction is very suggestive support.

Radiological investigations may be useful on two counts. First, they may be necessary to exclude other pathology. This is of particular importance where patients show evidence of a single spinal cord lesion which could reflect extrinsic cord compression, an intrinsic intramedullary tumour or a plaque of demyelination. Here myelography may be mandatory to exclude a potentially reversible cause of cord compression. Second, imaging techniques may demonstrate the presence of a lesion or lesions in the brain or spinal cord. This may be done with computerized tomography (CT) or better still MRI scans. CT scans, particularly with the most modern high definition apparatus, may show multiple lesions, usually low density, often enhancing, and sometimes cerebral atrophy. Such lesions are most common in the periventricular white matter. MRI scans give a much greater yield especially for posterior fossa plaques as well as periventricular white matter lesions. Using MRI many lesions can be shown which are not apparent on conventional CT scans. Again such scan appearances are not pathognomonic for MS but are strong supportive evidence. Multifocal vascular disease may also give similar signals.

Blood tests may be important in the exclusion of other diseases. Thus patients with a spastic paraparesis or an optic nerve lesion should have a serum B12 measurement, and serology with Wasserman reaction, fluorescent treponemal antibody, *Treponema pallidum* haemagglutination or equivalent (to exclude syphilis). A full blood count, erythrocyte sedimentation rate (ESR), chest X-ray and views of an appropriate part of the spinal canal may be indicated. Always recall that the adult spinal cord ends at about L1 so radiological investigation of a spastic paraparesis includes the spinal column above this level (views of the lumbar spine are inappropriate). Rarely, studies to exclude a parasagittal cerebral lesion damaging the motor strips on both sides, may be necessary in investigating causes of a paraparesis.

It is important to re-emphasize that if a patient's symptoms and signs could all arise from one site (e.g. the foramen magnum), then it is essential to exclude extrinsic neuraxis compression.

Treatment

There is no known cause and hence no specific cure. However, in patients with an acute florid attack there is good evidence that a course of steroids may halt progression and bring about an earlier remission. There does not seem to be a great difference in the ultimate recovery from a relapse whether steroids are used or not. Traditionally, injections of ACTH were used and a variety of regimens described: each has its supporters. One regimen includes injections of 80,60,40 and 20 units daily, each dose given for 5 days. Other steroids have been used: pulse injections intravenously of methylprednisolone 500–1000 mg daily for 5 days, and oral steroids (e.g. dexamethasone, prednisolone) in varying courses. Potassium supplements may be necessary. Not all patients respond to steroids and a very small number may develop an acute psychosis. The latter is a contraindication to further steroids. Prolonged steroid treatment or frequently repeated courses have little justification. They only produce long-term side-effects (e.g. weight gain, facial mooning, osteoporosis, proximal muscle weakness), and there is no evidence that they prevent relapses.

Because there is no definitive therapy for MS, numerous therapeutic claims have been made. These have not been shown by careful clinical trials to be statistically of benefit, although many have their supporters and even some trial evidence for a 'favourable trend'.

Special diets have been tried: low fat, low sugar, vitamin supplements, B12 injections, and the addition of polyunsaturated fatty acids (usually as sunflower seed oil or Naudicelle capsules). For a time a gluten-free diet was proposed. These dietary measures have no statistical support.

The use of hyperbaric oxygen with patients in decompression chambers has recently enjoyed a vogue, although a series of careful trials has shown no evidence of lasting benefit.

Immunosuppression using drugs such as azathioprine, cyclophosphamide and cyclosporin, has been tried. These are potentially toxic drugs and it would be important to have clear evidence of their efficacy before these are recommended. Statistical evidence to date is lacking. The latest substance that has been proposed is copolymer I, but more information is awaited.

In severe relapses rest is important and bedrest may be necessary if there is distressing vertigo, vomiting, severe limb weakness or bladder upset. Symptomatic treatment may include antiemetics, vestibular sedatives and analgesics. In many patients with mild relapses no treatment is necessary. Carbamazepine is particularly effective in the control of paroxysmal disorders (*see* p. 346) as well as in trigeminal neuralgia.

Chronically affected patients pose many problems, not least in the support they and their families may require. Spasticity may be helped with baclofen (Lioresal) 10–60 mg given in divided doses, often with the larger dose at bedtime. Care must be taken to titrate the effects of the drugs against the symptoms as too high a dose may cause flaccid weakness with floppy limbs which will not support a previously ambulant patient. Other drugs can be tried: diazepam (Valium) and dantrolene sodium (Dantrium). In all these drug treatments a low dose is used initially and then gradually increased depending on the response. If medical measures fail then, rarely, destructive methods can be used for severe spasticity with bad flexor spasms. These may include section of tendons or the use of intrathecal phenol to 'block' appropriate lumbar and sacral roots by chemical damage.

Neurogenic bladder disturbances may require expert urodynamic assessment. It is important to exclude infection particularly where incomplete bladder emptying may lead to a residual 'pool' of stagnant urine. Certain drugs such as propantheline (Pro-Banthine) or emepronium (Cetiprin) may reduce frequency and urgency. Constipation may be aided by bulk preparations, various aperients or enemas.

Depression may merit appropriate treatment with tricyclic antidepressants.

Provision of aids supervised by physiotherapists and occupational therapists may significantly help selected patients and their families. A home assessment visit may allow the provision of appropriate bathroom aids (e.g. a lavatory seat at the correct height with support rails, a shower for the disabled, a bath hoist) and a variety of other measures. Many such aids can be funded with the help of local authorities. Courses of physiotherapy sometimes with hydrotherapy may prove useful. Local MS societies may add helpful support.

Acute disseminated encephalomyelitis

This is a form of acute inflammatory disturbance, probably immunologically determined, which may follow certain infections or vaccination, arising as a monophasic illness. It has similarities to experimental allergic encephalomyelitis. It most often follows measles and is found in areas of the world where immunization has not been carried out. It may also follow rubella, chickenpox and, less often, mumps. The symptoms may start 2–5 days after the rash or sometimes some 10–40 days later. There is commonly a deteriorating conscious level, delirium, fever, meningism, convulsions and the appearance of focal neurological disturbances, movement disorders and cerebellar ataxia. Some patients may become comatose, others may show a transverse myelitis.

Pathologically there are scattered patches of demyelination throughout the white matter of the brain and spinal cord accompanied by prominent perivenous infiltration of mononuclear cells and lymphocytes. The CSF shows a lymphocytic pleocytosis and an elevated protein.

There is a high morbidity and mortality despite intensive treatment which includes high dose steroids.

Diffuse cerebral sclerosis (Schilder's disease)

This term probably covers a number of different disorders which may include the leucodystrophies, which are genetically determined disturbances of metabolism and of formation of myelin. These often lead to the widespread destruction of white matter accompanied by prominent gliosis. Some are associated with breakdown products of myelin, e.g. metachromatic or globoid bodies, which may give their name to the disorder, metachromatic leucodystrophy. One type, inherited as an X-linked recessive trait, is associated with adrenal failure, adrenoleucodystrophy. Some may be accompanied by a peripheral neuropathy. These are not strictly demyelinating disorders in the inflammatory context. Most can be diagnosed by estimating the levels of specific lysosomal enzymes in peripheral white blood cells or fibroblasts.

There is also a more specific entity, *encephalitis periaxalis diffusa*, which is not genetically determined and affects young adults or children, producing very extensive areas of myelin loss, maximal in the posterior parts of the cerebral hemispheres. The presentation is variable and may be acute or insidious. Visual impairment, mental deterioration, epileptic seizures or increasing unsteadiness are the most frequent early manifestations. These may be followed by a hemianopia going on to cortical blindness, a hemiplegia or quadriplegia and dementia. The CSF may be normal or show an elevated IgG and sometimes a lymphocytic pleocytosis. There is no specific treatment and most patients only survive a few months.

Transverse myelitis

This describes an acute spinal cord lesion which may appear to 'transect' the cord causing an acute loss of function below that level. In the most severe form the motor upset produces an acute paraplegia, initially flaccid but later spastic, with loss of control of bowel and bladder. There may be sensory loss for all modalities below that level with a clear line of demarcation. In less severe forms some sensory function may be preserved: the distribution of this may suggest that certain sensory tracts are predominantly affected (e.g. if pain and temperature sensation are lost this suggests spinothalamic damage). An acute paraplegia or tetraplegia with loss of pain and temperature sensation, but preservation of joint position and vibration also suggests a vascular myelopathy (cord stroke), particularly in middle-aged and elderly patients. Sometimes the myelitis may progress producing an ascending level and in the acute stage, with flaccid weakness, this may be difficult to differentiate from a Guillain-Barré syndrome.

The cause is most commonly acute demyelination of the white and grey matter of the spinal cord most often in the thoracic region. It may also arise as part of the initial presentation of MS, but may also be part of a postinfective acute disseminated encephalomyelitis, the brunt falling on the cord. This may follow the viral exanthemas (measles, rubella, chicken pox) or less often other viral infections. It may also follow vaccination, herpes-zoster infections and glandular fever. Rarely, it may follow spinal cord bacterial infections, or be part of a meningovascular luetic infection. Current interest has been aroused in that some forms of myelitis may be due to HIV infection: some forms of spastic paraplegia found in the West Indies have been shown due to human T lymphotrophic virus (HTLV) I.

The diagnosis is often made by excluding an acute cord compression by myelography and showing the CSF is abnormal with an elevated protein, and often a lymphocytic pleocytosis. The CSF IgG may be elevated.

Treatment is with steroids if there is no bacterial infection. In some patients recovery may be poor.

Devic's disease, neuromyelitis optica describes a myelitis with optic neuritis. Here a spinal cord lesion, transverse myelitis, is associated either together or sequentially with an optic neuritis. The optic neuritis may affect one or both eyes and both conditions usually arise within days or weeks. Pathologically the lesions show extensive demyelination, but there has been debate about whether this is a form of MS or a separate monophasic illness. Treatment is with steroids.

17

Degenerative diseases of the central nervous system

Motor neurone disease

This ranks as one of the worst of the degenerative diseases of the nervous system because it causes a relentless progressive loss of motor neurones in the anterior horns of the spinal cord, in the motor nuclei of the brainstem and the pyramidal cells of the motor cortex. This produces:

1. Progressive muscular atrophy from a lower motor neurone lesion involving the anterior horn cells.
2. Progressive bulbar palsy from the lower motor neurone lesion of the motor nuclei of the cranial nerves, particularly in the medulla.
3. Amyotrophic lateral sclerosis from an upper motor neurone lesion with pyramidal tract damage from neuronal loss in the motor cortex, which will cause spastic weakness of the limbs. Similar involvement of the pyramidal pathways to bulbar motoneurones causes a pseudobulbar palsy.

In most patients there is a combination of all these motor deficits.

The prevalence is about 5–7/100 000. Men are affected more frequently than women and the greatest incidence is in older patients, between the ages of 50 and 70. The cause is unknown although in about 5–10 per cent it may be familial with an autosomal dominant inheritance and often an earlier age of onset. There is also a curious geographic incidence with areas of increased frequency, e.g. Guam, the Kii peninsular of Japan. In a few patients with a past history of paralytic polio, features of progressive muscular atrophy may develop after a long interval, often 15–20 years. Familial progressive muscular atrophy may also be found to cause the spinal muscular atrophies in infancy and childhood (*see* p. 355).

The pathology of motor neurone disease (MND) is a loss of motor neurones in the brainstem, motor cortex and anterior horns. The anterior roots atrophy and there is evidence of degeneration in the lateral columns.

Clinical features

The onset is variable. It may be a predominantly lower motor neurone picture with asymmetric wasting and weakness of the small hand muscles, or a foot drop with wasting of the distal part of the leg. Fasciculation is common and patients may complain of cramps in the legs, particularly at night. The weakness and wasting may be accompanied by exaggerated reflexes and extensor plantar responses from the upper motor neurone involvement. Later, the weakness may be very widespread with increasing disability. Other patients may present with spastic weakness of the legs with a stiff dragging leg and difficulty running. Often this may be combined with obvious fasciculation or asymptomatic weakness in the arms. In time, widespread weakness with an admixture of upper and lower motor neurone signs becomes apparent.

In about one-third, presentation may be with bulbar symptoms, causing difficulty in speaking and swallowing. Pronounciation becomes difficult and the speech soft and more laboured. Chewing and swallowing weakens leading to choking, overspill and even nasal regurgitation. In such patients the muscles of the soft palate and tongue are weak, the tongue fasciculates, later showing atrophy. The motor side of the pharyngeal reflex may be lost. There may be associated upper motor neurone features with an increased jaw jerk. Emotional lability may occur.

Within months there is steady progression which may aid diagnosis, particularly if the presentation is with asymmetrical weakness in one limb. The absence of intellectual change, sensory signs or sphincter upset also point to the diagnosis. Within about 18–24 months many patients are confined to a wheelchair. The weakness may involve the trunk and neck muscles, so support for the back and head becomes necessary. Increasing bulbar weakness may lead to anarthria, and an unsafe swallow may require a semisolid diet. There is often marked weight loss and widespread wasting. Later the respiratory muscles weaken: this may lead to an aspiration pneumonia and weak cough. There is often breathlessness, particularly on lying, and terminally respiratory failure.

The condition progresses leading to death most commonly from a secondary chest infection within about 3 years. Patients with severe bulbar weakness have the worst outlook. About 10–15 per cent of patients with predominant progressive muscular atrophy may show a slower course, surviving 10–15 years.

Investigations and differential diagnosis

It is important to exclude potentially reversible conditions which may mimic MND in its early stages. These include certain muscle diseases, thyrotoxicosis and polymyositis, which may present with proximal muscle weakness, bulbar weakness and even fasciculation. Bulbar problems may also occur in myasthenia gravis, or local obstructive lesions in the oropharynx or upper oesophagus. A spondylotic cervical radiculomyelopathy or intramedullary spinal cord lesion, or even subacute combined degeneration, may produce a combination of lower and upper motor neurone signs. However, these are commonly accompanied by sensory signs and sphincter disturbance. A predominant motor neuropathy, e.g. lead poisoning, might mimic a progressive muscular atrophy.

Investigations should include blood tests to check thyroid function, creatine kinase (this may be slightly elevated with denervation but grossly elevated with polymyositis), and serum B12 level. An edrophonium test and estimation of anti-acetylcholine receptor antibody will eliminate myasthenia. Otolaryngological examination, endoscopy or a barium swallow may be necessary in patients with severe dysphagia. Electromyographic (EMG) studies and nerve conduction measurements will help to exclude a peripheral neuropathy, and confirm the presence of widespread denervation in the limb and trunk muscles. In selected patients myelography may be necessary. The CSF may be normal or show a slightly elevated protein.

Treatment

There is no specific remedy although symptomatic measures may be used. Baclofen and diazepam may help spasticity; simple analgesics may relieve discomfort, and antidepressants help some distress. Patients and their families need considerable support through this harrowing illness. Various walking aids such as frames, later wheelchairs, special beds, bath hoists, electric suckers may all help in the nursing of patients at home. Later respite care with short stays in hospital or a hospice allow the family some rest. In the terminal stages regular strong analgesics, with diazepam, may prove helpful.

Spinal muscular atrophies

These include a number of rare heredofamilial degenerative disorders affecting the motor neurones in infancy, childhood or adolescence. They have varied degrees of severity and differing patterns of progression. There is no specific treatment.

1. Infantile spinal muscular atrophy (Werdnig–Hoffmann disease)

This is the most severe condition often presenting as a floppy infant at birth or within the first few weeks, always before 6 months. It is usually inherited as an autosomal recessive condition. The baby appears limp and all the motor milestones are delayed. Feeding may be difficult and there is early respiratory distress. Clinically the baby may lie immobile with the legs splayed in a 'frog's legs' position. Fasciculation may be seen in the tongue but seldom in the limbs. The reflexes are lost. Most children die within 2–3 years.

The muscle enzymes are often slightly raised. EMG studies may show fibrillation (denervation features) and muscle biopsy reveals atrophic fibres interspersed with clumps of hypertrophic (type I) fibres.

2. Chronic spinal muscular atrophy (Wohlfart–Kugelberg–Welander disease)

This is a milder condition presenting later, between the ages of 2 and 17. It is also inherited as an autosomal recessive condition. The tempo of the progression is slower and many children remain ambulant. The later the onset, the better is the outlook. Occasionally, the illness may present in adult life. Various forms have been described relating to the distribution of the weakness. These include pelvic girdle and proximal limb muscles, scapuloperoneal atrophies and some facio-scapulo-humeral atrophies. There is appropriate muscle wasting and weakness often with fasciculation. Many children may show a kyphoscoliosis. Some patients show a tremor.

EMG studies will confirm denervation and this will be supported by muscle biopsy. The creatine kinase is mildly elevated.

The hereditary ataxias and related disorders

These are a group of uncommon degenerative disorders in which the brunt of the neuronal loss falls on the cerebellum, spinocerebellar or spinal pathways. They have a genetic link. Most frequently they are spinocerebellar degenerations.

Friedreich's ataxia

This is the most common of the hereditary ataxias with a prevalence of about one per 50 000. Most patients present with symptoms of unsteadiness of gait about the age of 10. The disease slowly progresses, many patients becoming confined to a wheelchair. It causes premature death, often between the ages of 30 and 40, most commonly from cardiac complications.

The disease leads to a shrunken spinal cord with the most prominent damage affecting the posterior and lateral columns. This accounts for position sense loss, absent reflexes and extensor plantar responses. There is also involvement of the spinocerebellar tracts, and neuronal loss is reported in the cerebellum in some patients. The inheritance is usually autosomal recessive, although in rare families a dominant form may be found.

The clinical picture is an ataxia of stance and gait. Later there is dysarthria, arm clumsiness and sensory symptoms and signs. Tremor is common. Nystagmus is present in some 20–40 per cent. There is often muscular weakness. Loss of vibration and position sense leads to a sensory ataxia with a positive Romberg's sign. The ataxia progresses and later this is accompanied by muscular wasting with increasing weakness, leading to patients being confined to a wheelchair. Musculoskeletal problems are common, particularly a kyphoscoliosis and pes cavus. A few children may present with scoliosis.

There may be a number of associated defects. The most important, a cardiomyopathy, is present in about 50 per cent. This may cause exertional dyspnoea and palpitations. It may also lead to premature death. The ECG will be abnormal with commonly extensive T wave inversion. About 20 per cent of patients develop diabetes mellitus. There may also be visual impairment with optic atrophy and also deafness in a number of patients.

Investigations

Routine blood tests are usually normal unless the patient has diabetes. The ECG may be abnormal. Nerve conduction studies are usually abnormal with absent or diminished sensory action potentials. Somatosensory evoked potentials may be absent or impaired. There may be slight slowing of motor conduction velocity. The CSF is usually normal. The CT brain scan is also normal.

Treatment

There is no specific treatment. Recognition of the disease is important to allow a clear prognosis and genetic counselling. With increasing disability, provision of appropriate aids may help to maintain mobility and independence. A variety of cholinergic drugs has been tried but the results have been conflicting. Cardiac arrhythmias and heart failure may require treatment. Deterioration in mobility is common with any intercurrent infection or illness.

Adult-onset ataxias

A number of families with a later onset of progressive cerebellar ataxia have been described: in many the inheritance has been autosomal dominant. Marie, Sanger-Brown and Holmes are the names of some of the neurologists who described these disorders. In many the major pathological changes arise from loss of the cerebellar nerve cells. Some have been described by the pathological

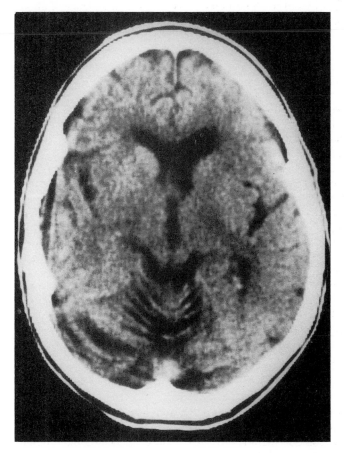

Fig. 17.1. CT brain scan to show primary cerebellar degeneration. Note the widened cerebellar folia, sometimes called 'tiger stripes'.

findings, e.g. olivopontocerebellar atrophy. Many affected patients also show increased tendon reflexes in the limbs, particularly the legs, unlike Friedreich's ataxia.

The clinical presentation is commonly after the age of 30, in some as late as 50 or more, with progressive unsteadiness of gait which will result in patients often being confined to a wheelchair after 10–15 years. Dysarthria is common and there may be clumsiness in the arms. In patients with symptoms of some duration, the ankle jerks may be absent and there may sometimes be posterior column sensory loss in the feet. Many of these patients show other signs. These may include an ophthalmoplegia, ptosis, optic atrophy, pigmentary retinal degeneration, dementia and extrapyramidal signs.

Most of these patients will show evidence of cerebellar atrophy on computerized tomographic (CT) brain scans (Fig. 17.1). Some may show abnormalities on nerve conduction studies. The CSF and blood chemistry are normal.

However, it is important to send blood for thyroid function tests, a lipid profile (to exclude abetalipoproteinaemia) and a vitamin E estimation. Chronic alcoholism may present with a cerebellar deficit and rarely cerebellar signs may be a non-metastatic or a metastatic manifestation of malignant disease. Hypothyroidism may cause cerebellar ataxia (*see* p. 415).

Abetalipoproteinaemia (Bassen–Kornzweig disease)

This is an autosomal recessive inherited disorder usually presenting in childhood (age 3–15) with limb weakness, sensory ataxia (positive Rombergism) and areflexia. Later cerebellar signs appear and there may be visual failure from pigmentary retinal degeneration (night blindness may be the initial symptom). Some patients may show pes cavus and scoliosis. There may even be steatorrhoea.

On the blood films patients show spiky red cells, acanthocytes, and a marked lowering of the blood lipids – cholesterol, β-lipoproteins. Electroretinograms are abnormal and motor conduction velocities may be slowed.

A low fat diet with vitamin A and E supplements may prevent deterioration.

Vitamin E deficiency

This is a rare condition which may cause a peripheral neuropathy and cerebellar ataxia, in part from sensory loss. Most commonly this occurs in patients with malabsorption of fat in chronic intestinal disorders.

Ataxia–telangiectasia (Louis–Bar syndrome)

This is an autosomal recessive inherited disorder commonly presenting in early childhood with delay in walking. By the age of 4–5, children may appear ataxic with an intention tremor and dysarthria. They may also show choreic fidgets, jerky eye movements and later rotatory nystagmus. As the disease progresses there is evidence of a decline in cognitive function. Many patients may also show features of a peripheral neuropathy with weakness and depressed or absent reflexes. The cutaneous manifestations include telangiectasiae of the outer parts of the bulbar conjunctivae, and on the bridge of the nose and cheeks in a butterfly distribution.

Pathologically there is loss of nerve cells in the cerebellum, anterior horns and degeneration in the posterior columns, spinocerebellar tracts and dorsal root ganglia. Patients also lack immunoglobulin, IgA, causing an immuno-deficiency.

The disease relentlessly progresses and most patients die within 10–20 years from secondary infection. About 20 per cent develop lymphomas.

Abnormal laboratory tests include liver function disturbances, a low IgA and often high levels of alpha fetoprotein. EMG studies are usually abnormal.

There is no specific treatment.

Hereditary spastic paraplegia

This is a rare condition with an autosomal dominant inheritance, first described by Seeligmuller and Strumpell. It often appears to be relatively benign causing a very gradual spastic weakness of the legs which insidiously deteriorates over many years. The age of onset is very variable but, if in childhood, there may also be shortening of the heel cords (tendo Achilles). The spasticity is often more striking than any weakness. The arms are often spared, although in time the hands may become impaired for fine manipulative tasks. The reflexes are exaggerated and the plantar responses extensor. There is usually no sensory disturbance. Pes cavus is common. Occasionally, families have been described with other neurological features, e.g cerebellar upset, optic atrophy, dementia, distal wasting.

Pathological studies have shown degeneration of the pyramidal tracts. In some cases the spinocerebellar tracts and posterior columns are also damaged. Investigations are normal. These include nerve conduction studies and CSF examination. Myelography may be necessary to exclude a compressive spinal cord lesion, although the absence of sensory changes or sphincter upset may suggest the diagnosis – a positive family history being the strongest support.

There is no specific treatment. Childhood cases may need surgical lengthening of the heel cords. Drugs such as baclofen or dantrolene sodium may reduce spasticity if this is severe. Physiotherapy may help to maintain mobility.

Phakomatoses

These are a group of diseases with a heredofamilial origin in which the patient is usually born with a cutaneous lesion often associated with neural lesions. As the child develops, these skin and neural lesions commonly progress, often producing benign tumours, although rarely these may undergo malignant change.

Neurofibromatosis (von Recklinghausen's disease)

This has a frequency of 30–40/100 000 and shows a dominant inheritance, although sporadic cases may arise. It produces abnormalities of the skin and numerous tumours of the peripheral nerves.

The skin lesions commonly include café-au-lait patches, often numerous and of large size, and also areas of depigmentation. Axillary freckles are common. Many cutaneous nodules may be apparent; some represent small neuro-fibromas arising from the small cutaneous nerve branches, others vary in size and shape, often feeling soft. Sometimes the neuromas may become very large causing gross disfigurement, e.g. plexiform neuromas.

At certain sites as the neuroma increases in size it may become trapped compressing local structures, e.g. in the spinal canal or exit foramina of the skull or spinal canal. This may produce pain with later loss of function in that compressed nerve. This may lead to a spinal root problem, cord compression, or deafness. About one-third of patients may need admission to hospital at some stage to treat such complications.

Other soft tissues may be involved and also bone. Scalloping of the vertebral bodies may arise and even an overgrowth of bone or an erosion. In the iris of the pupil Lisch's nodules may be present in some 90 per cent – these are small white hamartomatous spots. There is an association with other nervous system tumours, particularly meningiomas and gliomas. Sarcomatous malignant change may occur in 2–5 per cent of patients.

In some patients the disease seems to be much more aggressive with rapid increase in the size and number of the neurofibromas. Root problems in the limbs and trunk are fairly common. Spinal cord compression may lead to a myelopathy. The most frequently involved cranial nerves are the optic, auditory and trigeminal. Bilateral acoustic neuromas may occur and this pattern of disease has a much worse outlook. At the other end of the scale there may be patients with a forme fruste showing some pigmentary skin changes and a few nodules which do not seem to alter over a lifetime.

Investigations are radiological: X-rays may show clear bone erosion or widening of an exit foramen (*see* Fig. 14.12). Myelography, CT scanning or even magnetic resonance imaging (MRI) scanning may be necessary to demonstrate lesions within the spinal canal or cranium.

In selected patients, surgery is necessary to decompress affected nervous tissue.

Tuberous sclerosis, adenoma sebaceum, epiloia, Bourneville's disease

In this condition there may be hyperplasia of ectodermal and mesodermal cells leading to lesions in the skin, nervous system and other organs. It has an incidence of about 5–7/100 000 and usually a dominant inheritance, although sporadic cases attributed to mutations are found.

Clinically, there is a triad of skin lesions – adenoma sebaceum, epilepsy and mental retardation. The epileptic seizures arise from tubers within the brain. In about one-third there may be no significant mental changes.

The usual skin lesions are curious red to pink nodules on the cheeks termed adenoma sebaceum although they are actually angiofibromas (Fig. 17.2). Other skin lesions include shagreen patches, slightly elevated areas of skin like orange peel often found in the lumbosacral region, and subungual fibromas, fleshy nodules arising in the nail bed (Fig. 17.3). Many children may also show white patches of vitiligo in the skin.

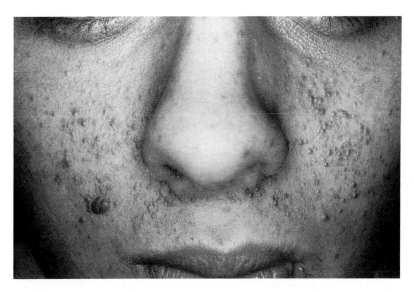

Fig. 17.2. Adenoma sebaceum – the typical skin lesions on the face in a patient with tuberous sclerosis

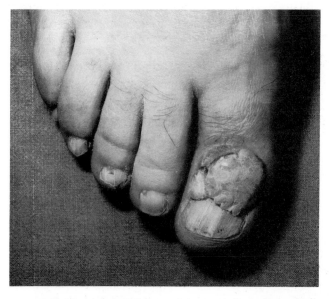

Fig. 17.3. A subungual fibroma of the great toe in a patient with tuberous sclerosis

Epileptic seizures are the common neurological presentation usually starting in childhood. In infancy the seizure pattern may include myoclonic jerks, salaam attacks (flexion spasms) but more commonly major fits or complex partial seizures. These may prove difficult to control with anticonvulsants.

The degree of mental retardation varies from mild to severe. In infancy this may be suggested by developmental delay.

Patients may also show retinal lesions, yellow plaques often near the optic disc. Pathologically the brain shows curious lumps, the tubers, both on the surface and within the cerebral substance. These may calcify and some 50 per cent may show this on skull X-rays. In the lateral ventricles these tubers may produce an irregular surface termed 'candle guttering'. They consist of abnormal glial tissue and rarely malignant gliomatous change may occur.

The condition may worsen with increasing age: in part from mental deterioration, in part from intractable seizures, and in a few from neoplastic change. Severely affected patients have a shortened life span.

The diagnosis rests on the clinical picture, abnormal EEGs and X-ray and CT scan appearances. The seizures should be controlled with anticonvulsants.

Sturge-Weber syndrome (meningo-facial angiomatosis)

These patients show an extensive port-wine stain birth mark (naevus flammeus) of one side of the face involving the eye. There may be an overgrowth of soft tissues at this site. Associated with this is an extensive intracerebral calcification with involvement of the underlying brain which may become atrophic. The cerebral changes lead to epileptic seizures, major and partial, with often an infantile hemiplegia. Many patients are mentally retarded. The affected eye may lose vision and develop glaucoma. The calcification seen on the skull films is characteristic (Fig. 17.4).

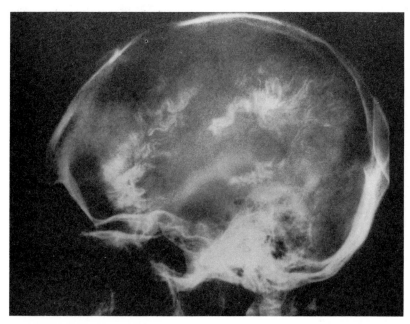

Fig. 17.4. Lateral skull X-ray to show intracranial calcification. This pattern outlining the folia is typical of Sturge-Weber syndrome

Retinitis pigmentosa

Tapeto-retinal degenerations are rare inherited disorders causing progressive visual loss. The inheritance is varied: recessive, dominant and occasionally sex-linked. Electroretinograms (ERGs) will detect these disorders at an early stage.

In most patients there is an insidious fall in visual acuity although this may be preceded by a loss of night vision. There is often an early loss of the peripheral visual field, the central vision being spared. This is one of the conditions which may produce tubular or constricted (gun-barrel) visual fields. Usually the optic disc appears pale and the retinal vessels attenuated. Black 'bone corpuscles' – spiky areas of pigment – are visible in the periphery of the retina (initially the pupil may need dilatation to see these).

Some forms of retinitis pigmentosa are associated with other inherited disorders, e.g. Refsum's syndrome, cardiac conduction defects, primary muscle disease, an ophthalmoplegia.

There is no specific treatment and many patients end up with severe visual impairment.

Lipidoses

These are a group of very rare disorders characterized by the abnormal deposition of lipid metabolites in the central and sometimes peripheral nervous system, usually arising from an autosomal recessive inherited enzyme deficiency. Most present in infancy or early childhood.

The most common neurological symptoms include a failure to thrive with delayed development, mental retardation, epileptic seizures (often myoclonic as well as generalized) and visual failure with retinal changes. Later, other damage becomes apparent with the appearance of motor deficits; initially the child is often hypotonic but later spastic with sometimes dystonic postures. These in time lead to total dependence and early death. In a few there may be associated skeletal abnormalities, and hepatic or bone marrow infiltration.

The diagnosis may often be established by the demonstration of enzyme abnormalities in the white cells in the blood, or by a positive biopsy which may be obtained from a number of tissues – rectum, skin, muscle, liver, marrow or brain. The EEG will be abnormal and if there is peripheral nerve involvement, nerve conduction studies will confirm this.

There is no specific treatment that is effective.

Some of the more common forms are given in Table 17.1.

Mucopolysaccharidoses

These are a group of rare autosomal recessive inherited disorders (although Hunter's type may be sex-linked) in which there is abnormal storage of lipids in neural tissue and of polysaccharides in connective tissue. The last may produce bizarre and marked skeletal abnormalities, e.g. dwarfism, gargoylism. An outline of the four most common types is given in Table 17.2.

Table 17.1 Heredodegenerative metabolic storage diseases

Name	Enzyme deficiency	Accumulation	Type	Epilepsy	Mental	Motor	Visual	Organs	Time to death
Tay-Sachs GM$_2$-gangliosidosis	Hexosaminidase A	GM$_2$-ganglioside	Infancy late juvenile	+	+	+	+ Cherry red 90%		6 months–3 years
GM$_1$-gangliosidosis	β-galactosidase	GM$_1$-ganglioside	Infancy (85%) before 6 months	+	+	+	+	'Hurler's'	6 months–3 years
Niemann-Pick	Sphingomyelinase	Sphingomyelin	Infantile	+	+	+	+ Cherry red 25%	Liver, spleen, marrow	1–2 years
Gaucher's	Glucocerebrosidase	Glucocerebroside	Infantile 4–6 months adult	–	+	+	0	Liver, spleen, pancytopenia	10–12 months
Fabry's angiokeratoma corporis diffusum	Ceramide trihexosidase	Trihexosyl-ceramide	Puberty	+	+	–	Corneal clouds	Skin lesions, Limb and abdominal pains	to 40 years +
Metachromatic leucodystrophy	Aryl sulphatase A	Sphingolipid sulphatide	1–4 years later	Rare	+	+	+	Peripheral neuropathy EMG High CSF protein	1–3 years
Krabbe's leucodystrophy	Galacto-cerebrosidase	Galacto-cerebroside	3–6 months	+	+	+	+	EMG Peripheral neuropathy	to 1 year

Table 17.2 Mucopolysaccharidoses

Name	Enzyme defect	Excess in urine	Clinical	Outcome
Hurler's	? α-iduronidase	Dermatan heparan sulphate	Skeletal *dwarfism*, odd facial features, large viscera, deformed thorax, heart abnormal, mental retardation, spastic, deaf, corneal changes	to about 10 years
Hunter's	?	Dermatan heparan sulphate	Overall milder and slower, mental deterioration, may be sex-linked	20–40 years (heart)
Morquio-Brailsford	?	Keratan sulphate	Skeletal *dwarfism*, normal intelligence, deaf, abnormal thorax, cardiac, atlanto-axial subluxation, poor odontoid	20 years +
San filippo	?	Heparan sulphate	Progressive *mental deterioration*, aggressive, mild physical signs, slight dwarfism	30–40 years

Two further types include Scheie and Maroteaux-Lamy disease

Aminoacidurias

These also represent rare inborn errors of metabolism with an autosomal recessive inheritance and presentation in infancy. They produce an enzyme deficiency which will usually lead to the accumulation of a metabolite in the urine.

The clinical features include failure to develop, mental retardation and seizures. Specific skin changes, ocular disturbances, or even episodic disturbances of consciousness or neurological function may occur in some.

The most common are the phenylketonurias where there is a failure to convert phenylalanine to tyrosine. Mental retardation, epileptic seizures and abnormal hair pigmentation may be the presentation. Recognition is important for dietary restriction of phenylalanine may prevent deterioration.

A number of other disorders can be identified often from a urinary amino acid chromatogram, e.g. homocystinuria. In Hartnup disease the urine contains an excess of amino acids and indicans. This may cause a red scaly skin, and episodic ataxia. Sulphonamides and sunlight may sometimes precipitate attacks.

18

Developmental disorders of the central nervous system

A number of uncommon neurological disorders may arise as a result of the failure of the tissues to form or grow. Such disorders are commonly present at birth, although their recognition may not occur until later when signs may present in childhood. Some 3 per cent of all live births show evidence of a malformation. Many of the severe abnormalities result in a stillbirth or early death within a few months.

Such developmental abnormalities may arise from:

1. Chromosome abnormalities, e.g. trisomy, Down's syndrome (mongolism).
2. Damage *in utero*
   (a) exposure to irradiation, e.g. X-rays
   (b) exposure to drugs, e.g. thalidomide, cytotoxics
   (c) infections, e.g. rubella, toxoplasmosis, syphilis, AIDS
   (d) malnutrition
   (e) trauma sometimes with placental haemorrhage.
3. Damage at birth: difficult delivery, particularly if premature.
4. Unknown – this is a large group.

In many instances faults arise from a combination of genetic and environmental factors.

Spina bifida

In normal development the spinal canal fuses around the spinal cord which has formed from the neural crest. Failure of the neural tube to close may be described as rachischisis and has led to the term spinal dysraphism. Commonly there is failure of the bony spinal canal to close posteriorly leading to a defect in the neural arches – spina bifida (Fig. 18.1). This arises most often in the lumbosacral region, but sometimes in the cervical region. The mildest form, which is often asymptomatic, is called spina bifida occulta. It may be picked up on a routine spinal X-ray and is said to be present in some 17 per cent of all spinal X-rays. There is usually a failure of fusion of the laminae of the neural arch with no visible abnormality of the overlying skin. In some instances there may be an abnormality of the skin with a visible pigmented birthmark, a dimple, a tuft of

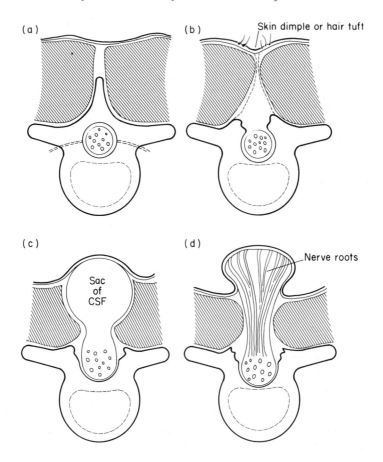

Fig. 18.1.   Spina bifida. Transverse sections through the lumbar region: (**a**) normal;
(**b**) spina bifida occulta; (**c**) meningocele; (**d**) myelomeningocele

hair (faun's tail), or even a swelling from a lipoma or other pathology.

In more major disturbances, neurological symptoms may be present and the defect is no longer silent, 'occulta'. In the lumbosacral region such defects may damage the lumbosacral nerve roots, less often the conus or lower part of the spinal cord. This may be associated with other congenital abnormalities which may result in a split spinal cord from a bony spur, diastematomyelia, in a cord with an unusually low termination (well below L1) or with tethering from a persistent filum terminale.

Symptoms include:

1. Gait problems with difficulty walking from wasting and weakness of distal muscles (below the knee) accompanied by depressed or lost reflexes. The weakness may be asymmetrical. There are commonly deformities in the feet. In severe forms there may be a flaccid paraplegia with 'flail' feet.
2. Sensory abnormalities with lost feeling in the feet, legs or saddle area. These

may lead to painless ulcers, or even neuropathic joints. Any skin lesion commonly proves difficult to heal.

3. Sphincter disturbances: most often incontinence with enuresis from impaired bladder control. Chronic retention may lead to back pressure on the kidneys with accompanying recurrent or persistent urinary infections, which if uncorrected, may lead to hydronephrosis and renal failure. Constipation may be present. Examination may show an enlarged bladder, a lax anal sphincter or loss of the anal reflex.
4. Associated skeletal abnormalities: these are varied and may include a scoliosis, talipes, pes cavus, tight heel cords.

Such symptomatic patients require investigation with X-rays of the spine, computerized tomographic (CT) or magnetic resonance imaging (MRI) scans and often myelography. Urological assessment should also be undertaken: urine cultures obtained, the blood urea measured and an intravenous urogram performed.

Surgical treatment may be possible in selected patients to prevent deterioration but management is often directed to coping with the various defects.

Spina bifida cystica

Between one and four per 1000 live births may show a cystic defect produced by herniation of the meninges, and sometimes neural tissue through the bony defect caused by failure of the bony canal to fuse. A meningocele is a sac of fluid (CSF) containing meninges and covered by skin (*see* Fig. 18.1(c)), a myelomeningocele contains neural tissue in addition (*see* Fig. 18.1(d)). Sometimes such defects may be open and, as such, are very liable to infection in the neonate. The more major defects are accompanied by much more severe neurological damage and the most marked may prove incompatible with survival. Many of these infants show multiple skeletal defects, e.g. talipes, and other congenital abnormalities.

Again, such cystic defects are far more common in the lumbosacral region and some 75 per cent of myelomeningoceles arise here. In this region they will be associated with:

1. Motor weakness.
2. Sensory loss.
3. Sphincter disturbances (*see* p. 368).

The most severe may show a flaccid paralysis extending as high as L1 associated with incontinence.

If there is a cystic swelling with herniation of brain tissue and meninges at the head-end this is termed a meningoencephalocele. This may appear in the frontal region, in the roof of the nose or orbit, or at the back of the skull. Many such patients show features of severe cerebral damage and seldom survive. Small defects may require surgical closure.

In many instances a spina bifida cystica may be associated with *hydrocephalus*. The infant's head may appear large at birth and rapidly expand in the first few weeks of life accompanied by splaying of the skull sutures and enlargement of the ventricles. It is probable that in many instances there is an obstructive hydrocephalus with blockage of the CSF pathways. This most commonly occurs at the craniocervical junction from a Chiari malformation (*see* p. 372) but may also arise from an aqueduct stenosis or even as the result of secondary infection (from meningitis through an 'open' meningocele).

Management

This will be determined by the severity of the condition and the presence or absence of other congenital defects. All mild or moderately affected infants will require radiological studies, spinal and skull X-rays and a CT scan.

Surgical treatment is aimed at closing any spinal defect and relieving any associated hydrocephalus. The latter is achieved by the insertion of a shunt, commonly ventriculo-atrial. Successful surgery will then allow the child to be treated by a combined team which will include physiotherapists, teachers, orthopaedic specialists in addition to the parents. Surgical fitters may help to provide various aids, splints and appliances. Preserved proximal limb strength allows walking in calipers: 'flail' feet may need below-knee 'irons'. Faulty bladder control with retention or abnormalities of the renal tract may require self-catheterization and regular urine cultures with treatment of any infections. Some children may benefit from the surgical fashioning of an 'ileal bladder' draining through an ileostomy bag. Bowel function may be regulated by regular 'potting', the use of aperients and enemas. Great care of the skin is necessary to prevent the appearance of trophic ulcers. In some selected patients, orthopaedic surgical procedures may prove helpful with tendon transplants, fusion of joints or the lengthening of the tendo Achilles.

The long-term management of such patients is a difficult task and families will need much help and encouragement as well as tangible support. However, in milder cases, over 80 per cent of affected children will be able to walk with treatment.

In the severely affected infant, where there are gross deficits often associated with other abnormalities, the decision about attempted surgery may be very hard. Very severe defects may technically be difficult to close: furthermore, the quality of life, particularly if associated with cerebral faults, may be bad. Such decisions may be strongly influenced by the infant's parents, and may be agonizing.

Hydrocephalus

'Water on the brain' describes the enlargement of the fluid-filled ventricular system. This is hydrocephalus and in the newborn about two per 1000 live births are affected, boys more often than girls. CSF is formed in the choroid plexuses of the ventricles circulating from the lateral ventricles via the third ventricle through the aqueduct to the fourth ventricle. It leaves the latter through the foramina of Magendie and Luschka, to circulate throughout the posterior fossa cisterns, ascending over the surface of the cerebral hemispheres, to be absorbed via the arachnoid villi in the superior sagittal sinus into the blood stream.

Hydrocephalus may arise from:

1. Obstruction of the CSF pathways. This may occur from developmental faults, e.g. a Chiari malformation, obstruction of the exit foramina, or an aqueduct stenosis. It may follow obstruction secondary to infection from meningitis or following a haemorrhage (spontaneous or traumatic). It may also follow blockage by tumours, particularly in the posterior fossa.
2. Increased CSF production. This may occur with certain forms of poisoning, e.g. by lead or vitamin A excess, and in some forms of meningitis.
3. Communicating hydrocephalus where there is no obstruction to CSF flow but there may be faulty absorption in the subarachnoid space, or faulty CSF production. Here the ventricles appear enlarged but there is no block. In adults this may be termed low or normal pressure hydrocephalus (NPH) (*see* p. 296).

Hydrocephalus in the infant will produce progressive enlargement of the head which will be more than the 97th percentile for the age. This may be associated with bulging fontanelles and difficulty with head control. As the pressure rises the infant will become irritable and often vomits. There is a delay in the milestones and a failure to thrive. Ocular signs appear with the

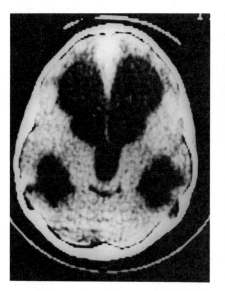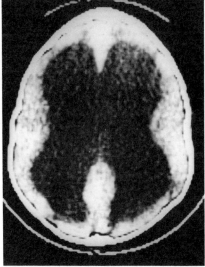

Fig. 18.2. CT brain scan showing gross hydrocephalus caused by an aqueduct stenosis. Note the enlargement of the lateral and third ventricles

sunset phenomenon – the eyes deviating downward while the upper eyelids retract. This may be associated with bilateral abducens palsies and lost upgaze. There may be swelling and later pallor of the optic discs which can lead to visual failure. Untreated further physical and mental retardation occurs.

Such children will require skull X-rays and a CT scan. Older children should also have psychometric testing. In many instances the scan will show gross ventricular dilatation and the site of any obstruction can be determined. Blockage of the outlets of the fourth ventricle (Dandy-Walker syndrome) causes dilatation of all the ventricles including the fourth. Dilatation of the lateral and third ventricles alone suggests an aqueduct stenosis (Fig. 18.2).

Treatment is usually by shunting: a ventriculo-atrial or ventriculoperitoneal shunt. Occasionally, where there is an obstructing mass responsible or a fault at the craniocervical junction (Chiari malformation) a direct surgical attack at the appropriate site may be made. Shunting may be associated with complications: about one-third of shunts run into difficulties largely from blockage, infection or the development of a subdural collection.

Chiari malformation, Arnold–Chiari malformation

This describes a developmental abnormality at the craniocervical junction with displacement of the cerebellar tonsils downward accompanied by an elongation of the medulla so that both pass down through the foramen magnum into the upper cervical canal (Fig. 18.3). This downward displacement impacts obstructing the CSF flow. This may be associated with hydrocephalus, with a spina bifida cystica, and with expansion of a cystic intramedullary lesion – a

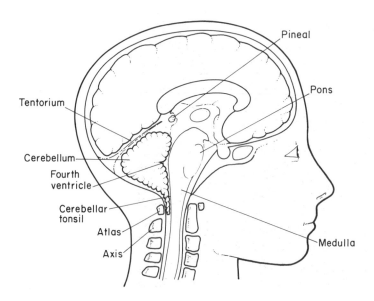

Fig. 18.3. A median sagittal section to show a Chiari malformation

syrinx (syringomyelia *see* p. 196). Some 60 per cent of patients with syringo-myelia have a Chiari malformation. In many patients Chiari malformations may be associated with multiple congenital abnormalities.

Symptoms include those from hydrocephalus (*see* p. 295), from a myelo-meningocele, if this is present, or from a syrinx (*see* p. 196). In older patients a Chiari malformation may cause occipital headache, neck stiffness, oscillopsia with nystagmus (often downbeat) and cerebellar ataxia with an unsteady gait. The lower cranial nerves may be involved, the accessory or hypoglossal and even the eighth. There may be long tract signs with spasticity in the legs and posterior column sensory impairment in the hands, or even a 'cuirasse' distribution of sensory loss.

Investigations include X-rays of the craniocervical junction, CT scanning and myelography, the latter with films taken supine to show any cerebellar displacement. MRI scanning however, is now the investigation of choice (Fig. 18.4).

If there is evidence of progressive deterioration then surgical treatment may be undertaken with decompression of the craniocervical junction.

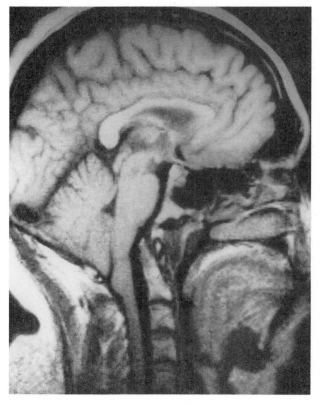

Fig. 18.4. Sagittal view MRI scan of the craniocervical junction showing cerebellar ectopia, *see* Fig. 18.3

Basilar impression

This is caused by upward displacement or protrusion of the cervical spine invaginating the base of the skull at the foramen magnum. It may arise as a developmental defect when commonly it may be associated with other congenital abnormalities e.g. Chiari malformation, or fused vertebrae in the Klippel-Feil syndrome (Fig. 18.5). It may be acquired with softening of bone as in Paget's disease.

Patients may be asymptomatic but often show a short neck and low hair line. Symptoms may arise from compression of the cerebellum with ataxia and nystagmus, or compression of the cord with the development of spastic weakness and sometimes posterior column sensory loss in the hands. Occasionally, an obstructive hydrocephalus may develop, producing headache and symptoms of raised intracranial pressure. The lower cranial nerves may sometimes be

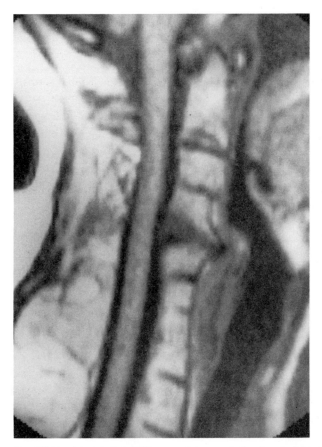

Fig. 18.5. Lateral view MRI scan of the cervical spine showing Klippel-Feil deformity with fused vertebrae. Note the prominent osteophytic spurs indenting the oesophagus anteriorly and the spinal cord posteriorly

affected with speech and swallow difficulties. Trauma may precipitate symptoms. Movements of the head and neck are often restricted and painful.

Plain X-rays of the skull will confirm the presence of basilar impression. On a lateral skull film normally the angle between the basisphenoid and the basilar part of the occipital bone lies between 110 and 140°. In basilar impression this angle is widened. A further X-ray finding is that if a line is drawn joining the back of the foramen magnum to the back of the hard palate this should normally lie above the cervical spine (Chamberlain's line). In basilar impression the odontoid process may lie above this line.

Treatment is surgical to decompress the craniocervical junction if the patient is symptomatic.

Other developmental abnormalities include fusion of the atlas and the foramen magnum, and atlanto-axial subluxation. The last may be congenital if there is an absent odontoid and this may be found in some disorders, e.g. Morquio's disease. Acquired forms of atlanto-axial subluxation are also found, particularly in rheumatoid arthritis (*c*. 5%) or less commonly in Down's syndrome or from a tuberculous retropharyngeal abscess. Such lesions cause compression high in the spinal cord with signs of a progressive spastic tetraparesis accompanied by marked discriminative sensory loss and position sense loss in the hands.

Modern surgical techniques to correct the malalignment of the spine, to decompress the cord, and then fuse the spine to achieve stability may now be undertaken in selected patients. These are major surgical procedures.

Myelodysplasia

This term is used to describe defects of closure of the neural tube which commonly affect the lumbosacral region of the spinal canal and are frequently associated with some form of spina bifida. The most common defect is *diastematomyelia* in which the spinal cord is split in two, either by a bony spur or a fibrous band. Other developmental faults may also be present and there may be an association with lipomas, or dermoids. Such affected children show evidence of weakness and wasting in the legs, with sensory impairment and sphincter disturbance (*see* p. 368). There may be associated skeletal abnormalities, e.g. scoliosis, talipes, a poorly developed lower leg. Myelography will confirm the diagnosis.

In many children there may be a slow deterioration and surgical treatment may arrest this, although this seldom allows full recovery. In a few patients there may be a familial incidence.

Prevention

Recently emphasis has increasingly been placed on the prenatal diagnosis of neural tube defects and major neurological developmental disorders. Alpha-fetoprotein may be found in increasing concentrations in the amniotic fluid of affected fetuses with neural tube defects *in utero*. Amniocentesis enables sampling of such fluid to measure the levels of alpha-fetoprotein. Ultrasound examination of the fetus during pregnancy may detect some structural abnormalities.

Cerebral palsy

This describes a congenital abnormality of motor function and affects about two per 1000 live births. Affected children will usually show a combination of weakness, incoordination and involuntary movements. A number of causes are recognized: these include pre-, peri- and postnatal brain injuries. Infections *in utero*, e.g. rubella, syphilis, or intoxication of the mother with drugs or alcohol, may also be responsible. In many children no specific cause may be identified.

Brain injuries may arise from a difficult birth with anoxia or haemorrhage: premature infants are particularly susceptible and some 10–20 per cent of low birth weight infants (less than 1.5 kg) develop a spastic diplegia. Severe neonatal jaundice, purulent neonatal meningitis, encephalitis, or the development of an obstructive hydrocephalus may also be responsible.

The clinical picture may be very varied but most commonly there is a spastic diplegia, Little's disease; the legs are more affected than the arms. This may be associated with delay in motor milestones and the appearance of a spastic gait. The legs tend to scissor and in time contractures develop, particularly of the tendo Achilles. There may be abnormal postures, clumsiness and incoordination and involuntary movements, often choreoathetotic. The affected limbs are commonly spastic with increased tone, exaggerated reflexes, clonus and extensor plantar responses. Many mildly affected children will show abnormal added movements in the arms, e.g. supination or odd postures, when attempting to walk on their heels or the outsides of their feet (Fog's test). A proportion of children with cerebral palsy may appear floppy and hypotonic.

Other children may show a different emphasis on motor faults so that a monoplegic, hemiplegic, ataxic, choreoathetotic, flaccid or mixed picture have been described. The mixed group is the largest. A number of other problems are commonly linked with cerebral palsy. Some 25 per cent may show a squint, usually convergent; about 30–40 per cent may have epileptic seizures; 5–10 per cent show deafness and nearly 75 per cent show an IQ below average. In about one-third there may be evidence of mental retardation, occasionally this appears gross. Older children often experience emotional and behavioural problems. Speech difficulties with a slow spastic dysarthria and dribbling are common. The more severely affected show multiple handicaps.

An acute infantile hemiplegia may develop in young children after a severe hemisphere insult, e.g. meningitis, haemorrhage, prolonged epileptic seizure. After the illness, the patient may be hemiparetic and in time there is a failure of the affected limbs to grow normally, remaining smaller, more spastic and weak. In some patients focal epileptic seizures may develop in the affected limbs. The skull X-ray may show the size of the cranial vault over the affected hemisphere is smaller than on the normal side.

Patients with cerebral palsy are best assessed by special units which have trained staff to look at all functions, including the senses, speech, psychometric state (IQ), and special tests looking at various motor skills. These may be combined with a number of investigations such as an EEG, blood and urine tests to exclude rare inherited disorders, infections, hypothyroidism (urinary amino acid chromatogram, Wassermann's reaction, thyroid function). More detailed investigations will be necessary if there is evidence of any progressive deterioration, in patients with optic atrophy or progressive visual loss, predominant ataxia, progressive loss of motor skills and if there is no obvious cause for their palsy.

Treatment

This may involve special schooling for the child and much support and guidance for the parents. Very severely affected children may need the skills of special units, often residential. Physiotherapy has been shown to benefit many children and a variety of regimens of differing intensity has been used. Less severely affected children should be encouraged to lead 'normal' lives, although allowances may be necessary for slowness or other motor problems. In selected patients orthopaedic procedures, e.g. tendo Achilles lengthening, or the provision of special appliances may help mobility. Other aids may be necessary for those with greater handicaps. Speech therapy is important in those with poor articulation. Epileptic seizures will need to be controlled with anticonvulsants. In a small number of patients with severe spasticity the use of baclofen or dantrolene sodium may reduce this. Of the children reaching adulthood with cerebral palsy, some 20–25 per cent are able to work but some 30–50 per cent end in some form of institutional care.

19

Cerebrovascular disease

Cerebrovascular disease represents a major cause of disability and death. It is the third commonest cause of death in the Western World, behind cancer and ischaemic heart disease. The death rate from stroke is approximately 100/100 000 of the population, an annual rate that is strongly age related, doubling for each 5-year increase in age.

Stroke is also the commonest cause of neurological disability in adults in the UK where 100 000 individuals will have their first stroke this year. Approximately 25 000 more will have a second or third stroke. Most stroke victims are over 65 years of age and the annual incidence rises to 20/1000 per year by the age of 85.

Risk factors

The risk of stroke is greater in the black community and in Japan and males are slightly more vulnerable even after adjustment for the age structure of the population ($\times$ 1.3). Other risk factors have been defined by prospective epidemiological studies such as that carried out over the last 25 years or so in Framingham, Massachusetts. Arterial hypertension, heart disease, atrial fibrillation, diabetes mellitus, smoking, obesity, hypercholesterolaemia, oral contraceptives, alcohol and an elevated haematocrit all emerge as independent risk factors, although only the first four make a major impact. Hypertension has the greatest effect and the chances of stroke are increased throughout the range of both diastolic and systolic blood pressure in both sexes and at all ages. Atrial fibrillation increases the risk by six, but if it is due to rheumatic heart disease, the risk is increased seventeen-fold. Diabetes increases the risk some threefold. Smoking has only a weak effect and hypercholesterolaemia only emerges as a risk factor in those under 55 years of age. Both these latter factors are much more strongly related to the risk of coronary heart disease. Binge alcohol drinking has been associated with strokes in young people. Although the risk of stroke is increased in women on the oral contraceptive ($\times$ 3), the absolute risk is very small (about one in 10 000) and probably reduced with the advent of modern low dose formulations. A high haematocrit is linked with stroke but some of the relationship appears to be due to the association of haematocrit with hypertension and smoking.

Some of the associations are thought to reflect a causal relationship as in the case of hypertension and embolism from rheumatic heart disease in atrial fibrillation. In other situations the 'risk' may relate to some shared underlying pathology, e.g. in the case of ischaemic heart disease with underlying widespread atheroma. Nonetheless, the 10 per cent of the population from which some 50 per cent of the strokes and heart attacks will come, can be predicted by attention to the whole range of risk factors, providing a theoretical basis for a preventative health care programme. The importance of such a strategy will become increasingly obvious as the limited scope for treatment of strokes once they have occurred emerges in the following account of the management of the disease. There is evidence from some countries that the incidence of stroke is falling, a welcome trend which some have attributed to the widespread introduction of treatment for hypertension.

Classification

Four out of five strokes are due to cerebral infarction in which there is loss of neurones and destruction of cerebral architecture due to ischaemia, usually as a result of arterial occlusion. About one in eight strokes is by contrast due to primary intracerebral haemorrhage, and one in twelve is a case of subarachnoid haemorrhage which may or may not be complicated by parenchymatous damage with focal deficit.

The time profile of the resulting focal clinical deficit varies widely. In transient ischaemic attacks (TIAs) little or no tissue necrosis occurs before blood supply is restored, and the symptoms last less than 24 h, usually 15–20 min or an hour or two. Completed strokes outlast this arbitrary 24-h rule and can usually be shown, e.g. by computerized tomography (CT) scanning, to be accompanied by permanent tissue damage. Those with complete recovery as judged by disappearance of symptoms in 3–4 weeks are sometimes called minor strokes or RINDS (reversible ischaemic neurological deficits) while longer lasting events are called major strokes. When a stroke is of unusually slow development it is referred to as a stroke in evolution or an ingravescent stroke. When, after a period of stability, a stroke patient's deficit increases, the term deteriorating stroke is often applied.

Finally, stroke can be classified by the territory of the cerebral injury either topographically referring to the site of any haemorrhage or infarct, e.g. capsular infarct, putaminal haemorrhage, or according to the vascular supply, e.g. middle cerebral territory infarct, vertebrobasilar transient ischaemic attack.

An attempt should be made in each case to define the time course, siting and pathological nature of the cerebral injury, as all three factors are relevant to the discussion of aetiology, prognosis and management.

Pathology

Transient ischaemic attacks

It is doubtful if brief attacks lasting only a matter of minutes can ever be due to cerebral haemorrhage, and as the name implies all such events are believed to be due to a temporary insufficiency of blood supply to a focal area of cerebral tissue. There is good evidence that most are due to temporary embolic occlusion of intracerebral arteries, the emboli emanating from atheromatous disease of extracranial arteries or the heart, and rarely due to haemodynamic crises in which cardiac output or systemic pressure falls. Such haemodynamic changes would be expected to cause the features of global cerebral ischaemia – the familiar changes of syncope with clouding of vision and consciousness. A focal deficit would only be expected if local circumstances led to one area of the brain becoming critically ischaemic before others. Such a situation can arise if there is a flow-reducing narrowing of say one internal carotid or middle cerebral artery. Under these circumstances brief focal deficits may follow postural hypotension, cardiac arrhythmias, exercise, getting out of a hot bath, etc. In practice these haemodynamic attacks are rare.

Much more commonly, patients reporting transient ocular or focal cerebral symptoms have evidence of atheromatous disease of the parent neck vessel or a cardiac condition that could be the source of embolism. Emboli may be seen in the retina; shiny refractile cholesterol crystals lodged at arteriolar branches, migrating pale platelet fibrin thrombi or white calcific debris from a heart valve. Auscultation of the neck may reveal a bruit over the carotid bifurcation, a sensitive but not very specific clue to the presence of arterial narrowing. Non-invasive Doppler duplex scanning of the carotid bifurcation, minimally invasive intravenous digital subtraction angiography, and potentially more hazardous arterial angiography may reveal the presence of atheromatous disease of carotid or vertebral arteries in patients with TIAs (Fig. 19.1). Clinical examination, ECG, chest X-ray and echocardiography may reveal a potentially relevant cardiac abnormality, such as atrial fibrillation with atrial thrombus, a recent myocardial infarction with ventricular thrombus, or valvular disease with valve related vegetation or thrombi. Rarely an atrial myxoma is the source of tumour emboli. One study found cardiac abnormalities in about 25 per cent of TIA patients, no cause in another 25 per cent and atheroma of relevant neck arteries in 50 per cent. Embolism from atheroma of the aorta or from neck vessels 'missed' by angiography probably accounts for many of the group in which routine investigation is unrewarding. Very rarely a prothrombotic state can be detected by investigation of platelet number or function, or attention to rare abnormalities of the clotting cascade (e.g. 'lupus anticoagulant', deficiencies of protein C, protein S or antithrombin III).

While the cause of atheromatous change in the neck arteries like that elsewhere is unknown, it it clear that the development of arterial lesions, and the growth of plaques, is related to hypertension, diabetes, hypercholesterolaemia and smoking so providing a possible link with some of the risk factors. TIAs are themselves sometimes spoken of as a risk factor as they carry an increased risk of stroke to their victims of four to five times. The reason for plaques to trigger artery-to-artery embolism is believed to relate to the turbulent blood flow downstream of an irregular narrowing and the tendency for plaques to rupture by a process analogous to metal fatigue. This exposes subendothelial components such as collagen III which causes platelet adherence and triggers platelet aggregation. As the clotting mechanism can also be triggered by the subendothelial exposure and by platelet activation, fibrin may form, stabilizing the

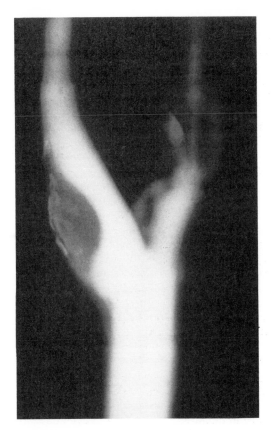

Fig. 19.1. Narrowing of internal carotid artery by atheromatous plaque (post-mortem angiogram)

mural thrombus. If the plaque has already caused a 50–75 per cent stenosis of the lumen, mural thrombus formation can cause complete occlusion of the vessel as well as or instead of being the source of embolism.

Completed strokes due to cerebral infarction

In many, the immediate cause of ischaemic destruction of cerebral tissue is thrombotic occlusion of a carotid artery already narrowed by a lipid laden atheromatous plaque (Fig. 19.2) or embolic occlusion of an intracerebral vessel such as the middle cerebral artery. Such emboli may arise from mural thrombus in a parent artery or commonly from a cardiac valve or chamber. Cardiac emboli are more often associated with cerebral infarction and completed strokes than with TIAs, perhaps due to their larger size. Especially in young individuals, when atheromatous changes of the vessels are unlikely to be marked, a cardiac source for cerebral embolism should therefore be sought.

Whether or not brain tissue will be infarcted with death of neurones after

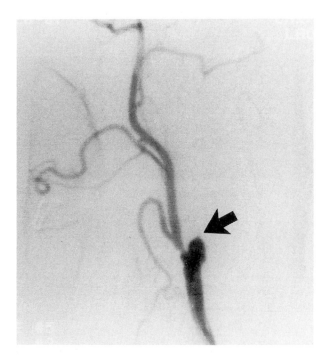

Fig. 19.2. Occlusion of internal carotid artery at bifurcation (digital subtraction angiogram)

vessel occlusion depends on both the depth and duration of ischaemia (Fig. 19.3). Cerebral tissue does not survive a complete cessation of blood flow for more than a few minutes (witness the rapidly destructive effects of cardiac arrest), but flow is rarely so reduced after occlusion of a single vessel due to collateral channels. If flow is adequately restored, although metabolism (and hence function) may have been temporarily suppressed, no infarcts may occur or only a few patchy areas show damage (TIA). If collateral supply is poor, if the perfusion pressure is low, if embolic occlusions remain fixed, then the flow may remain too low to sustain cellular integrity and necrosis results. For a time after ischaemic stroke, perhaps 6 h, there is evidence suggesting that a reversible state of ischaemia short of infarction exists. During this time there is an increased extraction of oxygen from arterial blood with increased desaturation of venous blood draining the area. Theoretically, at least, an increase in blood flow during this period could rescue tissue otherwise destined to infarction.

Many emboli break up and move on after minutes, hours or days. In contrast, occlusions of the carotid or basilar artery due to mural thrombosis rarely recannulate. With dissolution of an embolus, flow at high pressure may be restored to a necrotic area causing small petechial haemorrhages or frank haematoma formation. Some embolic strokes may thus be due to haemorrhagic infarction and some haematomas may be initially due to ischaemia.

With a large infarct there is consequent cerebral atrophy and a cystic cavity

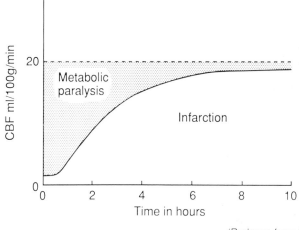

(Redrawn from Crowell)

Fig. 19.3. Relationship of severity and duration of reduced cerebral blood flow to cerebral outcome. (Redrawn from Crowell, In: *Cerebral Ischaemia Clinical and Experimental Approach*. Tokyo, Igabu-Shorin, 1982)

may mark the site of the original area of necrosis. Multiple infarcts, large and small, may cause a dementia due to overall loss of cerebral substance.

The American neurologist, Miller Fisher, described a further type of arterial change in stroke victims which was confined to small penetrating intracerebral arteries. The vessel wall was thickened by a process called lipohyalinosis which he found particularly common in hypertensive patients. The infarcts related to occlusion of these small vessels were small (4–8 mm) in size and slit like. Such lacunes were often marked clinically by the occurrence of a restricted neurological deficit that often recovered in a few weeks (RIND). Later studies have suggested that similar small deep infarcts can be due to embolic disease too, and may even be heralded by TIAs so their aetiology is more diverse than Fisher suggested.

Strokes in the territory of the vertebrobasilar arterial circulation are essentially similar to those in the carotid territory. There are one or two slight differences in the pathological description, however. Thus while the middle and posterior cerebral arteries share a propensity to embolism, the basilar artery, despite its intracranial site, is more often affected by atheroma and thrombosis *in situ*, a process that often appears to be gradual (and associated with stroke in evolution). Ulceration of plaques which triggers mural thromboembolism is believed to be rarer in the vertebral artery than in the carotid and the vertebral arteries are more vulnerable to mechanical effects of neck rotation and of trauma than are the carotid arteries. They are also more often affected by giant cell arteritis than are the carotids (*see* below).

Rarely, infarction may be due to a congenital abnormality of the neck arteries such as fibromuscular dysplasia, or to dissection of the vessel, not necessarily precipitated by trauma.

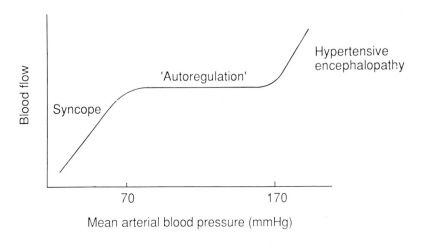

Fig. 19.4.   Autoregulation of cerebral blood flow

Stroke in evolution and deteriorating stroke

Normally the sudden embolic occlusion of a middle cerebral artery gives rise to the sudden onset of neurological deficit. When a comparable hemiparesis takes many days to evolve, the implication is that any occlusive thrombus is propagating, cutting off collateral channels or that a falling perfusion pressure is causing failure of the collateral flow. When deterioration occurs after a period of stability, repeated embolism or propagation of occluding thrombus can be the cause. So too can a systemic complication leading to cardiorespiratory failure or falling blood pressure. Normally cerebral blood flow is maintained by intrinsic homeostatic control over a wide range of mean arterial blood pressure (e.g. 70–170 mmHg) (Fig. 19.4). After ischaemic damage to blood vessels within the stroke area, such autoregulation fails either locally or sometimes throughout the hemisphere or whole brain. Under these circumstances any fall in blood pressure will lead to a fall in cerebral perfusion; blood flow has become pressure passive. Any injudicious lowering of a stroke victim's blood pressure may thus extend his or her infarct (Fig. 19.5).

The blood vessels in the ischaemic or infarcted territory are maximally vasodilated in response to the fall in intraluminal pressure and to locally generated vasodilating metabolites with local acidosis. This means that an elevation of P_aCO_2 due to chest infection may cause diversion of blood into the intact parts of the cerebral circulation, where dilatation can still occur (cerebral steal). It also means that drug induced vasodilatation is unlikely to be helpful (Fig. 19.6).

The failure of cellular pumping mechanisms as energy metabolism fails, and the damage to intracerebral vessels which become leaky, lead to cerebral oedema. This begins within 24 h and is maximal at days 3–6. Swelling of the infarcted area is the commonest cause of death of the stroke victim in the first week due to intracerebral shifts and subsequent damage to the brainstem. Deterioration of conscious level in the stroke patient is often due to oedema

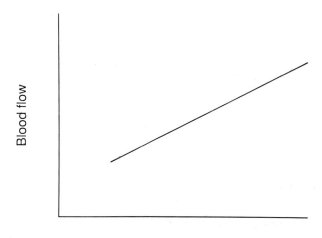

Fig. 19.5. Loss of autoregulation after stroke

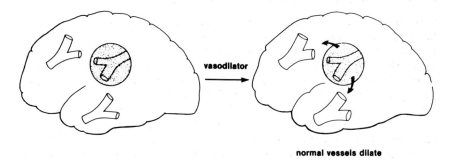

Fig. 19.6. Intracerebral steal. (Reproduced with permission from Hachinski, V. and Norris, J. *The Acute Stroke*. F.A. Davis, 1985)

formation and this too is aggravated by systemic changes such as hypercapnia and hyponatraemia due to inappropriate ADH secretion which can complicate stroke.

Cerebral haemorrhage

Although only a minority of strokes are due to spontaneous haemorrhage, their importance lies in their severity, high mortality and different management. The haemorrhage occurs as a result of rupture of a Charcot-Bouchard aneurysm, a microscopic aneurysm that develops in small vessels, usually as a response to sustained arterial hypertension. Some haemorrhages are due to rupture of penetrating arteries themselves. Rarely, arteriovenous malformations, mycotic

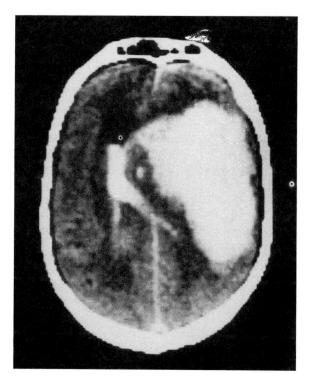

Fig. 19.7.   CT scan of hemispheric haematoma with blood visible in the ventricular system

aneurysms, amyloid angiopathy or the use of anticoagulant drugs is responsible. Abuse of amphetamines is another cause.

The rupture of a vessel or Charcot-Bouchard aneurysm causes the sudden development of a haematoma as the blood emerges at arterial pressure. Bleeding may be temporarily arrested but then continues leading to a slowly evolving clinical deficit. Intracranial pressure rises rapidly and severe headache and loss of consciousness may develop at the onset. The haematoma disrupts some tissue but the neurological deficit is also due to the acute displacement of fibre tracts and may not be permanent. Blood may escape into the cerebrospinal fluid causing blood staining and later xanthochromia of lumbar puncture fluid. The haemorrhage may also breach the ventricular wall with blood appearing in the ventricles (Fig. 19.7). The blood in a haematoma resolves over 10 days–3 weeks so its characteristic appearance on CT scanning may not be detected after that interval, reducing the chances of making such a pathological diagnosis in survivors.

Haematomas are mostly found in the basal ganglia especially in the putamen and thalamus, in the lobar white matter and in the cerebellum or pons. Rarely, a haematoma in the region of the external capsule slowly splits white matter fibres extending itself fore and aft, undercutting the grey matter of the cortex.

Such a process explains how a cerebral haemorrhage may deteriorate, although the usual cause for deterioration lies in the secondary effects of brain shift and herniation due to the mass effect of the haematoma and any associated oedema.

Subarachnoid haemorrhage

The victims of subarachnoid haemorrhage are younger than those of cerebral infarction or intracerebral haemorrhage, the average age being about 50 years. The causative arterial lesion is, in at least 80 per cent of cases, an aneurysm on one of the arteries of the circle of Willis (Fig. 19.8). The rapid onset of bleeding into the subarachnoid space causes the dramatically sudden onset of headache, and if the intracranial pressure rises rapidly, loss of consciousness. Meningeal irritation causes neck stiffness. Focal neurological deficit mimicking other types of stroke occurs either because blood tracks into the cerebral substance or because blood product provoked spasm of basal arteries leads to cerebral ischaemia. This may be focal causing local deficit or more diffuse causing a declining level of consciousness. Hypothalamic disturbance may cause

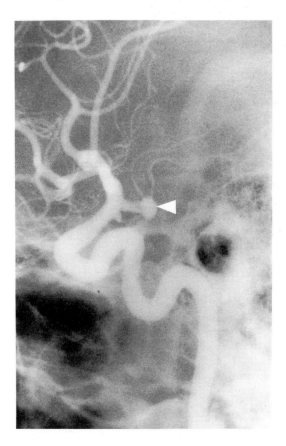

Fig. 19.8. Angiogram revealing cerebral aneurysm (*arrow*)

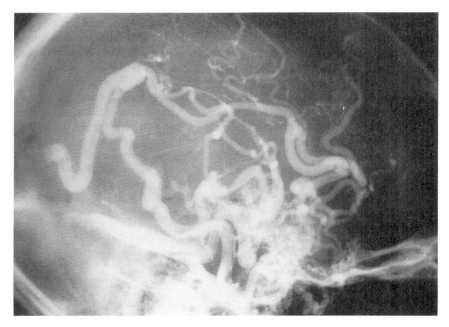

Fig. 19.9. Angiogram showing extensive cerebral angioma

systemic complications like inappropriate ADH secretion, pulmonary oedema or ECG changes due to subendocardial ischaemia.

In about 20 per cent the presence of blood in the cerebrospinal fluid tends to cause obstruction of the arachnoid villi with the rapid development of hydrocephalus. This frequently resolves but occasionally returns during the years after a bleed. The damaging effects of an acute bleed lead to death in about 25 per cent of cases with a similar number succumbing to the effects of recurrent bleeding or ischaemia in the next 2–3 weeks. The long-term risk of re-bleeding is about 2 per cent per annum.

An alternative source of subarachnoid bleeding is an arteriovenous malformation (Fig. 19.9). The mortality of bleeds from such anomalous vessels is less perhaps because the bleed is not always arterial and therefore not always at arterial pressure. Epilepsy and focal deficit other than that due to the bleed are more common than with aneurysms.

Blood disorders, the use of oral contraceptives, and anticoagulant medication are other rare causes of subarachnoid haemorrhage.

Cerebral venous thrombosis

Thrombosis of intracranial venous sinuses or cerebral veins can be provoked by infections, especially cranial sepsis (meningitis, scalp infection) or in debilitating dehydrating diseases. It may complicate the oral contraceptive, the puerperium, diabetes, ulcerative colitis, heart failure or haematological conditions such as sickle cell anaemia, paroxysmal nocturnal haemoglobinuria, haemolytic anaemia and cryofibrinogenaemia.

The occlusion can cause venous infarction which is usually haemorrhagic with some blood staining of the spinal fluid. Venous infarction often involves the cortex and epilepsy is likely. If sufficient venous drainage is impaired, intracranial pressure rises with impaired consciousness and papilloedema.

Clinical features

There are clues in the history and examination which can be used to deduce the pathological type of stroke and its location, information that can then be used when planning the appropriate management.

Transient ischaemic attacks

As defined, these are episodes of focal neurological disability lasting less than 24 h. Most last several minutes or a few hours. Their onset may suggest a haemodynamic mechanism. Thus patients may describe the development of weakness, incoordination, sensory changes or visual problems on getting out of bed, running up stairs, turning their head, etc. In these circumstances the deficit, e.g. the weakness of an arm, may take a few minutes to reach its maximum, and there may be associated symptoms of a syncopal nature. More often, implying an embolic mechanism, the onset is abrupt and the attack occurs out of the blue. When the territory of the internal carotid artery is involved, brief loss of vision in one eye (amaurosis fugax) may occur or the patient develops weakness and/or sensory disturbance in an arm, or arm and leg with or without a droop of one side of the face and dysphasia if the dominant hemisphere is affected. If the vertebrobasilar circulation is involved, attacks of brainstem ischaemia occur with bilateral visual disturbance, vertigo, diplopia, facial numbness, dysarthria and ataxia with or without limb involvement which may alternate in successive attacks or be bilateral. Isolated vertigo can be due to vestibular disorders and it is unwise to conclude that the vertiginous patient is having ischaemic attacks unless other brainstem functions are affected. Similarly isolated drop attacks and visual blurring may have other explanations, e.g. syncopal visual darkening. Patients with vertebrobasilar ischaemia are more likely to describe an onset related to exercise or head rotation than those with carotid disease, suggesting flow may be more important than emboli in many of their attacks.

The neurological examination will usually reveal no deficit unless a small area of infarction has occurred when minor signs of no functional importance may be detected, e.g. an extensor plantar response.

The neurovascular examination may reveal a potential cardiac source for embolism and auscultation should be supplemented by chest X-ray and a routine 12-lead ECG in that assessment. If these preliminaries reveal any abnormality or the patient is young (less than 45 years of age) an echocardiogram is advised. If a cardiac source for emboli is elicited, anticoagulants may well be indicated. More commonly the cardiac examination is normal but bruits may be heard over major vessels in the neck. The interpretation of neck bruits

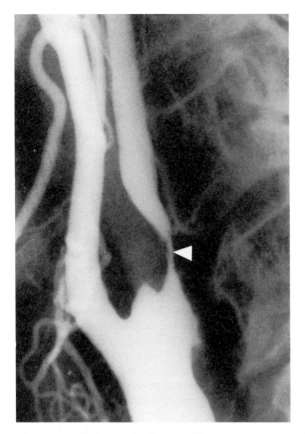

Fig. 19.10. Tight stenosis (*arrow*) of internal carotid artery in patient with TIAs

requires some care. Most are transmitted from the thorax when they will usually be audible in the suprasternal notch, and others are venous where they change with respiration and forced expiration against a closed glottis (the Valsalva manoeuvre). Local midcervical bruits arise in the carotid artery and reflect stenosis and turbulence in relation to atheromatous disease. As such bruits in this site are markers of atheroma they carry an increased risk of stroke and heart attack. In the patient with a TIA they direct attention to the carotid artery as a source for embolism. It is important to realize, however, that there may be no bruit over an occluded or even a tightly stenosed vessel and that the bruit may arise from the external and not the internal carotid artery.

It is logical to consider surgical repair of heavily diseased carotid arteries in patients with TIAs, to prevent embolization, to prevent occlusion by secondary thrombosis or plaque rupture, and thereby to reduce the risk of stroke (Fig. 19.10). Although randomized trials have not yet formally proved the efficacy of a surgical approach, the consensus view is that patients with TIAs due to a carotid stenosis at the bifurcation should be referred to an experienced surgeon who has proved his ability to carry out the operation with a low mortality and morbidity. To this end, patients who would be generally fit for vascular surgery are investigated by duplex Doppler scanning of the carotid bifurcation and by angiography.

In some 10 per cent of cases a carotid occlusion is revealed not amenable to endarterectomy, or the obstructive atheroma proves to be in the inaccessible carotid siphon or middle cerebral artery. The ingenious operation that anastomoses the superficial temporal artery to a pial branch of the middle cerebral artery through a burr hole or small trephine for such cases has been the subject of a recent multicentre randomized trial. It failed to prevent stroke when compared with medical care.

Since most emboli from the carotid artery are believed to be based on a platelet aggregate, inhibitors of platelet aggregation, such as aspirin, are employed to try to reduce the risk of subsequent stroke to those declaring themselves to be especially at risk by reporting a TIA. A dosage of 300 mg or 1200 mg of aspirin a day has been shown to reduce the risk of stroke, heart attack or vascular death in such patients by some 20 per cent and this is a valuable addition to the protection provided by risk factor management (treatment of hypertension, diabetes, hyperlipidaemia, cessation of smoking, etc).

In the case of vertebrobasilar TIAs, angiography is less commonly advised since surgical options are few and of unproven value. Some patients show a stenosis of the proximal subclavian artery causing retrograde flow down the vertebral artery into the supply to the upper limb. This haemodynamic situation, colourfully referred to as the subclavian steal syndrome, is rarely hazardous to patients and intrathoracic operations to repair a stenosed subclavian artery are rarely justified unless attacks of vertebrobasilar ischaemia are frequent, disabling and fail to respond to the medical regimen applied to carotid TIAs. In addition, a soft collar to limit head rotation may help those whose attacks are so provoked, the extreme position perhaps kinking off the larger of the two vertebral arteries.

Rarely, TIAs are due to haematological abnormalities with thrombocythaemia or abnormalities of coagulation, anaemia or polycythaemia so these should be sought when screening for risk factors is being carried out.

Unfortunately, although some 30 per cent of stroke victims in hospital describe a preceding TIA, community surveys reveal a lower figure (10 per cent) and most strokes occur without a TIA prompting preventative therapy.

Lacunar stroke

Many patients, particularly those with hypertensive small vessel disease, develop small deep lacunar infarcts which have characteristic clinical profiles. There may be a preceding TIA (in some 20 per cent) and the onset may be less than abrupt. Usually a sudden deficit develops, most often without headache, and since only deep structures are involved, dysphasia or other cortical problems are absent. A hemiparesis may be notable by the lack of dysphasia or visual field deficit, by sparing of the face, or by the total lack of accompanying sensory change (pure motor stroke). Alternatively, sensory change down one side of the body may develop without motor signs (pure sensory stroke). A combination of pyramidal and cerebellar involvement in the pons may cause a clumsy hand with dysarthria, or cerebellar ataxia may be seen on one side in which there is mild weakness apart from a more striking foot drop. Such deficits usually improve over a few weeks.

Although the majority of victims are hypertensive and/or diabetic, pure motor strokes may also develop from embolism from artery to artery, and it is prudent to examine such patients for neck vessel disease at least by non-invasive methods, especially if TIAs precede the event or a neck bruit is heard.

CT scans may 'miss' some of the smaller lesions especially in the brainstem where magnetic resonance imaging (MRI) is more sensitive due to the lack of bone artefacts in the posterior fossa. Nevertheless, CT scanning should be carried out if only to exclude a small haemorrhage in the hypertensive patient, and if it shows a cortical wedge-shaped infarct to reawaken interest in a possible source for embolism.

If repeated lucunar strokes are allowed to occur, dementia with pseudobulbar palsy may result. Prevention depends on treatment of hypertension, and aspirin in most cases.

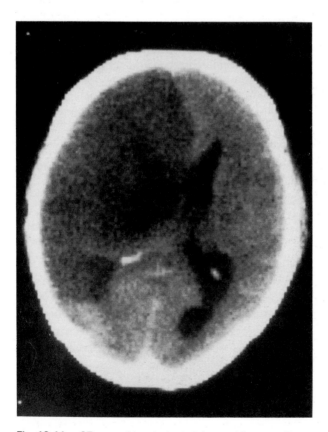

Fig. 19.11.   CT scan of hemispheric infarct with mass effect

Major strokes

The clinical picture can go some way to deciding whether the patient's hemiplegia is due to haemorrhage, or infarction, or if stroke is being mimicked by something else (tumour, subdural haematoma, arteriovenous malformation). If the acute event is preceded by TIAs, an infarct is likely, if by headache, mental changes or epilepsy, a tumour is suspected. If the onset is accompanied by severe headache, vomiting and coma, haemorrhage is very likely and the chances of haemorrhage are further increased if the patient is hypertensive and has neck stiffness on examination. Stroke in evolution may be due to extending infarction or a spreading and enlarging haematoma.

Only CT scanning can make the distinction between haemorrhage and infarction reliably, but must be carried out within 2 weeks as the distinctive high density of fresh blood fades and the low density area left in its wake is indistinguishable from an infarct. Haemorrhage is reliably detected; infarction may only be visible in 60 per cent (Fig. 19.11), although enhancement increases the yield, especially if carried out towards the end of the first week (Fig. 19.12). Infarcts may show some mass effect due to oedema in the first 3–4 weeks; later than this a tumour would be suspected. CT scanning also detects the other nonstroke causes of hemiplegia, etc, which would amount to some 1–2 per cent of those admitted with sudden deficits.

CSF examination for xanthochromia as proof of haemorrhage in stroke patients is not recommended. It is not sufficiently reliable and there is a risk of

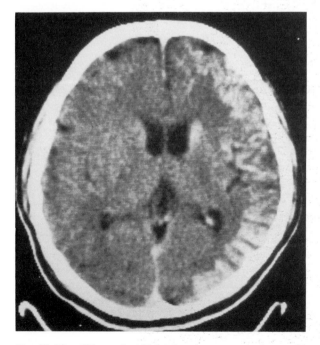

Fig. 19.12. CT scan in which infarction was only detected by the gyral pattern of enhancement after contrast injection

exacerbating pressure gradients and triggering brain shift if the haematoma or infarct is having mass effect.

The neurological deficit depends on the site of the haematoma or the territory of the infarction.

Putaminal haemorrhage

The usual clinical picture is of contralateral hemiparesis, hemisensory loss and conjugate deviation of the eyes to the side of the haematoma. Although the cortex is not affected, some higher cortical functions may be impaired, e.g. with some non-fluent dysphasia if the lesion is on the left but with preservation of the ability to repeat spoken phrases. If the haematoma enlarges into the capsule and its mass becomes critical, the conscious level falls and the ipsilateral pupil enlarges from pressure on the third nerve. The ipsilateral plantar may become extensor like that on the hemiparetic side from brainstem 'squeeze' which carries a poor prognosis. A more anterior lesion may affect sensation, a more posterior one causes a visual field defect. On the right side surgery is sometimes attempted, on the left the risk of dysphasia precludes exploration.

Caudate haemorrhage

This is much rarer and the haematoma rapidly gains access to the ventricular cavity. The general effects of haemorrhage (headache, vomiting and a stiff neck) are accompanied by little in the way of a hemiparesis unless the lesion is large, when the picture is like that of an anteriorly placed putaminal bleed.

Thalamic haemorrhage

Sensory changes in the contralateral limbs predominate sometimes with choreic movements or dystonic posturing rather than weakness. The eyes tend to be in forced downward gaze, often in a converged position with small poorly reacting pupils, signs all due to local pressure in the region of the quadrigeminal plate. Left thalamic haemorrhage may disturb speech with naming difficulties. Consciousness is often depressed because of the local effect on the upper brainstem. These haemorrhages are surgically inaccessible.

Lobar haemorrhages

These subcortical surgically accessible haematomas produce signs appropriate to their localization. In the frontal lobe, apathy, eye deviation and a contralateral hemiparesis can be expected. In the central region, hemisensory loss is also found and on the left dysphasia. Parietal lobe haemorrhages cause hemisensory loss and inattention in the visual half field, while a lobar bleed in the temporal lobe causes fluent aphasia with poor comprehension and little or no limb signs. Occipital haematomas cause severe hemianopias with or without sensory inattention.

Pontine haemorrhage

The classical picture is of coma with lost horizontal eye movements, pinpoint reactive pupils and quadriparesis. Hyperpyrexia and irregular breathing patterns may develop. Smaller haematomas may cause lacunar syndromes (*see* later). The large ones are invariably fatal (Fig. 19.13).

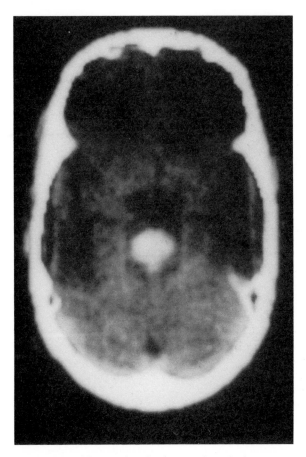

Fig. 19.13. CT scan showing haemorrhage in the pons

Cerebellar haemorrhage

This eminently operable lesion accounts for some 10 per cent of haemorrhages. When unilateral ataxia develops in the setting of headache and vomiting it is not difficult to suspect the diagnosis. The patient may not be seen before local pressure on the pons has produced coma or a picture like that of pontine hae-morrhage. Sometimes conjugate deviation of the eyes without an accompany-ing hemiparesis is the only clue.

Infarction in the territory of the middle cerebral artery

If the main trunk of the middle cerebral artery is occluded by an embolus and the whole vascular territory is infarcted, the patient shows ocular deviation, hemiplegia, with hemisensory loss, hemianopia and global aphasia, lacking comprehension or speech if on the left side. The infarct swells and the added features of brainstem compromise may be seen with a third nerve palsy and coma.

Embolism into upper branches causes infarction above the Sylvian fissure with contralateral hemiparesis, hemisensory loss, ocular deviation and a non-fluent aphasia with relative preservation of comprehension if on the left.

The territory of the lower branches includes the temporal cortex, so infarction produces fluent aphasia with minimal comprehension on the left, dyspraxia if on the right, but little or no limb changes. There may be a visual field defect, often an upper quadrantanopia, from involvement of the lower fibres of the optic radiation.

Smaller cortical lesions may cause a deficit restricted to the contralateral hand and face with difficulties in calculation and writing (on the left) or with visuo-spatial tasks if on the right. Deep infarcts cause contralateral limb findings, hemiparesis and hemianaesthesia, but little if any speech defect or other abnormality of 'higher function'.

Anterior cerebral artery

Emboli less often enter this vessel. When infarction is produced in its territory the clinical picture reflects its role in supplying the paramedian frontal lobe, the caudate and anterior perforating substance. Patients have a contralateral hemiplegia, most marked in the leg. The hand may be normal but there may be weakness at the shoulder. Any sensory loss is restricted to the lower limb. Apathy and incontinence are common. Speech can be reduced in amount as in a Broca's aphasia but, by contrast, the patient can still repeat well.

Posterior cerebral artery

This is the commonest target of emboli in the posterior circulation. An isolated hemianopia is common. It may spare the macular region of the central vision if the patient's occipital pole (where the macular is 'represented') has additional blood supply from posterior parietal branches of the middle cerebral artery. When an infarct is located in the occipital lobe, difficulties with colour appreciation, facial recognition and in naming objects presented visually may be seen. When the infarct is more parieto-occipital, the visual defects may be of neglect or inattention and may be accompanied by hemisensory neglect, the patient failing to appreciate bilateral cutaneous stimuli in the absence of sensory loss. Higher function abnormalities on the left may include selective difficulty in reading (infarction in the angular gyrus), naming difficulties (posterior thalamic infarct), and verbal memory problems (temporal lobe infarction).

If both posterior cerebral artery territories are infarcted from an embolus at the top of the basilar artery, cortical blindness with confusion arises. The patient cannot see but may describe visual scenes in a confabulatory way. Pupillary reflexes are normal but optokinetic responses are lost in all directions. These are defined in Chapter 3, p. 69. Memory loss may be severe.

Vertebral artery

Occlusion of one vertebral artery may produce no neurological symptoms or a TIA may occur. If collateral flow is inadequate (vestigial other vertebral artery), infarction in the brainstem occurs, usually in the territory of the posterior inferior cerebellar artery. The complex resulting deficit (Wallenberg's syndrome) reflects involvement on one side of the nucleus ambiguus, the trigeminal nucleus, vestibular nuclei, cerebellar peduncle, spinothalamic tract and autonomic fibres. Thus the patient has a Horner's syndrome, dissociated (pain and temperature) sensory loss on one side of the face and the other side of the body, nystagmus to either side, ataxia of the ipsilateral limbs, palatal and vocal cord paralysis.

If the medulla is involved, paralysis of the tongue and a hemiparesis result. If the cerebellar hemisphere is infarcted, a picture like that of cerebellar haemorrhage may be seen but without severe headache and vomiting (Fig. 19.14). Sometimes only vertigo mimicking a labyrinthine lesion results. These latter problems usually result from intracranial occlusion of the vertebral artery.

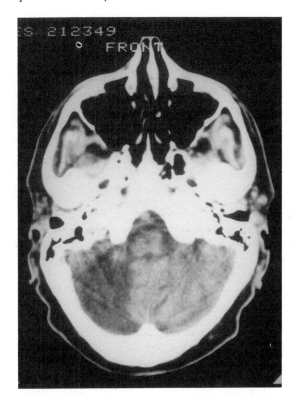

Fig. 19.14. CT scan showing infarction of the left cerebellar hemisphere

Basilar artery

While arteries like the middle and posterior cerebral are often affected by embolism and rarely by thrombosis, the opposite is true of the basilar artery which is often severely affected by atheroma on which an occluding mural thrombus can form. TIAs involving diplopia, vertigo and weakness of the legs are often reported before occlusion causes infarction, when quadriparesis and cranial nerve defects are seen.

A number of clinical pictures can be encountered. The lower cranial nerves (IX–XII) may be affected with paralysis of lower motor neurone type (bulbar palsy) affecting speech and swallowing. Alternatively, upper motor neurone impairment of the same structures causes a pseudobulbar palsy with brisk jaw and facial reflexes and a spastic tongue. This is often accompanied by excessive laughing and crying. Pontine infarction may cause a sixth nerve palsy, gaze paralysis or an internuclear ophthalmoplegia in which damage to the medial longitudinal bundle causes lack of adduction of one eye during lateral gaze. As with pontine haemorrhage the pupils may become small (Fig. 19.15).

Cardiac emboli may lodge at the top of the basilar artery and cause loss of vertical eye movement, pupillary abnormalities and stupor.

Lacunar infarction

These small deep infarcts in the capsule or pons cause characteristic clinical syndromes which were described above. Pure motor hemiparesis without sensory or speech disturbance, pure sensory hemideficit, the clumsy hand-dysarthria syndrome and homolateral ataxia with crural paresis, are the commonest. Hemiballismus from a small subthalamic infarct is rare.

CT scans often fail to visualize the small infarct but are important since small haemorrhages and larger embolic infarcts can be mimicked, especially in the case of the pure motor hemiplegia. The lacunar infarct causes equal involvement of face and leg. Disproportionate involvement of arm, or face and arm, is more likely from a middle cerebral embolus.

Investigation for a source of embolism in heart or neck vessel is usually reserved for those with bedside pointers such as atrial fibrillation or a carotid bruit, since the yield is much lower than in other types of stroke.

Management of completed strokes

If a primary intracerebral haemorrhage has been diagnosed, there may be a role for neurosurgical intervention. Aspiration of clot with relief of local distension of fibre tracts and shift of structures may improve the conscious level and the neurological deficit. This is true of external capsular haematomas and some large superficial lobar haemorrhages. Smaller clots probably do not need surgery, and deep haematomas in the basal ganglia are unlikely to be helped. In the posterior fossa pontine haemorrhage is rarely operable but a clot in the cerebellar hemisphere that is producing coma by obstruction of the aqueduct and pontine compression may respond dramatically to surgical decompression.

The treatment of blood pressure in patients with stroke is problematical. It

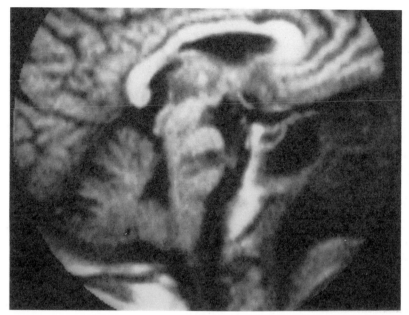

(a)

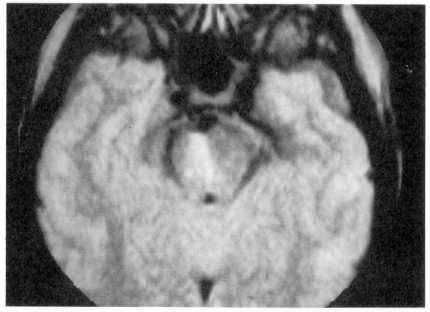

(b)

Fig. 19.15. Magnetic resonance images showing small infarct in pons; **(a)** of low density in T_1 images of sagittal section, **(b)** of high signal in T_2 images of axial view

will be argued that it is better to delay the institution of treatment in most patients with infarcts because of the temporary paralysis of autoregulation rendering blood flow pressure passive with a real risk that induced hypotension will extend the volume of infarction. There is a comparable disturbance of blood flow in cases of haemorrhage but the head of pressure may be relevant to the risk of continued bleeding, so some slight reduction in blood pressure is usually advised if levels are high.

The recurrence of stroke after haemorrhage, whether a recurrent haemorrhage or infarction, is reduced by treatment of blood pressure over the long term. Aspirin is probably contraindicated.

If an ischaemic stroke is suggested by the clinical and CT findings, a cardiac source for embolism should be sought as for TIA, especially in the young. If none is suspected, disease of neck vessels should be considered. The risks of carotid endarterectomy in the aftermath of a major stroke are much greater than in patients with TIA so angiography is rarely indicated, since even an operable carotid stenosis will not be tackled at that time. If the patient makes an excellent recovery it may then be considered as part of the long-term strategy to limit the risk of recurrence. To this end, risk factor management and aspirin will be advised.

If a cardiac source for emboli is found in the form of atrial fibrillation, anti-coagulants are normally advocated, though there is as yet no proof of their efficacy as judged by a good trial. If the cerebral embolism follows a recent myocardial infarction anticoagulants for 6 months may be advised, to be followed by long-term aspirin.

If the patient's stroke is evolving during the period of inpatient observation, CT scanning is urgently needed to distinguish non-vascular causes of a rapidly progressing deficit, a potentially operable haematoma and evolving infarction. If the latter is suggested by the absence of mass effect or blood on the scan, heparinization may also help stabilize the deficit which is assumed to be due to propagation of thrombus or embolism off the top of a more proximal occlusion, although again there is no proof of the advisability of this approach. Large infarcts may become haemorrhagic as embolic occlusions recannulate, so there is a risk of inducing haemorrhage.

If stroke deterioration appears to be due to oedema, hypertonic solutions may be used, e.g. glycerol or mannitol. Dexamethasone even in very large doses has not been found to relieve the oedema of infarction despite its success in the case of superficially similar swelling around brain tumours. Often deterioration is due to systemic factors and treatment of cardiac decompensation or a chest or urinary infection may restore stability.

Subarachnoid haemorrhage

The patient is suddenly struck down by a headache which may be of dramatic severity. Its onset is so abrupt that it is described by the patient with a click of his fingers or as though he had been struck on the back of the head by a sledge hammer. Vomiting and drowsiness are common. Neck stiffness and photophobia develop mimicking meningitis, but fever does not complicate a bleed unless later on an infection of chest or urine complicates the picture. As blood tracks down into the spinal theca the patient may complain of backache.

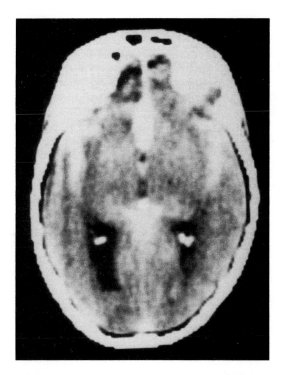

Fig. 19.16. CT scan showing blood in the CSF spaces after subarachnoid haemorrhage

CT scans detect the presence of blood in the subarachnoid space (Fig. 19.16) confirming the diagnosis without the need for a lumbar puncture which is not without risk but must be carried out if there are no facilities for emergency scanning. If a haematoma causes a focal deficit, CT scanning must precede any thoughts of CSF examination for fear of promoting brain shift.

The site of the bleeding aneurysm may be suggested by the clinical picture. A third nerve palsy from onset suggests an aneurysm of the internal carotid artery or the posterior communicating artery. More extensive paralysis of eye movement on one side suggests the aneurysm is in the cavernous sinus. Hemiparesis and aphasia suggest a middle cerebral aneurysm, leg weakness and bilateral extensor plantars an aneurysm of the anterior communicating artery. An isolated hemianopia would implicate a rare aneurysm of the posterior cerebral artery. Vertigo and nystagmus imply a posterior fossa aneurysm. Those at the top of the basilar artery tend to cause amnesia and quadriparesis.

Alert subjects will be investigated by angiography and referred for clipping of any aneurysm(s). If early operation is possible, the subsequent development of focal ischaemic problems due to spasm of basal arteries exposed to shed blood can be treated energetically with induced hypertension, something that would be hazardous before the aneurysm is clipped. Inhibitors of fibrinolysis are successful in reducing the risk of rebleeding but add to the risk of ischaemic changes, so are rarely advocated.

If no aneurysm is found and no arteriovenous malformation revealed by the angiography, rare causes including blood dyscrasias should be reviewed. Bleeding from a vascular malformation too small to show up on angiography probably explains some of the angiographically normal cases. As there is no way to predict who will rebleed, all patients without operable aneurysms are treated with sedation and bedrest.

Arteriovenous malformations may be surgically accessible on the surface of the brain. When deep in the hemisphere they are more safely dealt with by embolization procedures in which a small balloon is manipulated into the main fistulous connection between arterial and venous components and lodged there reducing the vascularity and size of the malformation. These lesions often cause epilepsy and may cause focal deficit without bleeding.

Unusual causes of stroke

Giant cell arteritis

This inflammatory condition of medium-sized arteries affects the elderly. Most victims are over 55 years of age and have an erythrocyte sedimentation rate (ESR) over 55. They complain of severe headache often accompanied by scalp tenderness and by systemic malaise, perhaps with claudication pain in the masseter when eating. The internal elastic lamina of the artery becomes fragmented and invaded by inflammatory cells and giant cells. The intima is thickened. The vessel may occlude. The superficial temporal artery is often affected and may be tender, red and thrombosed. Involvement of the ophthalmic or ciliary arteries can cause infarction of the optic nerve and blindness is a much feared complication of the disease. The diagnosis, strongly implied by the elevated ESR, is confirmed by biopsy of the superficial temporal artery. High daily doses of steroids (80 mg/day prednisone) are reduced after the first few weeks and monitored by the suppression of both symptoms and the ESR. It is rarely possible to wean patients off their steroids in much less than 12 months. The condition may relapse (or start) in the form of polymyalgia rheumatica, when malaise is dominated by aches and pains around the hips and shoulders. This lower grade activity can usually be contained by a low dose of prednisone, e.g. 10–15 mg/day.

The disease does not affect intradural arteries which lack elastic laminae which appear to be the target organ. Strokes may occur from involvement of extradural vessels, usually the vertebral artery, with brainstem infarction. Rarer complications of the disease include isolated cranial nerve palsies, progressive dilatation of the aorta, mesenteric claudication, gangrene of the scalp and peripheral neuropathy.

Other arteritides

A panarteritis with nodular changes in the vessels underlies the condition known as polyarteritis nodosa. This affects mostly men who may suffer from abdominal pain, asthma, fever, pericarditis, renal disease and hypertension. Fifty per cent have involvement of the peripheral nerves with a diffuse neuropathy or a mononeuritis multiplex due to infarction of nerve trunks consequent upon thrombosis of an inflamed vasa nervorum.

Similar small vessel occlusions may cause fleeting central nervous system manifestations with seizures or focal deficits, but the damaged vessels may rupture so subarachnoid haemorrhages and cerebral haemorrhages can develop. These central nervous system complications are fortunately rare, since they are difficult to manage. Muscle pain due to polymyositis or a neuropathy may respond to steroids after the diagnosis has been suggested by an elevated ESR with leucocytosis and eosinophilia and confirmed by biopsy of muscle, nerve or kidney.

An even rarer necrotizing arteritis is associated with granuloma formation (Wegener's granulomatosis). The upper and lower respiratory and the renal tract are usually involved with nasal ulceration, pulmonary infiltration and/or glomerulonephritis. The granuloma in the nasopharynx may damage cranial nerves by direct spread or they and peripheral nerves may be affected by the vasculitic small vessel disease (mononeuritis multiplex). The renal lesion can be lethal but immunosuppression with cyclophosphamide offers a good chance of inducing a remission.

Meningovascular syphilis and tuberculous meningitis may cause vasculitic strokes.

Cerebral venous thrombosis

On the background of sepsis, dehydration or a predisposing condition such as the puerperium, the oral contraceptive agents or sickle cell anaemia, a young patient develops headache, drowsiness, fits and a rapidly evolving focal deficit, e.g. hemiplegia. The patient is found to have papilloedema. CT scans show haemorrhagic infarction and angiography is diagnostic as long as late films showing the venous phase are specifically obtained. If there is no infarction on scans, anticoagulants may be used as they would be expected to limit spread of the thrombotic process. In the presence of haemorrhagic infarction they are contraindicated.

Hypertensive encephalopathy

This is a very rare condition. Very high arterial pressures may exceed the upper limit of autoregulation of cerebral blood flow. Segments of intracerebral vessels no longer contract in the face of rising intraluminal pressure but give way and become leaky. Patchy congestion and oedema develop. The patients have headache, fits, focal problems like aphasia and become unconscious. The examination reveals papilloedema and very high systemic arterial pressure, e.g. 250/150 mmHg. The hypertension is often of renal origin and the rate of rise in blood pressure often rapid. Slower elevations of pressure cause some shift of the autoregulatory curve to the right with a higher breakthrough point with hypertrophy of the muscular media of intracerebral arteries.

Blood pressure must be lowered promptly, although there is still a danger of inducing infarction if the patient becomes hypotensive while still having raised intracranial pressure from oedema. Short-acting drugs should be used so that blood pressure control can be regulated (e.g. labetalol or hydralazine).

Watershed infarction

The areas of brain on the boundary zones between the territories of supply of the main intracerebral vessels are vulnerable during periods of systemic collapse with hypotension (Fig. 19.17). The far field of a vessel's territory is most likely to infarct in these situations. The site most often damaged in this way, during cardiac arrest or after blood loss, is the parieto-occipital cortex between the field of supply of the middle and posterior cerebral arteries. The patients develop

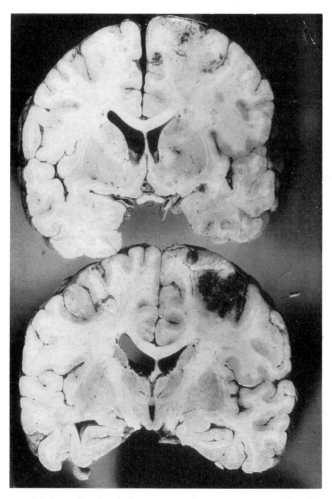

Fig. 19.17. Post-mortem brain slices revealing haemorrhagic infarction in the watershed between the anterior and middle cerebral artery territories due to severe hypotension

complex visual problems with visual disorientation and sometimes difficulty in seeing more than one thing at a time. They fail to make sense of a picture or scene even though they can identify components. There may be confusion, memory difficulties and apraxia of the hands which despite adequate strength and coordination cannot execute skilled tasks.

Multi-infarct dementia

The net result of multiple infarcts whether lacunar or large embolic lesions, is loss of brain substance with atrophy. The patients become demented. The illness can often be distinguished from the slowly evolving dementia of Alzheimer's disease by the clinical features (p. 235).

The patients retain some insight and give a history of a sudden onset of memory and cognitive difficulty that has deteriorated in a stepwise fashion, associated with the occurrence of strokes, usually on a background of hypertension. Physical complaints are common and evidence of previous hemiparesis usually found, perhaps with the dysarthria and brisk facial reflexes and extensor plantars of a pseudobulbar palsy.

Treatment largely depends on control of blood pressure and other risk factors.

Rehabilitation

Rehabilitation begins with the care of the acute stroke and continues through the course of any inpatient stay and on into the period after return home, to work or in retirement. Stroke affects all the family since someone will have to take on the role of carer if the patient is left with deficit. The impact should not be underestimated. Finances will be strained by the loss of a wage earner and/or the need for a carer to give up work to be with the patient. Relationships are stressed by the new roles in the family, the frustration and sometimes the personality change of the patient, the nature of the disability including incontinence or severe communication difficulty, and the depression that sets in after stroke in some 30 per cent.

Much can be done to anticipate and minimize these difficulties by providing support, expert guidance and practical aids. Physiotherapists, speech therapists, occupational therapists, nurses and social workers all have roles to play. In different cases one or other will be most heavily involved, becoming the natural team leader.

Although trials have shown that formalized speech therapy achieves little more than enthusiastic volunteers in helping patients communicate, the expert has a valuable role to play in instructing the family and other carers how best to deal with the speech difficulties, identifying the more unusual kinds of dysphasia and dysarthria and helping with related problems like dysphagia. Physiotherapists and occupational therapists are more directly involved in assessing and treating physical disabilities. No one special kind of physiotherapy has been proved superior to another but passive movements in the early stages are important to prevent later shoulder problems and contractures and active exercise helps motivate the patient towards physical recovery thereafter.

Bad postures and inefficient use of the limbs are likely to develop if the patient's recovery is unsupervised.

Various aids may be necessary or adaptations to the home may be required. Mobility is crucial to preserve a social life, so attempts must be made to arrange for the patient to be got out and about one way or another. Patients may be unable to go back to driving because of epilepsy or a visual field defect, but weakness of a limb is not necessarily a bar and the patient can be specifically reassessed about this.

Most recovery occurs in the first 6 months and most of this in the first 2 months. Some 10 per cent further improve after 6 months, but when dealing with patients it is best to view this as an unlikely bonus.

The prognosis can be gauged to some extent. Incontinence persisting after the first 2–3 days is usually a sign that the patient may not regain independence. Its disappearance in a severely hemiplegic patient can be a clue to a recovery that otherwise looks unlikely. If good arm function is to return, a fair grip develops within 3–4 weeks. If the patient is not walking normally by 5–6 weeks, the patient is unlikely ever to walk at a normal speed. If the patient can only lift his leg off the bed in the same time course, he will nonetheless walk, though not normally.

Vascular disease of the spinal cord

The blood supply of the spinal cord leaves it vulnerable to the effects of aortic dissection or surgery when the chief arterial supply (which is often a branch of the ninth or tenth thoracic artery) is obstructed. The resultant infarct affects the anterior two-thirds of the cord as collateral channels tend to protect the dorsal columns. The resulting paraplegia is striking for the sparing of joint position sense in the face of severe weakness, sphincter paralysis and a 'level' to pain and temperature appreciation in the lower thoracic region. Partial lesions often recover well but total infarction may leave a permanent paraplegia.

The cord damage associated with cervical spondylosis is partially compressive in origin, but a vascular component is often suspected. When cord compression at the foramen magnum or at C3/4 produces wasting of small hand muscles, it is suggested that vascular compromise has caused some ischaemic damage at T1. This is thought to be a watershed in the vascular supply to the cord or due to venous engorgement.

Haemorrhage into the spinal cord is only likely in the presence of an arteriovenous malformation. If this bleeds a sudden paraplegia develops. It may also cause the insidious development of mixed upper and lower motor neurone signs in the legs with symptoms which are worse on exercise. This is thought to be due to changes in the venous drainage of the arteriovenous malformation. Such lesions can be suspected by the appearance of vessels on myelography but angiographic injection of selected thoracic vessels is needed as a prelude to surgery or embolization of the malformation in an attempt to prevent progression.

20

Metabolic disorders

Vitamin deficiencies

Many of these result from the effects of widespread malnutrition, e.g. starvation, or from severe malabsorption. A few may reflect dietary fads or the substitution of food in the diet by alcohol.

Wernicke's encephalopathy; Wernicke-Korsakoff syndrome

In this condition multiple small areas of necrosis and haemorrhage are found in the midbrain, the peri-aqueductal region, the paraventricular areas of the thalamus, the hypothalamus, the mammillary bodies and around the fourth ventricle. The cerebellum may also show neuronal loss. This damage is due to thiamine deficiency and if treated early many of the clinical features can be reversed.

The presentation is usually acute with the combination of mental confusion (Korsakoff's psychosis) with an ophthalmoplegia and ataxia. The confusion includes amnesia for recent events, loss of recall and often confabulation. Many patients appear apathetic, muddled and drowsy. A few may show the more florid hallucinations of alcoholic withdrawal.

The ocular signs include single or bilateral abducens palsies (54 per cent), disturbances of conjugate gaze (44 per cent), and often horizontal and vertical nystagmus (85 per cent). The ataxia is a reflection of cerebellar damage and may be so severe as to prevent walking unaided. There may also be signs of a peripheral neuropathy, present in some 80 per cent.

The condition is most commonly found in alcoholics, but also in other malnutrition states particularly if there is protracted vomiting.

Thiamine deficiency can be determined by a significant reduction in the red cell transketolase level. Untreated the condition is fatal and in severe cases some nervous system damage may prove irreversible. Treatment is with intravenous thiamine 50–100 mg daily for 5 days, accompanied by the restoration of a normal diet (or adequate parenteral feeding where indicated). Glucose administration, by itself, can dramatically worsen the effects of thiamine deficiency.

Vitamin B12 deficiency

This may cause a peripheral neuropathy (*see* p. 135), subacute combined degeneration (SACD) from spinal cord damage, optic atrophy and even dementia. Commonly the presentation is with sensory symptoms in the feet. The deficiency may arise after total gastrectomy, in vegans, after some parasitic infestations of the gut and from the failure to absorb B12 in the stomach from a lack of intrinsic factor (pernicious anaemia).

B12 deficiency is accompanied by a macrocytic megaloblastic anaemia and low serum B12 level. The CSF is normal. Nerve conduction studies usually show some neuropathic changes, and some patients may show abnormal visual evoked potentials. A Schilling test measuring the absorption of radioisotope-labelled B12, with and without intrinsic factor, may confirm the diagnosis and its mechanism.

Treatment is with injections of hydroxocobalamin, initially 1000 μg daily for 10 days, then monthly for the rest of the patient's life. Providing severe damage has not occurred symptoms usually improve over the first few months of treatment.

Pellagra

This is a deficiency of nicotinic acid (niacin) which may affect the nervous system to cause fatigue, apathy, drowsiness and even confusion. It may damage the pyramidal tracts producing spastic weakness of the legs, or more widespread neurological disturbance with extrapyramidal and peripheral nerve signs. Occasionally an acute confusional state with deteriorating conscious level arises. Many patients also show skin changes with a dermatitis, mucocutaneous lesions and gastrointestinal disturbances, particularly diarrhoea and even malabsorption. A scarlet painful tongue is common.

Pellagra was originally described in vegans from poor maize-eating countries and in deprived prisoners. It is probable that many of these patients were suffering from multiple vitamin deficiencies as well as an inadequate diet.

Nutritional and toxic amblyopia

Certain deficiency states may cause optic nerve damage leading to visual failure and optic atrophy. These include B12 deficiency (*see* p. 161) and thiamine deficiency: the latter may have some links with the toxic effects of alcohol and/or tobacco to which many of these patients are also exposed.

There is an insidiously progressive impairment of vision affecting both eyes. The acuity falls and the optic discs appear pale. Often there are centrocaecal scotomas most easily detected by a red target.

Abstinence from tobacco and/or alcohol is essential and most patients are also given hydroxocobalamin injections, although it is equally important to ensure a good diet with thiamine and other vitamin B supplements.

Tropical amblyopia and neuropathies

These again result from the combined effects of malnutrition and vitamin deficiency, most often found in deprived areas associated with starvation or in prisoners. Many have combinations of beri-beri, pellagra and their neurological manifestations. These include a peripheral neuropathy with complaints of sensory symptoms and sometimes 'burning' in the feet, with weakness and clumsiness of the extremities: in a few this may be combined with a spastic paraparesis. Usually the signs are of a sensorimotor neuropathy with prominent muscle wasting and marked ataxia. There may also be signs of visual upset with blurred vision leading to optic atrophy and sometimes deafness. Many patients also show mucocutaneous lesions and some complain of abdominal pain.

It is thought in some instances that cyanide intoxication from excess cassava in the diet may be responsible and a number of patients may show raised plasma cyanide and thiocyanate levels. In others malnutrition is responsible. The CSF is normal and the B12 level commonly normal.

Treatment is by a full diet, extra B vitamins and avoidance of cassava. In some patients the condition seems irreversible.

Toxic effects

Alcohol and the nervous system

Most doctors are only too familiar with some of the effects of alcohol, particularly acute self-poisoning. Alcohol is an inhibitor depressing cerebral function and this is well illustrated in *acute intoxication*. As the blood level rises patients will show a confusional state with slurring dysarthria and clumsiness (blood levels of 100 mg/100 ml), which will lead to a depressed conscious level and then coma (blood levels of 300–400 mg/100 ml). This can prove fatal. There will be accompanying peripheral vasodilation and a tachycardia.

Chronic habituation

Abstinence syndromes

Patients habituated to alcohol will develop acute withdrawal symptoms if their intake stops suddenly. This cessation may be precipitated by injuries, an acute infection or surgical emergency leading to admission to hospital with the loss of their regular supply.

The first stage, the *shakes*, consists of irritability, restlessness and tremors, with an exaggerated startle response. Patients appear overactive with a tachycardia, are inattentive and sometimes febrile. Such symptoms commonly start the morning after cessation and last some 24–48 h. They may be relieved by further alcohol.

The next stage may include confusion and sometimes auditory and even visual hallucinations accompanied by considerable amnesia. The *blackouts* of the alcoholic consist of gaps in their memory, often of hours' duration, for which they have no recall but may show some automatic behaviour. Mild hallucinatory states may be described as 'bad dreams' but when severe may merge with delirium tremens (DTs).

Withdrawal seizures or *rum fits* start 8–48 h after the cessation of drinking, most often in the second 12 hours. The seizures are usually generalized tonic-clonic attacks, either single or a cluster in series. About one-third of such patients may go on to develop DTs.

The final withdrawal stage is *delirium tremens* which has a mortality. A coexistent infective illness or injury may increase the risks of DTs. There are vivid hallucinations, often frightening (seeing animals), marked confusion, anxiety and overactivity, leading to insomnia. DTs are likely to start 2–4 days after stopping drinking, and usually last 2–3 days, but occasionally may last much longer.

Treatment of DTs involves adequate sedation, rehydration and usually parenteral feeding with glucose solutions and thiamine given intravenously. Any concomitant infection or injury should be treated appropriately. Sedatives used include chlordiazepoxide, diazepam or a chlormethiazole drip. Phenothiazines have also been used but may precipitate seizures. Paraldehyde may sometimes be useful to sedate and control seizures.

Alcoholic damage

Alcohol may produce damage to the nervous system by its direct toxic effects. These include:

1. Peripheral neuropathy (*see* p. 134).
2. Cerebellar degeneration with ataxia.
3. Cerebral degeneration with dementia.
4. Myopathy and cardiomyopathy (*see* p. 112).

Other rare disturbances are central pontine myelinolysis (self-descriptive) and Marchiafava-Bignami disease (primary degeneration of the corpus callosum). Alcohol may also precipitate the Wernicke-Korsakoff syndrome (*see* p. 407).

Cerebellar degeneration

Here there is loss of cerebellar neurones leading to atrophy. This may present with clumsiness, slurred speech and ataxia, difficult to differentiate from the effects of acute intoxication, although these signs persist even after 'drying out'.

Cerebral degeneration

Chronic alcoholics may have evidence of a diffuse global dementia, with cerebral atrophy indicated by ventricular dilatation and widened cortical sulci on CT brain scans. However, such radiological findings do not always correlate with a dementia. In older alcoholic patients (aged more than 45) with dementia, there is a much smaller chance of improvement with abstinence.

The management of alcoholic dependence is covered in the Chapter 21.

Toxic effects of drugs

Many drugs may affect the nervous system. Drug toxicity includes the unwanted side-effects of those used in therapy, e.g. a peripheral neuropathy (*see*

p. 134), or those due to self-poisoning, e.g. a depressed conscious level leading to coma as a result of overdosing with tranquillizers or antidepressants. These effects are dose-dependent. The effects of habituation to opiates and other powerful analgesics are described later.

Habituation to barbiturates and other sedatives, e.g. benzodiazepines, may produce slowing, apathy, slurred speech, clumsiness and ataxia like a drunk. These features may be linked with emotional lability and personal neglect. Such signs may fluctuate greatly. Withdrawal states from such habituation may lead to restlessness, tremors, insomnia, agitation and even withdrawal seizures.

Phenothiazines and butyrophenones, used particularly in the control of the chronic schizophrenic patient where depot injections of long-acting preparations are employed, may cause extrapyramidal symptoms and signs (*see* p. 207). These predominantly are rigidity, slowed movements and a shuffling gait. Such symptoms may be reduced by the use of anticholinergic drugs, e.g. benzhexol. Phenothiazines and butyrophenones may also provoke involuntary movements, dyskinesias, dystonic postures and even restlessness (akathisia). Many of these symptoms reverse with the cessation of therapy and the use of anticholinergics. However, a group of *tardive dyskinesias* may arise, particularly affecting the muscles of the face, mouth, neck and trunk, which prove very resistant to treatment.

A rare complication is the *malignant neuroleptic syndrome* which may occur in patients treated with a variety of psychotropic drugs, most commonly haloperidol and depot injections of fluphenazines. Here rigidity and akinesia develop acutely accompanied by a depressed conscious level, fever, and an autonomic disturbance with an unstable blood pressure. It is associated with massive rises in the serum creatine kinase level and often abnormal liver function tests. In many there has been a fatal outcome, although treatment with bromocriptine and dantrolene sodium has been effective.

Heavy metals

These may damage the nervous system. They may be used therapeutically, e.g. gold injections in rheumatoid arthritis which may cause a thrombocytopenia and bleeding resulting in peripheral and central nervous damage.

Lead poisoning

This is far less common now lead has been removed from paint. Previously, children were more often affected presenting with irritability, confusion, clumsiness, and seizures with a relatively acute encephalopathy causing a deteriorating conscious level and grossly swollen brain. There was associated anorexia, vomiting and abdominal pain. In adults a peripheral motor neuropathy (*see* p. 134), anaemia and abdominal pain are the common symptoms.

Plasma lead levels will be raised, usually greater than 50–70 μg/dl. There will be an associated anaemia with basophilic stippling of the red cells and 'lead lines' may be present on X-rays of long bones in children.

Treatment is by the use of chelating agents.

Other metals also are toxic: manganese poisoning may produce an encephalopathy and extrapyramidal signs; mercury poisoning produces tremors, confusion and cerebellar disturbance.

Organophosphates, used as insecticides and in certain mineral oils, have had recent prominence when they have been used as cooking oils. These have produced a severe peripheral neuropathy with axonal degeneration. Acute poisoning will produce headache, vomiting, pinpoint pupils, profuse sweating, and abdominal cramps (i.e. anticholinesterase effects) which may be relieved by atropine.

Physical insults

Anoxia

The brain requires a rich oxygen supply. If the circulation is arrested, within 2–3 min the normal function fails. Consciousness may be lost even more quickly and if there is asystole the patient will become unconscious within 15 s. Over the next 5 s there may be twitching, rigidity or clonic jerks which can be mistaken for an epileptic seizure. Within 4–5 min of circulatory arrest cyanosis appears, the pupils dilate and become unreactive, the plantar responses become extensor and the breathing may appear stertorous. Providing oxygenation and the circulation are restored to the brain within 5 min, recovery usually occurs: beyond this irreversible damage may follow.

A respiratory arrest or an obstructed airway may produce acute respiratory failure, but more often the picture is a combination of hypoxia and ischaemia with concomitant circulatory failure.

The cardiopulmonary mechanisms producing acute anoxia most often follow heart attacks with ventricular arrest or fibrillation, from acute respiratory failure, e.g. in drowning and asthmatic crises, from severe trauma or from anaesthetic mishaps. A fall in cerebral perfusion may occur during operations particularly on the open heart, or where there is massive blood loss leading to shock. More chronic hypoxia may arise from ventilatory muscle weakness, e.g. Guillain-Barré syndrome, certain myopathies, and obstructive airways disease or fibrosis.

With a slower onset, hypoxic symptoms include restlessness, agitation, tremors, headache, clumsiness and confusion. Blood gases will confirm a low PO_2 and high PCO_2 (*see* p. 43). Ventilatory muscle weakness in the adult may be accompanied by a low vital capacity (1.0 litres or less).

Patients who have sustained anoxic brain damage, but who have survived may show a variable picture with a depressed conscious level often with some preservation of the brainstem reflexes, but commonly twitching or myoclonic jerking of the limbs, sometimes repeated seizures, decerebrate or decorticate postures and extensor plantar responses. A variety of deficits may persist in less severely damaged survivors. These include cognitive deficits, extrapyramidal and pyramidal signs, visual field defects, involuntary movements, ataxia and action myoclonus.

Electric shock

This may cause death often from cardiac arrest. Commonly, at the site of contact, whether from an electric cable or lightning, there may be extensive burns with destruction of tissue. The nervous system may be damaged directly, e.g. shock to the head producing a hemiplegia, or the damage may involve the spinal cord or peripheral nerves. In survivors a delayed myelopathy has been reported with slowly progressive damage leading to muscular atrophy or even a transverse myelopathy.

Hypothermia

Prolonged exposure to cold can cause damage although, under experimental conditions, very low temperatures are necessary to produce conduction block in a peripheral nerve. Deep body temperatures of less than 35°C which may follow cold exposure, particularly in the elderly, in patients with hypothyroidism, or after drug overdoses, may lead to impaired cerebral function—confusion, stupor and coma. The respiration and metabolism are slowed generally. Treatment is by gradual re-warming but there is an appreciable mortality largely due to cardiac arrhythmias and metabolic upsets.

Heat stroke

This most often follows vigorous exercise in very hot temperatures. It may be aggravated by impaired sweating, e.g. in patients with Parkinson's disease on anticholinergic drugs, or in patients with tetanus and autonomic disturbance. As the body temperature rises (rectal temperature of more than 41°C) agitation and confusion may appear with later a deteriorating conscious level. Patients may convulse and status epilepticus may itself lead to hyperpyrexia with further brain damage. Death is usually due to circulatory collapse and renal failure. Survivors may be left with cognitive deficits, spastic weakness and a severe cerebellar deficit. The latter often persists.

Malignant hyperthermia

Malignant hyperpyrexia is described in Chapter 4.

Decompression sickness

This is also termed *the bends*. Too rapid decompression causes nitrogen under pressure in the blood to produce gas emboli and microinfarcts which provoke acute pain in the limbs and trunk. The thoracic spinal cord is most often affected producing a paraparesis or posterior column disturbance, but brain damage leading to a hemiplegia, vertigo or visual upset may arise. These deficits usually recover slowly. Recognition of decompression symptoms, with recompression and then much slower decompression, may help to prevent this.

Mountain sickness

Symptoms arise as low-level dwellers climb to considerable heights quickly and start some 24–48 h after the ascent. These include headache, nausea, vomiting, lethargy, dizziness, impaired balance, irritability and insomnia. In some instances acute pulmonary oedema may develop and even cerebral oedema with papilloedema, stupor and a flaccid paralysis. The acute symptoms can be relieved by breathing oxygen. Slow acclimatization to height allows a gradual increase in haemoglobin concentration, which will largely prevent such symptoms.

Endocrine disturbances

Hypopituitarism

Most often this follows the destruction of the anterior part of the pituitary gland by a chromophobe adenoma (*see* p. 303), or from haemorrhagic infarction, pituitary apoplexy.

The earliest symptoms are secondary amenorrhoea and infertility in young women, and impotence in men. Later symptoms of hypothyroidism appear and even those of Addison's disease. Some young women may show a combination of amenorrhoea and galactorrhoea. In time, the secondary sexual features of men may be affected with the loss of the need for regular shaving. These endocrine symptoms may be accompanied by headache and visual symptoms and signs (*see* p. 303). Patients often show a rather smooth skin, pallor and fine hair. The sudden loss of consciousness in a patient with a pituitary tumour may be due to apoplexy of the gland which may cause visual loss, oculomotor signs and often meningism.

The introduction of reliable measurements of the pituitary hormones by radioimmunoassay has shown that many of these tumours are prolactin secreting. A very small number secrete excessive growth hormone (GH) leading to features of acromegaly, or ACTH with the features of Cushing's disease. Hormone assays may also be helpful in the recognition and assessment of the patient with an 'empty sella'.

To assess underactive pituitary function, blood should be taken to measure diurnal cortisol levels, TSH, LH, FSH, GH and prolactin. If there is diagnostic doubt about the presence of panhypopituitarism, a triple bolus stress test is carried out using hypoglycaemia (produced by a small dose of insulin) to stimulate the gland. Thyrotrophin releasing hormone and FSH/LH releasing hormone are used in the same test to stimulate these aspects of gland function. Baseline values and then samples of blood are taken at 20, 30, 40, 90, 120 and 180 min to measure the glucose, GH, prolactin, cortisol, ACTH, TSH, FSH and LH levels. In hypopituitarism these values do not rise.

Posterior pituitary function (failure causes diabetes insipidus) can be assessed by fluid balance studies and a water deprivation test. Fluids are restricted for 8 h and in normal patients the urine will concentrate as the plasma concentrates. This will cause a rise in urine and plasma osmolalities. In diabetes insipidus the plasma osmolality will rise (often more than 300 mosm/kg) but the urine remains dilute with an osmolality of less than 270 mosm/kg.

Thyrotoxicosis

Most patients with hyperthyroidism have evidence of a mild *proximal myopathy* with muscle weakness (*see* p. 111); a few have bulbar muscle weakness. These symptoms may sometimes be the presentation.

Dysthyroid eye disease, particularly in middle-aged women, may cause symptoms (*see* p. 163). Thyrotoxic patients may show a proptosis (exophthalmos) with lid retraction and lag. Less often infiltration of the external ocular muscles (the medial and inferior recti) may lead to restricted abduction and upgaze with complaints of diplopia. The conjunctiva may appear oedematous and injected. The thickened and restricted eye muscles can be demonstrated by a forced duction test (showing the eyeball is restricted in its range of movements) or with a CT scan of the orbital contents.

Conventional thyroid function tests, T_4 and T_3 resin uptake may be raised but, if equivocal, a tri-iodothyronine (T_3) suppression test may be helpful. Treatment is by drugs such as carbimazole and propranolol, therapeutic doses of radioiodine or even surgery.

Myxoedema

This may produce a progressive decline in mental function with the appearance of dementia, confusion, delusions, hallucinations and even paranoid suspicions. There may be physical and mental slowing and sometimes a slow decline of conscious level ending in coma. A few patients may present with an acute psychotic state, myxoedema madness.

Hypothyroidism may also produce a cerebellar ataxia with increasing unsteadiness. Muscle aching and fatigue are common complaints. A carpal tunnel syndrome occurs frequently in myxoedema.

Many patients show coarse features, thinned hair, evidence of physical and mental slowing, deafness and ankle jerks with slowed relaxation. There is often a bradycardia and the appearance of swelling and odema. Many of the patients are older women. Hypothermia is a risk in winter.

Thyroid function tests will confirm low T_4 and T_3 values with a very elevated TSH. Treatment is with thyroxine, starting with a small dose.

Adrenal disturbances

Cushings's syndrome

Here, excess cortisol is produced most commonly from a pituitary microadenoma (with excess ACTH), from an adrenal adenoma or hyperplasia, or from ectopic ACTH production due to a malignant tumour. Another common mechanism is iatrogenic from the excess administration of steroids.

Symptoms and signs include a proximal myopathy, obesity of the trunk (with a buffalo hump), thin skin, striae, easy bruising and oedema. About one-half of the patients are hypertensive and one-third diabetic. Osteoporosis is common and this may lead to vertebral collapse and pain. Depression may also occur.

The diagnosis is confirmed by elevated urinary cortisol levels, and loss of the usual diurnal rhythm in plasma cortisol levels; the normal fall (less than 250–300 nmol/litre) at night is not present.

Treatment is by removal of the excess steroids or their source.

Addison's disease

Originally tuberculous destruction of the adrenal glands was the most common cause but now this appears to arise more from an autoimmune self-destruction, or occasionally from carcinoma or metastases.

The symptoms are commonly insidious with weight loss, weakness and malaise. Addisonian crises may be precipitated by infections or surgery. Sometimes these may be accompanied by abdominal pain, vomiting and/or diarrhoea. Patients appear ill, hypotensive (this may be postural), feeble and often show skin pigmentation in scars, skin creases or inside the mouth.

There is usually hyponatraemia with an elevated blood urea and potassium. The plasma cortisol may be low or normal but the best confirmatory test is to measure the cortisol level 45 min after the intramuscular injection of 250 μg of tetracosatrin. In normal patients a rise above 600 nmol/litre occurs.

Acute treatment involves rehydration with saline, glucose and the intravenous injection of cortisol hemisuccinate 100 mg stat and then 200 mg/24 h. Replacement steroid therapy with cortisol 30 mg daily will be necessary and this may need to be increased if the patient is ill.

Hypoglycaemia

This most often occurs in insulin treated diabetics, less commonly from the use of oral hypoglycaemic drugs, and very rarely from insulin-secreting tumours (insulinomas). It is important that it is not missed as prolonged uncorrected hypoglycaemia will produce irreversible brain damage.

Symptoms appear as the plasma glucose falls below 2.5 mmol/litre and this fall will stimulate the adrenals so that pallor, sweating, tremor, tachycardia, anxiety and a light-headed feeling may apear – symptoms often recognized by diabetics so they can heed this warning and take sugar. The low plasma glucose affects the brain causing confusion, disordered behaviour (occasionally aggressive), slurred speech and unsteadiness. These symptoms may be mistaken for alcoholic intoxication. Continuing hypoglycaemia will then cause focal neurological signs, a hemiplegia, epileptic seizures, a deteriorating conscious level and coma.

If there is clinical suspicion, take blood for a glucose estimation and immediately inject 20–30 ml of 50 per cent glucose intravenously. The therapeutic response should be immediate unless hypoglycaemia has been prolonged or the diagnosis is incorrect. Plasma glucose levels less than 2.0 mmol/litre confirm the diagnosis. An insulinoma may be difficult to diagnose but a prolonged fast with estimation of glucose, insulin and plasma-C peptide levels will usually give the answer.

Hyperglycaemia

This may cause a deteriorating conscious level leading to coma from:

1. Diabetic ketoacidosis.
2. Hyperosmolar non-ketotic hyperglycaemia.

Diabetic ketoacidosis is the common cause of diabetic hyperglycaemic coma and usually is precipitated by an acute infection, poor diabetic control or both. Often the patient becomes ill over a few days with complaints of headache, weakness, vomiting and abdominal pain. There is dehydration with acidotic breathing and ketones may be present on the breath. Gradually there is increasing drowsiness accompanied by confusion which leads to coma. Often the blood pressure is low and the pulse rapid.

Hyperosmolar coma arises in elderly diabetics who become haemoconcentrated with a high plasma osmolality, high blood glucose but no ketosis. Some patients present in shock with features of dehydration.

Investigation

Ketotic patients show urinary glycosuria and ketonuria. The blood glucose is usually very high, the pH low with acidosis and a low bicarbonate, the potassium high and the sodium normal. The urea may be raised if there is considerable dehydration.

Treatment is an emergency with intravenous rehydration with saline, intravenous insulin and correction of acidosis. The electrolytes will need to be monitored regularly to maintain values, particularly potassium, within the normal range. The insulin dose will need to be titrated against the glucose value.

Hepatic failure

Liver failure may develop acutely, e.g. from hepatitis, or after self-poisoning with paracetamol, or more chronically leading to a portosystemic encephalopathy (where substances not properly detoxified by the failing liver may be released into the circulation to disturb brain function). The latter is found most often in the cirrhotic patient who may decompensate acutely in response to an infection, a gastric haemorrhage (often from oesophageal varices), to certain drugs, potassium loss or to protein excess. This decompensation is often episodic so patients may show a fluctuating conscious level, irrational behaviour, delusions, hallucinations and confusion. These may lead to a deteriorating conscious level with stupor and coma. Initially there may be prominent muscle twitching, a flapping tremor of the outstretched hands, and epileptic seizures may occur. Focal or bilateral pyramidal signs, rigidity, primitive reflexes and extensor plantar responses may appear. In coma the pupils may dilate. There may be associated stigmata from the liver disease with a fetor hepaticus, hepatic enlargement, spider naevi, jaundice, ascites, and oedema of the feet.

Many patients show an elevated blood ammonia; normally this is less than 50 mmol/litre but with hepatic failure it may rise well above 100 mmol/litre; in addition, there are abnormal liver function tests with particularly elevated enzyme levels; and a prolonged prothrombin time (which may lead to bruising and haemorrhagic complications). The CSF may be normal or show a slight protein rise. The EEG may show paroxysmal slow wave activity mirroring the depressed conscious level: sometimes triphasic delta waves appear in stuporose patients.

Treatment involves the elimination of any precipitating cause, the maintenance of a correct fluid balance with restriction of protein and its replacement by intravenous glucose. Coagulation defects will need correction. Nitrogenous products in the bowel and responsible organisms may be treated with neomycin. In selected patients haemodialysis may be life-saving.

Reye's syndrome

This is a rare form of encephalopathy arising in children aged 5–15, characterized by acute brain swelling with fatty infiltration of the liver. It appears often to be triggered by an acute viral infection, and in some instances perhaps by treatment with salicylates. The onset is acute with preceding symptoms of an upper respiratory tract infection, then profuse vomiting and a deteriorating conscious level ending in coma, seizures, rigidity and signs of cerebral damage.

There may be a low blood and CSF glucose, abnormal liver enzymes, a prolonged prothrombin time and a raised blood ammonia. The EEG shows diffuse slow activity.

Many children die but the prompt recognition with treatment to reduce the raised intracranial pressure, intravenous glucose and correction of any metabolic disturbance, allows some survivors, although a few may show signs of residual damage.

Renal failure

As the blood urea rises patients will become increasingly confused and drowsy, stuporose and eventually comatose. Associated with the depressed conscious level there may be hallucinations, twitching, tremors, asterixis, restlessness, tetany, myoclonic jerking and even tonic-clonic seizures. Very commonly these symptoms fluctuate. Patients with a depressed conscious level may show acidotic breathing which later may wax and wane (Cheyne-Stokes). There are often associated features with initial complaints of anorexia, nausea, vomiting, a haemorrhagic state and, in acute renal failure, oliguria.

Electrolyte disorders are common with hyperkalaemia, hyponatraemia and a rising blood urea and creatinine.

Treatment depends on the cause, but dialysis relieves the uraemia, and allows reversal of many of the neurological symptoms. Convulsions are usually controlled with low doses of anticonvulsants.

Two clinical states are recognized in dialysis patients.

Dialysis dementia

This occurs in patients on long-term dialysis and may be associated with mental clouding, myoclonus, tonic-clonic seizures and speech disturbance. It is accompanied by a diffuse EEG disturbance. It has been suggested that aluminium toxicity from the dialysate may be responsible.

The dysequilibrium syndrome

This also affects patients on dialysis who complain of headache, nausea, agitation, irritability and even seizures. The symptoms often come on within a short time of starting dialysis and it has been suggested that they may arise from too rapid dialysis. They usually last some hours.

Patients with uraemia may develop a peripheral neuropathy (*see* p. 135). After renal transplantation patients on immunosuppressive treatment are more prone to unusual infections e.g. cryptococci, listeriosis (*see* p. 337).

Electrolyte disturbances

Hyponatraemia

This may arise from water 'intoxication' without a sodium deficit, but there may also be loss of sodium from the gut (diarrhoea and vomiting) or from renal disease. Most water intoxication occurs in sick patients who are being fed by nasogastric tube or intravenously. Hyponatraemia may also be found with inappropriate secretion of antidiuretic hormone (ADH).

With a falling plasma sodium patients complain of anorexia and headache, and may become apathetic, drowsy and confused. Muscle cramps, twitching and seizures may appear. Patients may pass into coma. Later oedema of the limbs and even the face may appear.

A plasma sodium of less than 120 mmol/litre usually causes some symptoms and values of less than 110 mmol/litre may lead to fits and a significant decline in conscious level. It is important to measure carefully the patient's fluid input and output, the urine and plasma electrolytes and osmolalities.

Causes of inappropriate ADH secretion include:

1. Malignant disease, particularly carcinoma of the lung and lymphomas.
2. Nervous system disorders:
   trauma, head injuries, subarachnoid haemorrhage
   meningitis, tuberculous meningitis, strokes
   polyneuritis, e.g. Guillain-Barré, porphyria.
3. Infections, pneumonia.
4. Drugs, e.g. carbamazepine, chlorpropamide, cyclophosphamide.

In patients with inappropriate secretion of ADH there will be a continuing excretion of a concentrated urine despite a hypotonic plasma with falling osmolality (often less than 270 mosm/kg) so the urine osmolality will be greater than that of the plasma.

Recognition of the mechanism is important. Correction of dilutional fluid overload is necessary in water intoxication. In excess ADH states fluid will need to be restricted to 500–1000 ml/day. Treatment of the cause is also important, e.g. meningitis.

Hypokalaemia

A low serum potassium, less than 3 mmol/litre may be associated with complaints of fatigue and muscle weakness. With values between 2.0 and 2.5 mmol/litre there may be flaccid paralysis with depressed or absent reflexes. There may be associated bowel involvement leading to an ileus. Hypokalaemia may precipitate cardiac arrhythmias. Sometimes there may be thirst and polyuria.

Certain medical conditions causing hypokalaemia may present with muscle weakness; these include aldosteronism (Conn's syndrome), Cushing's disease, and some forms of periodic paralysis (*see* p. 109). Other causes of potassium loss include diuretics, renal causes, and gastrointestinal upsets (diarrhoea and purgative abuse, pyloric stenosis and vomiting). The agents used to reduce intracranial pressure such as mannitol or urea by a diuresis may lead to potassium loss.

Treatment involves correction of the cause and potassium supplements.

Calcium metabolism

Hypocalcaemia

This will produce neuromuscular irritability with a calcium level of less than 2.0 mmol/litre, accompanied by complaints of tingling in the extremities and around the mouth, twitching, carpopedal spasm, tetany and even epileptic seizures. In many patients there may be complaints of lethargy: in a few psychotic features and even stupor. Patients may show skin changes, a dry coarse skin with brittle nails, cataracts, and even papilloedema. Tapping over the facial nerve will provoke twitching of the facial muscles (Chvostek's sign) and inflation of a pneumatic cuff around the arm above arterial blood pressure may produce a *main d'accoucheur* from carpal spasm (Trousseau's sign).

The serum calcium will be low and the ECG may show a prolonged QT interval.

Hypocalcaemia is most often found following surgery to the neck with the removal of the parathyroid glands (often during thyroid surgery), in severe malabsorption, renal failure, with prolonged use of certain anticonvulsants, and even from primary failure of the parathyroids.

Treatment is usually with calcium and vitamin D supplements. In the acute situation 20–30 ml of 10 per cent calcium gluconate injected intravenously over 10 min is effective.

Hypercalcaemia

This presents with 'stones, bones and abdominal groans', from renal stones (50 per cent), bone pain and abdominal pain. In about one-third of patients hypercalcaemia may be found in an asymptomatic subject.

Hypercalcaemia may cause anorexia, nausea and vomiting, constipation, polyuria and thirst. Fatigue, a proximal myopathy, confusion and behaviour disorders may herald neurological upsets. In a few patients there may be collapse with coma. Patients sometimes show a conjunctivitis from corneal calcification.

The serum calcium will be high, greater than 3 mmol/litre, but it should be remembered that venous sampling below an inflated tourniquet may give an erroneously high calcium value.

Hypercalcaemia is most often found in primary hyperparathyroidism (where high levels of parathyroid hormone will be detected), in patients with widespread bony metastases, sarcoidosis or vitamin D intoxication.

Treatment depends on the cause. In an emergency high serum calcium levels can be lowered by a combination of a diuresis with frusemide, and either calcitonin intravenously (100–200 units) or mithramycin (25 μg/kg).

Behçet's disease

This is a rare multisystem disorder of unknown aetiology which classically leads to recurrent orogenital ulceration often associated with ocular lesions, most commonly a uveitis or iridocyclitis, but which may include an optic neuritis, retinal vasculitis, hypopyon and loss of vision. Skin lesions include a tendency to furunculosis and erythema nodosum, and there is often a polyarthritis. Deep vein thromboses and superficial thrombophlebitis are common.

In about one-third the nervous system may be involved leading possibly to a meningoencephalitis, cranial nerve palsies, a hemiplegia, cerebral sinus thrombosis and even dementia. Pathologically there is perivascular and meningeal infiltration with lymphocytes, plasma cells and macrophages with multiple foci of softening and necrosis in the white and grey matter often found in relation to blood vessels.

The CSF may show a lymphocytic pleocytosis in acute relapses but may be normal in quiescent disease. The erythrocyte sedimentation rate (ESR) is usually elevated and there may be a leucocytosis. Other treatable causes of meningitis should always be excluded, e.g. tuberculous meningitis, fungal infections.

There is no specific therapy although steroids and immunosuppressives appear helpful in acute relapses. CNS involvement implies a bad prognosis.

Sarcoidosis

This is another multisystem inflammatory disease of unknown aetiology leading in many instances to granuloma formation. It has similarities to tuberculosis although no infective agent has been identified. Over 85 per cent of cases show lung changes with hilar gland enlargement and often diffuse lung infiltration. Other common features are skin involvement with erythema nodosum or sarcoid infiltration, and arthropathy. Ocular changes with a uveitis arise in 15–25 per cent. Liver biopsy will be positive in 70 per cent and about 30 per cent may show palpable enlarged lymph glands, and 15–25 per cent an enlarged spleen.

Histologically there are non-caseating granulomas containing epithelioid cells and multinucleate giant cells surrounded by lymphocytes. In time hyaline fibrosis may develop.

The nervous system may be involved in 5–10 per cent. Most commonly there may be multiple cranial nerve damage, often a bilateral facial palsy, or a peripheral neuropathy, symmetrical or a mononeuritis multiplex. Sarcoid granulomas may also present like mass lesions in the brain, or a sarcoid angiopathy may produce a stroke-like picture. Occasionally, hypothalamic lesions may present with drowsiness and diabetes insipidus. Meningitic involvement may lead to the development of an obstructive hydrocephalus.

The CSF may show a mild pleocytosis, a mild to moderate lymphocytic rise, a low sugar and an elevated protein: cultures being sterile. CT scans may show granulomatous masses. Biopsy of an affected lymph gland, liver, muscle, skin lesion, ocular lesion or even a central nervous system mass may give the diagnosis. Most patients show an abnormal chest X-ray with hilar gland enlargement. About two-thirds have a negative tuberculin skin test. A Kveim test (intradermal Kveim antigen injection followed by biopsy) is positive in 80–90 per cent of patients with active disease. Serum angiotensin converting enzyme (SACE) levels may be elevated with active disease and can be used to monitor activity. In up to 20 per cent there may be hypercalcaemia.

Treatment is often symptomatic but steroids may be helpful in patients with nervous system involvement. Prednisolone 20–40 mg daily for 2 weeks and then reduced to a maintenance dose for 3–6 months is one regimen that has been used.

21

Psychiatric disorders

While it is clear that neurology and psychiatry should be considered in an integrated way, the historical development and clinical attitudes associated with each speciality have tended to produce separation. Thus, the enormous influence of Freud from the beginning of this century tended to unify psychiatry and separate the subject from medicine in general because of the dominating view that psychiatric disturbances derive exclusively from internal emotional conflicts and social stresses. This is in total contrast to the causes of neurological abnormalities which involve the concept of 'physical diseases', thus following the medical model.

However, psychiatry began to revert to being a medical speciality again with the remarkable chance discoveries in the 1950s of medication having completely new psychotropic properties. Chlorpromazine was a new compound with antipsychotic activity, an effect not known before. Only a few years later both the tricyclic compounds (the first was imipramine) and the monoamine oxidase inhibitors (the first was iproniazid which is no longer available) were found to have antidepressant actions, i.e. they effectively relieved some cases of depression without stimulation. Up to this time the amphetamines, which produce non-specific stimulation, were sometimes used as an unsatisfactory treatment for depression. Antidepressant activity, again, was entirely new. A third group of novel drugs was also introduced, the benzodiazepines. These had antianxiety properties with less sedation than the barbiturates and they seem to be virtually without danger in overdose. So the benzodiazepines came to replace the barbiturates completely.

These new compounds were then used in animal experiments to investigate their properties. As a result, we now know that all drugs which are antipsychotic block dopamine receptors, while all drugs which are antidepressant increase the availability of some monoamine neurotransmitters, of which noradrenaline and 5-hydroxytryptamine (5HT) are probably the most important. From these findings it can be deduced that both schizophrenia and mania, which both respond to antipsychotic medication, involve dopamine overactivity, while certain types of depression are associated with a reduction in neurotransmitter activity. Integration with neurology becomes apparent with the observation that an antipsychotic drug used to block dopamine as a treatment for schizophrenia also produces dopamine antagonism in the basal ganglia, causing parkinsonism as a side-effect.

Nonetheless, parkinsonism requires a different diagnostic approach on the part of the clinician when compared with diagnosing schizophrenia, and herein lies the particular problems of dealing with neuropsychiatric presentations. Neurological abnormalities are detected, often with considerable precision, by the use of objective signs. Psychiatric conditions are diagnosed almost exclusively by subjective means (e.g. symptoms such as thought disorder, delusions, flattened emotions) and the physician may find it difficult to change from one diagnostic approach to the other, although they really need to be used together.

Furthermore, the brain can be affected by a very wide range of influences which tend to produce relatively few cerebral presentations. Thus, delirium may result from infections, trauma, tumours, drugs, poisons and disorders of various systems such as cardiac, renal and hepatic (*see* Table 21.3). Even this list is not complete. So flexibility and diligence are required in taking the history and for the adequate investigation of such cases.

Finally, psychiatry introduces the extremely important dimension of emotion, which is of considerable relevance to all the ills of man, no matter how apparently organic they may be. Ignoring this aspect can cause major problems in understanding and managing a case. Depression and anxiety tend to increase the experience of pain and reduce tolerance of disabilities of purely physical origin. Some psychiatric states result in the elaboration and fabrication of physical symptoms and sometimes physical symptoms derive directly from emotional disorders.

Psychiatric diagnosis

A scheme which does not claim to be comprehensive, is given in Table 21.1 in order to demonstrate some principles.

Table 21.1   Types of psychiatric disorders

Personality disorders	Neuroses	Psychoses
Immature	Anxiety states	Schizophrenia
Inadequate	Depressive neurosis	Organic
Antisocial (psychopathic)	Obsessional neurosis	Affective disorders (manic-
Obsessional	Hysteria	depressive disease)
Hysterical (histrionic)		

Personality

The personality is the sum of all those various characteristics that make an individual unique. Included are the individual's personal way of behaving, reacting, relating and feeling, to name some aspects. To what extent the personality is disordered is more relative than absolute and depends upon the presence of a greater or lesser degree of tension or incongruity between the individual and his social environment. For example, a highly inadequate individual may enjoy a life of emotional stability nonetheless because of an understanding, protective, capable spouse. The precise, rigid, punctual, controlled obsessional person may be happy working in a bank, but could be badly misplaced as an actor, and there may be destabilizing social stresses in these circumstances: professional failure being one possibility. In addition, the personality type may modify the presentation of complaints. The patient with hypochondriacal personality characteristics may elaborate complaints of a true organic disorder so that it is obscured. The hysterical patient may experience complaints in an exaggerated way and over-respond to them emotionally. The immature person may become helpless, dependent and anxious when physically ill. Personality disorders make the individual vulnerable to neuroses if there are sufficient stresses, either internal or in the environment or both. Neuroses often produce social incapacity and they are likely to produce symptoms that frequently require medical investigations.

Anxiety states

Anxiety can be a normal experience and it may be an adaptive response to environmental threats (preparation for fight or flight). However, there are those who frequently respond with distressing anxiety, which does not easily settle down, whenever there are problems, even quite minor ones. The symptoms of anxiety are well recognized and include palpitations, tremor, dyspnoea, urinary frequency, diarrhoea, sleep and appetite disturbances. Sometimes only one anxiety symptom dominates the clinical picture so that urinary frequency, say, is the main complaint and it is thus a physical symptom caused by a neurosis, although this may need to be established by appropriate investigations.

Phobic anxiety is a particular form of anxiety. The anxiety experienced, which is often almost intolerable, is specifically associated with a situation or object not normally producing such an extreme response. Even with normal individuals, with whom the anxiety is usually unpleasant but not severe, phobic anxiety is frequently associated with snakes, lifts or heights. Phobic anxiety states quite often follow frightening car accidents even when there has been no physical injury and despite a stable personality. The individual may thereafter suffer intense and intolerable anxiety on even trying to enter a car and so driving is avoided and considerable social inconvenience may be caused. It needs to be emphasized that this is a real and distressing condition which may have medicolegal significance in the case of accidents. It often settles in time but may need skilled behaviour therapy. If the symptom does not improve spontaneously specialized help should be sought without too much delay because treatment becomes more difficult the longer the symptom is present. This condition should not be confused with compensation neurosis, when there may be enhancement or prolongation of symptoms specifically associated with the anticipation of financial advantages (*see* below).

Depressive neurosis

The relationship between depressive neurosis (often called reactive depression) and endogenous depression, which is one of the affective disorders, seems to be endlessly controversial (Kendall, 1976). It is true that research does not support a clear-cut differentiation between these two forms of depression but a separation seems to be clinically useful because the treatment is different. The neurotic illness occurs mainly in young adults, it is always reactive to stresses and it does not usually respond to antidepressant medication. The endogenous type has highly characteristic symptoms, it is often inherited, the onset is in the second half of life, it is sometimes associated with stresses and usually responds well to antidepressant medication. What seems certain is that the presence or absence of a precipitating stress (the depression being reactive to this) is not a reliable differentiating feature. It is mainly the symptoms which clearly identify endo-genous depression and the age of the patient is likely to be important.

Of course, as with anxiety, depression can be an entirely normal experience. It is then perhaps better given a separate name, such as 'grief'. Grief is not only a natural emotion, it seems to be a necessary experience to facilitate the indi-vidual's adaptation to the causal event. This usually involves loss that threatens the individual; it may be the break up of a close relationship or loss of self-esteem on failing an examination or with sudden unemployment. The difference between grief and clinical depression cannot be rigidly defined. It is to do with the extent to which the individual is incapacitated by, and suffers from the depression that makes the condition a neurosis and not a normal reaction, e.g. everyone becomes depressed to some extent at the death of a parent. In these circumstances the bereaved person may need a week or two off work. But if a bereavement causes someone to be incapable of work for a period of months, then the response is to be regarded as maladaptive and this then constitutes a neurotic reaction requiring treatment.

The symptoms of neurotic depression are not very specific. There is depressed mood and there may well be suicidal ideas, sometimes potentially dangerous in intensity. But the depression tends to vary so the patient becomes more cheerful in congenial company. Probably for similar reasons the indiv-idual feels worse in the evenings when he may be alone in the absence of the act-ivities of the day which take his mind off the depressing event. Appetite is impaired but there is usually no weight loss and there may be difficulty in getting off to sleep. There are never depressive delusions. These symptoms should be compared to those of endogenous depression (*see* Table 21.2).

Obsessional neuroses

It should be made clear that the observation, 'he is obsessed with his health', does not describe an obsessional condition. In this case the person is pre-occupied with his health and therefore may be hypochondriacal. Obsessional symptoms involve ruminations (repetitive thoughts) and compulsions (repeti-tive actions). The characteristic quality is that the symptoms are recognized by the patient as intrusive, unwanted and alien to him. Hence the patient attempts to resist the ideas but the resistance causes increasing anxiety until the obsessional activity is carried out. Anxiety then reduces until the idea occurs again. Thus the patient may feel very strongly that there is no need to keep counting in sevens in his head, or to wash his hands for long periods of time, and he tries not to do so, but the anxiety soon becomes intolerable as a result so he gives in to obtain relief. In this way the repetitious behaviour is maintained.

Obsessional symptoms include persistently repetitive counting, checking, touching, cleaning and washing, to list the most common. Obsessional illnesses may be primary neuroses which fluctuate over the years depending on the level of stress under which the patient is living. The symptoms worsen as the individual goes through periods of increased anxiety and improve when the person is feeling more calm and secure. However, obsessional symptoms, especially when they appear suddenly for the first time in the second half of life can be associated with an endogenous depression and the obsessional symptoms will then be likely to respond well to antidepressants or electroconvulsive therapy (ECT) as does the underlying affective disorder. Obsessional symptoms often appear after head injuries when the patient's unavoidable preoccupation with them may cause much distress and is liable to impede rehabilitation.

Obsessional symptoms can be very difficult, and sometimes impossible, to treat adequately. They can cause more incapacity than most psychiatric illnesses and some patients spend their whole waking-life driven by the rituals or continuously preoccupied by the ruminations which they are totally unable to control. One feels that neurosciences and psychiatry should meet here under concepts such as reverberating circuits and conditioned behaviour, especially with the production of obsessional symptoms by brain damage, but this so far remains an association only to be hoped for because so little is known about the development of obsessional symptoms, other than their association with raised anxiety levels and with depressive illnesses.

Hysteria

However, this *is* an area where neurosciences and psychiatry meet, and frequently overlap. It might not have been expected that a psychiatrist (Slater, 1965) once advocated the abolition of this diagnosis while a neurologist (Walsh, 1965) reinstated it. It should be noted that there is often confusion between the hysterical personality and hysterical behaviour, on the one hand, and hysteria as a neurosis on the other. The hysterical personality is associated with hysterical behaviour and both are characterized by flamboyance, exhibitionism, high drama, suggestibility, attention seeking and exaggeration. An audience is essential. It seems accepted that those with hysterical personalities are especially prone to hysteria as a neurosis but hysteria may well occur in those with other types of personality.

It should also be made clear that 'hysterical' means more than a symptom that is psychological and not organic in origin. Hysteria involves a state of dissociation or conversion, unconsciously determined for emotional gain. This definition tends to be met with suspicion, especially by those who are not psychiatrists, who wonder whether these symptoms can ever be really unconsciously determined when the motivation may be so selfish. But the gain is usually not a simple desire to manipulate others or obtain financial reward, it is often an attempt to reduce intolerable anxiety – controlling anxiety is a frequent theme among the neuroses in general.

Conversion is a concept whereby anxiety is 'converted' to a physical symptom and the anxiety is relieved in the process. Thus, if an individual finds life alone to be intolerable, perhaps because of a crushing bereavement, his solitary situation may produce an anxiety state or there may be a depressive neurosis, or both. But if so predisposed, there may develop hysterical symptoms mimicking physical ones, e.g. there may be paralysis of a limb. This is likely to require admission to hospital, giving the patient, to an extent, security and companions. If this mental manoeuvre succeeds in reducing anxiety as a result of the admission, there may follow the characteristic mood of hysteria which is called 'la belle indifférence,' a state of incongruous emotional calm in the presence of an apparently major physical abnormality. Of course neurotic solutions to problems, as in this example, are always maladaptive. The protective effect is often incomplete and it does not last. The price paid for the increased security resulting from the paralysed limb is an inability to function which is going to be unacceptable to the patient in the longer term. Conversion symptoms can be motor, such as disturbance of gait, loss of speech, muscle weakness or paralysis and abnormal movements. Sensory symptoms include pain, anaesthesias, blindness and deafness.

Hysterical dissociation involves altered awareness which may diminish or remove the patient's appreciation of anxiety-producing situations, hence protecting him. Characteristic is the hysterical fugue ('flight'). The patient loses his awareness of a major stress occurring at home and often randomly travels away from the disturbance. Typically, these patients get on any train that comes along and when they arrive at the terminus they complain that they do not know who they are or where they are. Nonetheless, some sort of selective awareness has allowed them to travel without difficulty. Other examples of dissociation include amnesias, twilight states, stupor and pseudo-psychosis.

Hysterical symptoms may mimic almost any medical condition and the diagnosis is even more difficult when there is an 'hysterical overlay'. In these cases there is a psychological use made of a real physical abnormality so that the discomfort may be enhanced and the disability exaggerated for emotional advantage. The presence of an emotional advantage is essential for hysteria. However, it is likely that the diagnosis of hysterical overlay is excessively used. Sometimes all that is meant is a physical condition complicated by psychiatric symptoms, an altogether different concept. For example, the presence of anxiety will increase the experience of pain of entirely physical origin.

While hysteria is becoming less common, increasing popular knowledge of medicine means that the presentations are now likely to be more sophisticated. Hysterical anaesthesias and paralyses are now rare in practice but many physicians, rather than psychiatrists, are likely to encounter chest and low back pain ('heart trouble' and 'slipped discs' are common) with hysterical causes.

With hysteria it is essential that the diagnosis is made on positive psychiatric grounds and not simply because of the absence of a physical cause. Even then, establishing this psychiatric diagnosis should not thereby imply that further physical investigations need never be undertaken. Slater's (1965) attempt to dispense with the diagnosis was because of the frequency with which significant physical illnesses subsequently occurred among those initially diagnosed as hysterical.

Hysteria and epilepsy

We would not now accept the close association between epilepsy and hysteria which was Charcot's concept of hystero-epilepsy. But, in contemporary context, the term usefully identifies a common problem which can be difficult to manage. Epilepsy, especially if poorly controlled for long periods, is often associated with personality abnormalities and much social disability. Hence these patients are frequently under considerable stress and it is not difficult to understand how anxiety can be 'converted' into an hysterical fit. That is, increasing fits demonstrate the presence of illness which elicits care and sympathy from others, and admission to hospital may be arranged so that an isolated, rejected epileptic person is given society's protection by becoming an inpatient. Those who experience true epileptic fits may well produce hysterical fits that are difficult to differentiate from those which are physically determined (Trimble, 1983).

Again, there may be true epileptic fits with an 'hysterical overlay'. The patient's over-response to the fit will perhaps induce desired behaviour in friends and helpers. So it is frequently not clear which fits are of entirely epileptic origin, which epileptic fits have psychogenic associations or causes, and which fits are entirely hysterical. Clearly, rigid differentiation may not be valid anyway, although the doctor will want to limit and calculate his caring attitudes to the hysterical fit while helping in every way with an epileptic fit.

By way of differentiation, the hysterical fit may fail to show the features of the epileptic fit and its form may, atypically for epilepsy, vary from time to time. A tonic-clonic phase will not occur and cyanosis or pallor are unlikely. Incontinence, tongue-biting and self-injury of any severity will not occur with hysterical fits which are almost exclusively produced in the presence of witnesses and there will be no changes in the reflexes immediately afterwards. However, if a fit follows an episode of acute distress, this is no indication that it is necessarily hysterical. True epileptic fits can have psychogenic trigger factors. Management will aim to control epilepsy by medication while attempting to introduce better self-understanding in those with hysterical fits and perhaps minimize unrealistic attempts at emotional gains. In practice, the differential diagnosis may be difficult and it may be that medication has to be reviewed and personal help arranged as seems appropriate for the individual case without an accurate diagnostic assessment being possible. Skilled psychiatric help is likely to be needed when there are major psychiatric aspects present.

Compensation neurosis and the post-concussion syndrome

Compensation neurosis tends to become confusingly entangled with 'post-traumatic neurosis' and the 'post-concussion syndrome'. First, it seems accepted that following quite minor head injuries characteristic symptoms are found which include headache, dizziness, irritability, depression, emotional instability, poor concentration, impaired memory, sleep difficulties and fatigue. Some authors have regarded this presentation as a neurotic reaction to injury or the fright of the accident. Others have considered that the symptoms arise from subtle brain damage which is very difficult to detect. This then, describes 'post-concussion' or 'post-traumatic' neurosis, if this is indeed a neurosis.

In some cases, the complaints persist for long periods when this would not be expected from the nature of the injury. Many of these are inevitably associated with legal action for compensation, which itself motivates towards persisting and augmented symptoms. However, compensation neurosis requires a wider view. After accidents, considerable social pressures may build up urging the victim towards compensation, and this does not necessarily involve neurotic motivation. Family doctors may continue to issue sickness certificates for unnecessary periods, often to avoid being autocractic about a patient's presumed suffering, and this tolerance confirms to the patient that he has a significant problem even if he has not. Unions, lawyers and colleagues encourage legal action, usually for different reasons. The patient may well feel angry about someone's negligence, real or supposed, and he wants retribution accordingly. So there are many factors contributing to compensation neurosis and it can be understood that the condition is not well-named. It is only in so far as the symptoms are exaggerated, become unexpectedly prolonged and the disabilities are excessive, because of an unconscious motivation for reward, that this is a form of hysteria.

It is often thought that there is a difficult clinical differentiation between those deliberately accentuating symptoms, which would involve malingering, on the one hand, and supposed unconscious accentuation produced by hysteria, on the other hand. These two aspects of a complex interaction of factors are probably best considered as a continuum rather than two separate concepts and there are clinicians who would consider that an individual who maintains symptoms deliberately and consistently for a number of years up to a Court hearing has a very abnormal personality anyway. It is usually assumed that the complaints resolve when compensation is agreed but this is not always so. Sometimes there is an angry need by the injured person for the other party to suffer in some way as the patient has suffered because of the accident, and compensation may not serve this end because it will probably be paid by an insurance company. However, it is generally agreed that psychiatric treatment will not succeed, and the patient may well not cooperate with it, while the legal case is pending. When the case has been decided, whatever the patient's motivation, he must come to adjust to a situation that is finalized, and he may need help with this (Steadman and Graham, 1970).

Treatment of the neuroses

This is best carried out by a psychiatric team. Current practice is that this includes a nurse, psychologist, social worker and occupational therapist, as well as doctors. It allows for a diversity of professions using a wide range of therapy, particularly required by neuroses and personality disorders. These conditions are best treated in day hospitals, rather than by admission, because this maintains the patients' social contacts and avoids undue dependence on the supportive therapeutic environment.

The social worker will facilitate contact with the family and may be involved in therapy in a family setting. This member of the team may also help to relieve social problems by assisting with financial management, housing and so on. As well as psychotherapy, the psychologist can offer behavioural techniques including anxiety management with the teaching of effective relaxation. Phobias and obsessional states are also dealt with by behavioural means, including response prevention (encouraging the patient to resist the obsessional demands by maintaining continuous preoccupation with other activities), and desensitization (the patient slowly coming closer to the phobic situation as anxiety subsides). For example, with phobias of cars after accidents, the patient is encouraged to get used to only sitting in a stationary car at first. Then to drive a distance of yards a few times, and then proceeding in this way gradually.

Repeated avoidance of phobic situations tends to increase the conditioned anxiety and the same will happen with an abrupt reintroduction to the phobia. However, 'flooding' has been used and can be successful, but it can be extremely disturbing. This involves the spider-phobic patient being kept isolated in a room with a spider. The anxiety rises rapidly but it often gets to a maximum and then it spontaneously subsides, leaving the patient tolerant of spiders. But patients tend to be reluctant to accept this rather extreme approach. A middle course of gradually overcoming the anxiety is best. Psychotherapy, either in a group or individually, aims to clarify personal difficulties and social problems. More realistic and effective solutions are worked out between the patients and the therapist.

Medication does not have a prominent role in the treatment of neuroses. The benzodiazepines (e.g. diazepam, lorazepam) are effective antianxiety drugs and may be used for a strictly limited period, never more than 4 weeks, usually to help the patient through an acute crisis. If used for long periods dependence will occur. Hysterical symptoms can sometimes be understood better by the use of intravenous diazepam (narco-analysis). With the dose carefully adjusted so that the patient does not go off to sleep, it can reduce the inhibition of disturbing thoughts and the patient may talk more freely about his problems which will then lead to better informed attempts to deal with them.

There is some evidence, which is not unanimously accepted by psychiatrists, that monoamine oxidase inhibitors (MAOIs) have a special place in the treatment of neurotic depression. These preparations therefore might be used for resistant cases but, as has been shown, depressive neurosis is usually a situational condition and it is preferable to encourage better adjustment rather than use medication passively. In general, MAOIs are drugs to avoid because of the adverse reactions with foods of high tyramine content and with some medicines, especially anaesthetics, pethidine and cough cures containing ephedrine. The effects of MAOIs last for 2 weeks on stopping these drugs.

Neuroses and psychoses

The older opinion, still advocated by some psychiatrists, is that the two conditions are on a continuum, with psychoses at the more severely disturbed end. This was originally the Freudian view. However, it is often stated that loss of insight offers an important differentiation between the two. Patients with neuroses are only too well aware of their symptoms, while often, but not always, patients with psychoses are unaware of being mentally abnormal. For example, the schizophrenic totally accepts his delusion of being controlled by the television as completely true and real; the manic patient is absolutely certain that he is the richest person in the world.

It was the discovery of antipsychotic and antidepressant medication that led to the possibility that there may be fundamental differences between the two groups of illnesses. The new medication has led more specifically to the possibility that the two 'functional' psychoses, i.e. schizophrenia and the affective disorders, have the characteristics of inherited neurotransmission disorders that spontaneously relapse and remit, although this does not offer a total explanation by any means. Furthermore, symptoms occur among all three psychoses (i.e. including organic psychoses, *see* Table 21.1) such as delusions and hallucinations, that are not found with neuroses, except that hysteria may produce mimicry. So a psychosis implies a metabolic abnormality, a disturbance with greater ramifications throughout the personality and potentially more disruption of social adjustment than is the case with neuroses.

The neuroses are usually clearly related to stresses and they appear to be only quantitatively different from normal experience. For example, it is easy to empathize with anxiety and depression, which everyone experiences, while some individuals have obsessional traits and others have hysterical aspects to their personalities, occurring as normal variants. Medication is only of secondary value for the neuroses and the main treatments are psychological.

With the psychoses, most symptoms are quite outside normal experience, that is they are qualitatively different. Medication is the essential treatment and has relatively specific effects. Antipsychotic drugs do not simply sedate disturbed patients they completely suppress the symptoms of schizophrenia and mania in most cases.

Considered in this way, it is remarkable that a number of groups of apparently quite dissimilar disorders have traditionally been classified together within a single speciality. The neuroses seem, on present evidence, to be true psychological conditions, implying the presumed absence of a metabolic abnormality. The two functional psychoses have largely 'medical' (meaning with an important physical component) rather than purely 'psychological' aetiologies and the organic psychoses are entirely medical with only secondary psychological presentations.

The psychoses

Symptoms

Because a few symptoms are prominent and frequently occur in all three psychoses, they are best considered at the beginning.

Delusions

These are false beliefs. The patient is totally convinced of the belief and it does not change despite persistent attempts at logical persuasion. Thus, arguing with the patient about his delusions, often done with the best intent, cannot succeed and may result in a hostile and uncooperative patient. The belief must also be out of context with the patient's social background. There are perfectly reasonable but socially unsophisticated groups of individuals whose culture causes them to believe that there are gods on mountains. There are many highly socially sophisticated individuals who believe unalterably in a virgin birth, so in these circumstances the beliefs are not delusional. Delusions occur in all psychoses, including organic states. 'Paranoid' means delusional, but it is usually used to refer to delusions of reference, i.e. the patient thinks he is being talked about or watched.

Hallucinations

These are false sensory perceptions with an absence of appropriate external stimuli. All five modalities can be involved and so patients may experience gustatory, visual, auditory and olfactory hallucinations as well as hallucinations of touch (tactile), e.g. a feeling of water or ants on the skin. These symptoms occur mainly in schizophrenia, auditory hallucinations being common and visual hallucinations unusual, and the organic psychoses when visual hallucinations are more often found.

Illusions

In this case sensory stimuli are perceived but misinterpreted. They are nearly always visual and sometimes auditory. For example, a shadow is seen but it is thought to be a person. An elaborate wallpaper pattern is thought to be animals crawling on the wall. Illusions occur with normal individuals as well as with organic syndromes, such as confusional states. They are not characteristic of schizophrenia and the affective disorders.

Schizophrenia

The popular view, which is quite wrong, is that schizophrenia involves a 'split personality' as in Stevenson's *Dr Jekyll and Mr Hyde*. Indeed, people are now derogatorily called schizophrenic when they voice views that seem to contradict each other. *Dr Jekyll and Mr Hyde* is a fictional account of an hysterical dual personality (a dissociative state) and the story has nothing whatever to do with schizophrenia. This serious illness involves 'shattering' rather than 'splitting' into two parts.

This diagnosis undoubtedly includes a number of related conditions rather than a single entity, but our knowledge so far is insufficient to classify them with reliability. However, there are recognizably at least two forms, the acute and the chronic. The acute illness is usually associated with much disturbed behaviour and obvious symptoms but it responds to medication and in time the patient returns to live in society, although often requiring a protected, supportive environment. The chronic form has mainly negative symptoms, such as limited communication, absence of emotions, social withdrawal and apathy. The sufferers usually are completely unable to care adequately for themselves and so they usually cannot manage outside hospital. These cases respond in only a limited way to antipsychotic medication. It seems likely that the chronic illness is associated with some sort of cerebral degeneration and these cases tend to have significant cerebral atrophy, seen on the CT scan.

The symptoms of schizophrenia are as follows.

Disorders of thinking

There is a breakdown in logical sequence so that one idea does not follow reasonably from another ('knight's move' thinking). When severe, one word apparently randomly follows the last without any meaning at all, giving what is expressively called a 'word salad'. This symptom emphasizes the shattering of associations involved.

Disorders of emotion

The abnormality is usually an absence of emotion so that schizophrenic patients have an emotional coldness or flatness. Emotional display and warmth in communication are not present. A related symptom is emotional incongruity. This is when the emotion expressed is inappropriate for the topic of conversation. The patient may laugh wildly when describing his concern about other people trying to harm him.

Catatonic symptoms

These are motor and they will vary from gross overactivity (catatonic excitement) to mutism and complete inactivity (catatonic stupor). There may be endlessly repeated mannerisms or the patient may remain in peculiar postures. With the famous 'waxy flexibility' (flexibilitas cerea), which is not often seen now that cases are treated more effectively and earlier, a limb is placed by the clinician into an awkward position and it then stays there for some time, it may be moved to another position, where it will remain again.

Delusions and hallucinations

These are described above.

It will be observed that these symptoms may occur in wholly organic states such as, in particular, abnormalities of the temporal lobes. But most forms of cerebral pathology may cause schizophrenic-like states which may sometimes be difficult to differentiate from true schizophrenia. Of course, behaviour disturbances and social peculiarities can also occur as a result of organic cerebral disorders as well as with schizophrenia.

Treatment

This has transformed the outlook for schizophrenic patients, many of whom, before the 1950s, were admitted to hospital for life. Although the illness tends to show apparently spontaneous relapse and remission, an attack can last for long periods of time, sometimes 10 years or more. With remission after such a long untreatable illness the patients frequently became institutionalized and socially helpless, so discharge was impossible: the so-called 'burnt-out' schizophrenic. Although their symptoms reduced in time, their personalities were irreversibly impoverished by the long illness and admission. Episodes of schizophrenia seem to have an increasingly adverse effect on the personality. So long attacks of uncontrolled illness, or frequent shorter attacks, are both associated with personality deterioration in the form of increasing introversion, eccentricity and social withdrawal.

Nowadays an attack can be controlled by antipsychotic drugs within a few weeks or months and earlier discharge is now usual. But this does not apply to the minority of patients with the chronic illness which is largely unresponsive. The use of depot medication, given by intramuscular injection every few weeks, has also been a major advance in that compliance can be easily monitored and the bioavailability of the drug is improved. Relapses of the illness are now most often due to a patient's refusal to continue with the injections. This is complicated by the fact that schizophrenic patients, because of defective insight, rarely understand clearly that they have been severely ill and are likely to relapse without regular medication.

However, the antipsychotic drugs frequently cause dyskinetic side-effects including akathisia, tardive dyskinesia and parkinsonian symptoms. These conditions may occur because of dopamine receptor blockade and some may be associated with the development of receptor super-sensitivity, as a result of the blockade. The side-effects usually improve with reduced doses but this may not be clinically desirable because there will be a risk of relapse. The parkinsonian symptoms usually respond to anticholinergic medication but tardive dyskinesia is difficult to deal with and it can become irreversible. It is presumably a commentary on the refractory nature of these side-effects that so many drugs have been advocated for them; including tetrabenazine, oxypertine, sulpiride, bromocriptine and amantadine.

Affective disorders

This group of illnesses involves abnormalities of emotional stability. 'Affect' refers to emotion. The name has replaced 'manic depressive disease' largely because most sufferers experience only episodes of depression and are never abnormally elated (i.e. manic). In the past, mania has been differentiated from a lesser state of hypomania, but these two words are now mostly used interchangeably. The depressed mood of the affective disorders is called 'endogenous' or 'psychotic'. Sometimes 'psychotic' means an endogenous depression which is severe and involves delusions.

The most common form of this group of illnesses involves recurrent episodes of endogenous depression and is called unipolar depression. Then there are patients who experience both episodes of depression and mania, and these are termed bipolar illnesses. The rarest form is when mania only occurs, and never depression (unipolar mania). Usually there are several years between attacks and so quite a long time needs to elapse before it is known whether a given illness is unipolar or bipolar. For example, there may be several attacks of depression, thus suggesting unipolar depression, before an episode of mania occurs which then makes the illness bipolar.

However, treatment of a case in practice is not much altered by these niceties of diagnosis, the main interest of which is genetic. It has been suggested that two inheritances are involved. In some families only depression occurs and never mania, while other families are prone to mania and depression, i.e. either

unipolar mania or bipolar illnesses. It is usually considered that unipolar mania
is the limited presentation of a bipolar illness.

It is not possible to account for the apparently spontaneous relapses and
remissions so characteristic of these illnesses. Indeed, affective disorders are
almost unique among both psychiatric and medical illnesses in that they often
show remarkable rhythmicity. Most patients with endogenous depression
report diurnal variation of mood. This occurs in association with early morning
waking, when the patients feel at their worst, and the mood gradually improves
to a greater or lesser degree as the day goes on. Thus, with these cases there
seems to be a circadian rhythm. Quite often the attacks have a seasonal quality
so that the illnesses may be more likely at a particular time of the year (seasonal
affective disorder). A number of cases show persistent, regular and rapid swings
such as 3 weeks of depression, one week well, then 2 weeks in mania; and this
can continue for years at a time if the cycle is not disrupted by treatment, and
sometimes treatment is unsuccessful in doing so.

Endogenous depression

Patients who have experienced spontaneous attacks of endogenous depression
and also severe grief after a distressing bereavement, for example, usually describe the two as different, although they often have difficulty in describing how
they are different. Probably as a result of the inability to describe the
experience, a number of patients do not mention depression when they seem to
be suffering from endogenous depression. Some tend to use such words as 'feelings of hopelessness', 'everything seems grey', 'feelings of desperation and
dread', and sometimes only 'I feel awful', without being able to say why.

It is possible to consider endogenous depression, not primarily as depression,
but as a wide-ranging functional abnormality, probably involving the limbic

Table 21.2   Symptoms of endogenous depression

---

*Depressed mood which does not vary; 'I can enjoy nothing'
  Characteristic feeling of wanting to cry with inability to do so
*Suicidal thoughts, which can be intense if the illness is severe and which must always
  be asked about
*Early morning waking at 4–5 a.m.
*Diurnal variation of mood; worse in the early morning and improving later
  Loss of energy, of general interests and sexual interest
  Loss of concentration, unable to take in a story in a newspaper or remember the plot
  as a television play develops
  Loss of appetite, usually with significant weight loss
  Impaired sleep, disturbed during the night with nightmares
*Increased anxiety, often with a sense of dread
  Epigastric 'churning'. This is often described in terms of the common 'butterflies in
  the stomach' but seems to be more unpleasant
*Feelings of worthlessness and pessimism. 'I will never get better', 'There is no future
  for my family and they would be better dead'
*A minor indiscretion many years previously may assume extreme importance and
  become a delusion associated with a certainty that extreme punishment is inevitable
  and deserved
*Hypochondriacal delusions. These are mainly alimentary with the bowels blocked and
  the insides rotting or diseased

---

*These are symptoms especially associated with suicidal risk.

system and hypothalamus, in which depressed mood is usually prominent but need not be, and including the major effects on energy, appetite, sleep, and some biological clocks. As a result, the illness has 'masked' presentations as discussed later. Mild attacks may have only a few of the characteristic symptoms, of which there are a number as shown in Table 21.2.

The clinical picture of the more advanced illnesses is one of either retardation or agitation. In the former there is a gradual slowing down of thinking and moving so that activity and communication may actually stop: a state of depressive stupor. Retardation reduces suicidal risks because of impaired motivation and reduced activity. Note that antidepressants and ECT tend to improve retardation before the depressed mood lifts so the initiation of medication may be paradoxically associated with suicidal behaviour which may be fatal, so the patient dies at the time when appropriate treatment has begun. Alternatively, there may be agitation, which is a state of restless misery in which the patient paces about wringing his hands and preoccupied by his distress.

There are two important aspects to bear in mind with this illness. First, it is very liable to be associated with suicidal behaviour. Suicidal intent should always be asked about tactfully so that the risk can be assessed ('Do you sometimes feel that life is not worth living?'). Suicidal risk is best seen as a continuum from mild thoughts to intense preoccupation, it is not well assessed as either 'genuine' or 'only' being threatened. Second, the illness can present in limitless ways and its presence is frequently 'masked' by atypical presentations or atypical symptoms.

For example, pain can be a purely depressive symptom in the sense that it may disappear when antidepressant medication is given. This symptom will usually require medical investigations, quite reasonably, but an underlying readily treatable psychiatric disorder may not be suspected and thus suicidal behaviour can occur unexpectedly. The pain is most commonly in the face or head and may also occur in the abdomen and chest. Asking the patient about depression often elicits the response that anyone would be depressed who suffers so much pain. Hence the primary problem has to be clarified and questions asked about appetite, weight loss, early waking and concentration difficulties may point to a primary depressive illness with pain as a symptom, rather than vice versa.

Similarly, depressed patients may complain mainly of loss of energy, or of anorexia with loss of libido or mental confusion and memory disturbances, abnormal bowel function or many other symptoms which strongly point to physical rather than psychiatric causes, but the symptoms may be due to an affective disorder nonetheless. Depression also considerably worsens the experience of many chronic medical disorders and makes them intolerable. Treating the depression allows the patient to accept the physical symptoms more easily.

There are also a number of other psychiatric disorders which do not suggest the presence of a depressive illness but which occur on the basis of endogenous depression. This diagnosis is more likely when the symptoms occur for the first time in the second half of life. Although some of the syndromes appear to be neuroses, primary neuroses are much less common during the later adult years. These presentations include phobic anxiety states, obsessional neurosis and even senile dementia. This assertion again depends on the observation that these conditions may clear up with antidepressants when, as true neuroses, they would not be expected to respond. There is no doubt that some apparent cases of definite senile dementia respond well to ECT, which may make a true dementia worse because confusion could be added. Obviously it is extremely important to detect these pseudodementia cases, but it seems that even with psychological testing reliable differentiation is not possible. Cases of pseudodementia can sometimes be separated by establishing the presence of a previous depressive illness and family history of depression. If there is doubt, a limited course of antidepressants can be tried, and a trial of ECT should also be considered.

The main treatment of depressive illnesses is by the use of the wide range of antidepressants now available. These have resulted in the decreasing use of ECT but this treatment, which is both potent and quite rapid in action, still has an important place for the more severe forms of depression and when there is considerable suicidal risk.

Mania and hypomania

It has already been pointed out that these two names, originally more clearly defined with one as a lesser disturbance than the other, tend to be used more or less interchangeably now. This is a difficult condition to manage because, uniquely in medicine, the patient feels pathologically *too well*, which seems a contradiction but is a clinical reality. Therefore patients almost never seek advice with this illness, although a small minority find the experience frightening because they feel unnaturally excited and there is a sense of imminent loss of self-control.

However, the majority feel in excellent health, they have limitless confidence and so they may embark on wild financial schemes totally beyond their means, they may cause havoc at work e.g. by attempting to take over from superiors or inviting the Board of Directors out to a meal in order to give them advice about running the company.

In depressed phases patients tend to lose their ability to cope with their job, so they soon take sick leave and hence there is less likely to be an adverse effect on their employment record, unless they have tried to carry on when they could not manage. However, manic patients, unless their illness is brought under control at an early stage, may become so disruptive at work that they are likely to lose their jobs. This is a tragic eventuality because they have a treatable illness, although their lack of cooperation and insight, which are symptoms of the disorder, makes management very difficult. Similarly, much harm may be done to the marital relationship because spouses find the grandiose schemes, the resulting major financial problems and the patient up all night perhaps singing to loud music, are quite intolerable if at all prolonged or if recurrent.

Some manic patients are jocular and amusing but many are more overbearing, irritable, intolerant of others and sometimes violent. Manic patients tend to be affronted by the suggestion they are ill and need admission to hospital when they have never felt so well and so sure of themselves. So most manic patients need compulsory admission and treatment, but implementing this can prove difficult. In order to force issues, the clinician must assemble adequate help.

Mania involves increased energy and therefore, perhaps in some metabolic way, the manic patient has 'the strength of ten' and the unreasonable psychotic anger to go with it.

There is also disinhibition and distractability, with pressure of speech, so that the patient rarely lapses into silence and may talk continuously for long periods. Sleep is decreased and sexual activity enhanced. With schizophrenia there is thought disorder, shown by a breakdown in the logical associations of ideas. In mania there is a rather similar symptom called 'flights of ideas'. This describes many different topics pouring into the patient's mind. Logical association is maintained for a given idea, but another idea then replaces it, one after the other in a rapid and bewildering succession. Grandiose ideas occur which are delusional so the patient may insist that he is God, or the greatest scientist ever known, or the head of an important family with international influence, and so on.

Of course, when the patient recovers from the episode of illness and has regained insight he is appalled by what has happened. Indeed, in the worst circumstances he may have lost his job, his spouse and his savings. He then enthusiastically agrees to seek medical advice the moment another episode of elation begins. But with the next occurrence of elation, inevitably there is increasing well-being and confidence, experiences which would not cause many to seek help. It is inevitable that insight is lost at the very onset of an attack, so is the chance of the sufferer's cooperation.

Differential diagnosis

The considerable social disturbance associated with this illness requires it to be effectively managed as soon as possible, and thus accurate diagnosis is needed. The presence of an affective disorder will be suggested by a previous episode of either depression or mania, and there may be a positive family history. Alternative causes, nowadays especially, are illicit drugs, including amphetamines, cocaine and some appetite suppressants. In addition, antidepressants, which although not stimulants, may switch those of unstable mood from depression to mania. Organic psychoses may be associated with mood changes and with disturbed behaviour. But there may be memory disturbances and impaired consciousness in these cases. With organic psychoses the mood is more likely to be one of fatuous euphoria rather than excited elation and the mental symptoms will usually fluctuate, unlike the sustained elated mood of mania.

The relationship between affective symptoms and tumours in particular parts of the brain remains unclear. In general, the commonest sites producing mood changes are frontal, when there is likely to be apathy and inappropriate behaviour; and temporal, when there tend to be schizophrenic-like symptoms.

The immediate treatment involves the use of antipsychotic medication in progressively increasing doses given by mouth or parenterally. The aim is to bring the excited state under control as rapidly as possible. The most commonly used drugs are haloperidol (Serenace) because of its considerable potency, and chlorpromazine (Largactil) because it is both potent and it has sedative properties. Lithium is a useful drug but it tends to take at least 2 weeks or more for the blood levels to rise to effective values. Therefore, as the illness settles with antipsychotic drugs, they are replaced after a time by lithium, which is also prophylactic and may be continued for a number of years if necessary. If lithium is undesirable for any reason, carbamazepine can be used instead. Because the control of these patients is often extremely difficult, mania should only be treated on psychiatric wards. Lithium blood levels need to be regularly monitored and the usual range is 0.4–1.0 mmol/litre. Lithium can cause hypothyroidism and, in the long term, renal damage.

Organic psychoses

With these disorders the psychiatric symptoms are generally non-specific and always secondary to a physical abnormality. This may be cerebral in origin but it can equally be associated with a systemic pathology. Thus, organic psychoses can be caused by both brain damage and electrolyte disturbances (Table 21.3).

Table 21.3   Acute confusional states

1. Infections
       systemic e.g. pulmonary, urinary
       neurological
           meningitis, tuberculous meningitis
           encephalitis
           meningovascular syphilis
2. Trauma
       head injuries
       subdural haematoma
3. Vascular
       thrombo-embolic infarction
       subarachnoid haemorrhage
       transient ischaemic attacks
       heart failure
4. Toxic
       drugs
           polypharmacy in the elderly
           hypnotics
           anticholinergics
       alcohol: acute, chronic
5. Metabolic
       uraemia
       hepatic failure
       hyponatraemia (inappropriate ADH secretion)
       thiamine deficiency (Wernicke's encephalopathy)
6. Endocrine
       hypopituitarism
       hypothyroidism
       hypo/hyperglycaemia
7. Epilepsy
       post-major epileptic seizures
8. Tumours
       primary
           glioma
           frontal, callosal
           obstructive hydrocephalus
       multiple metastases

A few physical illnesses are associated with characteristic psychiatric symptoms, such as the Korsakoff syndrome. Because the symptoms are generally non-specific, the presentations are rather incompletely divided into acute and chronic.

The acute syndromes are usually florid and include delirium, clouding of consciousness and confusional states, but these symptoms are likely to be mixed and often fluctuate in severity and vary in type. The most important feature is impairment of consciousness, although it may not be the most prominent. In addition, there may be confusion, disorientation, visual hallucinations and delusions of reference. Behaviour may become disturbed and there is often anxiety and perplexity.

The chronic state is dementia. The presentation develops slowly and includes intellectual impairment (cognitive deficit) with recent memory loss, disorientation, and personality deterioration without impairment of consciousness. Dementia may occur as a result of an acute condition which causes major and irreversible cerebral damage, but more commonly there are widespread, slowly progressive changes, as in senile dementia (Chapter 10). The acute confusional states are reversible while dementia often is not.

With the slow progression of dementia, it may be present for quite a long time before it is detected. Other people at work or in the home, who have close contacts with the patient, tend automatically to adapt, without awareness, to gradual personality change. The patient may also try to counter his increasing limitations by keeping within his familiar environment and assisting his deteriorating memory by using a notebook. Of course, with more severe dementia there is gross social disorganization and the patient will be unable to manage outside hospital.

Symptoms

Disturbances of consciousness involve a variable impairment of the normal state of being clear-minded, aware and alert. There is difficulty with understanding and thinking. Alertness may be lost even to the point where drowsiness occurs. In more extreme cases there may be stupor or coma. The level of consciousness often varies, even from hour to hour. Consciousness is preserved in dementia.

Disturbances of intellectual functions also called 'cognitive impairments' are shown by defective comprehension, an impaired capacity to learn and the reduced availability of common general knowledge. Psychological testing will give detailed information about the intellectual deficits present, if this is particularly needed.

Abnormalities of thinking involve slowing, impoverishment of ideas and a tendency to repetition. As a result, social judgements are poor and the patient lacks insight into his limitations.

Memory disturbance is often the earliest sign of the onset of dementia. It may begin with apparent absent-mindedness and there is subsequent progression with short-term memory most affected, while remote memory remains intact. There will also be disorientation, particularly in time. Confabulation may occur, which is when the patient gives a false account of his activities for a period which he is unable to remember. This is not deliberate lying but a pathological phenomenon.

Disorientation involves disorganization in the location of the patient in his environment. It should be tested for time, place and person, because all need not occur together.

Emotional disturbances are common and anxiety or depression can occur, which may be severe. Emotions may also become poorly controlled, so that excessive swings from depression to elation occur easily and transiently. This is called emotional lability. Sometimes there is emotional blunting, when emotional emptiness, flatness and absent emotional responses are observed.

Suspiciousness and delusions. Irritability and associated hostility are found and the uncertainty the patient experiences in understanding his environment can cause perplexity and suspiciousness, even amounting to delusions of reference (i.e. delusions referring to the patient: people are talking about him, watching him or following him; the television may give out messages to him).

Changes in personality and behaviour produce restriction of interests, greater rigidity and a tendency to increasing social coarseness. Personality function is partly expressed by behaviour, which becomes inappropriate and inconsistent, but the patient lacks insight into his behavioural disturbances. The onset of disinhibited sexual behaviour, stealing or other antisocial activities for the first time in later life, often involving legal action, may be the first presentation of an organic psychosis.

Management

The two frequent problems are first, to recognize a case as possibly an organic psychosis. This then leads to investigation of the underlying illness. If the clinical picture is mistaken for a primary psychiatric illness such as schizophrenia or an affective disorder, and there can be similarities, then investigations may be inadequate and the true pathology will not be discovered.

The second problem is the management of these cases in hospital where their disturbed behaviour may make it difficult for them to be tolerated on a general ward. This can lead to demands for transfer to a psychiatric ward. Most cases of organic psychosis can be managed on a medical or neurological ward if there is regular advice from a psychiatric team.

When a patient is unusually difficult he may need to be nursed in a psychiatric bed with visits by a physician who is supervising investigations. This is facilitated when both specialities are in a general hospital. But if the psychiatric bed is in the usual distant and isolated psychiatric hospital, where specialized investigations are much more difficult to arrange, then the transfer should be avoided and more psychiatric input on the general ward will be necessary.

The psychiatric treatment of an organic psychosis, as opposed to treatment of the causative physical abnormality, is symptomatic and supportive. The aim is to obtain the patient's cooperation as far as possible by his developing a relationship with nurses who get to know him; the use of antipsychotic drugs will reduce disturbing symptoms such as threatening delusions and will tend to control aberrant behaviour. In the case of untreatable dementia, transfer to an appropriate psychiatric ward will be needed. Nonetheless, the patient can be helped in a positive way by sensitive management involving suitable activities, methods of maintaining the patient's contact with his environment and regular help with meals and with attention to fluid intake and excretory functions.

Some other psychiatric disorders

There are a few other diagnosis which should be mentioned because of their potential importance in neuropsychiatric assessments.

Dementia in old age

See Chapter 10.

Anorexia nervosa and bulimia

It should be remembered that anorexia nervosa is potentially a life-threatening illness. The clinical characteristics are that most sufferers are women but men can have the condition. It usually begins in adolescence, mostly at about 16–17 years, and the onset often follows a normal attempt at dieting by an individual who is overweight. There develops an intense desire to be thin so that food is persistently refused and there is often deliberate vomiting and purging as well, in order to achieve this end. Curiously, it has been shown that these patients actually perceive themselves in a mirror as being fatter than they really are. In addition, there is amenorrhoea and this may precede the weight loss. The patients tend to be strangely energetic despite their emaciation. In both males and females there is reduced or absent sexual interest.

With about half the patients there are also episodes of gross overeating, called bulimia. In these binges large amounts of foods are eaten which are otherwise strictly avoided, such as bread, butter and jam. This causes a bloated feeling, then guilt and much remorse. So vomiting is induced and subsequently anorexia recurs.

It seems possible that there is a hypothalamic abnormality involved, but this probably becomes associated with certain types of family stress together with particular family responses to the refusal to eat. Thus a psychosomatically significant association of pathology and psychopathology causes the illness to become manifest, and then persistent.

There are important physical associations. Starvation will produce bradycardia, hypotension, constipation and hypothermia. There may be disturbed fluid balance, while repeated vomiting and the use of laxatives can result in hypokalaemia and alkalosis. Various endocrine abnormalities have been reported.

In the absence of clearer knowledge about the role of possible metabolic causes, treatment remains largely psychological. It is essential for the patients to be managed by experienced nurses who can avoid the many arguments the patients use to forgo food and who can be understanding but entirely firm about a previously agreed programme for progressive increases in weight; about

0.5–1 kg per week is usual. Over years, the disorder is episodic. Some become free of the problem while others continue to experience episodes of anorexia, sometimes with overeating as well. A few die.

Alcohol dependence

While the psychiatric effects associated with longer term and excessive alcohol intake are essentially organic psychoses, the problem begins with dependence. This is a phenomenon that is not well understood. There is the view that only certain individuals are liable to become seriously dependent, perhaps because they have a genetically determined predisposition. Others think that the incidence of dependence relates mainly to the ease with which alcohol can be obtained. Thus, public house employees will have particularly high risks and, now that expense account meals have become more lavish and more common, those who enjoy these privileges will also have a high risk.

Essential aspects include, once drinking has started the individual is often unable to stop until he is incapable of continuing. The drinker takes a similar amount of alcohol each day, whereas the unaffected person varies his intake from day to day, and on many days there will be no drinking. Drinking comes to take priority over other activities, including employment and home life. Tolerance to alcohol increases and so the intake rises in association with an increasing need for alcohol. Repeated withdrawal symptoms occur, usually following a fall in consumption. These symptoms of tremor and apprehension are countered by the dependent person taking more alcohol. This increasing intake produces early morning drinking which is diagnostic of the alcohol-dependent person, if he reveals it. Rapid resumption of dependence tends to occur after a period of abstinence, which has relevance for the longer-term management of these patients (Edwards *et al.*, 1977).

Alcohol problems occur most commonly among single or divorced young men but even adolescents are now increasingly convicted for drunkeness. This problem is less common in women but the prevalence is increasing.

Those who have an alcohol problem are notoriously unreliable in reporting accurate details, so assessment can be difficult. Alcoholic patients admitted to hospital for other reasons are likely to be deprived of their regular drink and severe psychiatric symptoms may be suddenly precipitated which could well confuse the doctor, especially if the patient has not revealed the alcohol problem (*see* p. 409).

Diagnosis is helped by liver function tests, especially for gamma glutamyl-transpeptidase and the mean corpuscular volume (MCV). These may be raised but abnormal results are not invariably due to excessive drinking. Alcohol has widespread adverse effects which include gastritis, cardiomyopathy, dementia, peripheral neuropathy and hepatic cirrhosis. In addition, drinkers are prone secondarily to many various problems such as head injuries, road accidents, vitamin deficiencies and tuberculosis.

One of the main psychiatric presentations is an acute organic psychosis or toxic confusional state, traditionally called delirium tremens (*see* p. 410). This occurs about 2 days, even up to 2 weeks, after long alcohol intake falls. There is agitation, restlessness, vivid illusions and hallucinations which are usually visual. Distorted animals are described and contribute to anxiety and confusion. Clouding of consciousness occurs, with disorientation and memory disturbances. There may also be marked autonomic effects such as sweating, fever and hypertension. Treatment is required urgently and is best carried out in a general hospital (*see* p. 410). Sedation with a benzodiazepine or chlormethiazole should be used, and anticonvulsants and vitamins may also be needed.

The other important psychiatric presentations are those of more chronic psychoses. In the case of alcoholic hallucinosis, in the early stages vague noises are heard. This auditory hallucination becomes more intense and with increasing paranoia, i.e. the noises become voices and the voices become accusatory until the patient cowers in his home, which he insists is surrounded by a crowd shouting accusations and threatening danger to him. The other chronic condition, alcoholic dementia, has a slow onset and, especially with the disingenuousness of these patients, it may not be suspected for a long time. It is likely to be irreversible and many require permanent hospital care.

Dependence on drugs

This problem has increased considerably during the past two decades. A large number of young people now take various illicit drugs on a casual basis and this renders them at risk for episodes of acute behavioural disturbance and also of becoming dependent. Older patients are more likely to be dependent on sleeping tablets, mainly benzodiazepines.

The common presentations in neurological practice will be episodes of strange disturbed behaviour, and there may be a real risk of the patient injuring himself or attacking others. With lysergic acid diethylamide (LSD), patients have jumped from a height in the belief that they had special powers of flying. Those taking amphetamines, especially over long periods of time, may show aggressive behaviour because of the onset of amphetamine psychosis resulting in paranoid fears. As with amphetamines, cocaine may be associated with overactivity, antisocial behaviour, confusion and sometimes rebound depression.

Diagnosis cannot be aided by specific aspects of the disturbed presentations and any young person can be involved. But much drug taking is found among those with abnormal personalities which may be suggested by a disorganized life style, social isolation within groups of similar individuals, a very poor work history and perhaps a police record. However, many young adults in and around big cities, while not socially unstable, experiment with drugs and adverse effects may suddenly appear. Suspicions about drug taking may arise from finding needle tracks, thrombosis of veins and multiple abscesses.

With acutely ill patients the most reliable diagnostic indicators will come from urine testing for drugs, a wise precaution in most cases where the diagnosis is unclear, especially in younger patients, although this will not give early information. If control of disturbed behaviour is urgently needed then parenteral chlorpromazine is probably the drug of choice, although the less potent benzodiazepines might be of value with some cases. It should be noted that the Mental Health Act (1983) does not allow an individual to be compulsorily admitted 'by reason only of . . . dependence on alcohol or drugs'. However, compulsory admission would be appropriate when an acute psychotic reaction is precipitated.

Mental handicap

Various names have been used to provide a collective noun for disorders associated with intellectual impairment starting in early childhood. Thus, 'deficiency', 'retardation' and 'subnormality' have now largely given way to 'handicap'.

In recent years there has been a quite fundamental reappraisal of the care of the mentally handicapped. First, many of these individuals are not in any way ill in a medical sense. They can be considered to have problems with self-management and social adaptation, and help with this is now more the responsibility of psychologists and social workers rather than doctors and nurses. It follows that the majority of those with mental handicap should not be in a hospital and they are best supervised in a community setting.

Another change concerns the much reduced importance of the intelligence quotient ($IQ = \dfrac{\text{mental age}}{\text{age in years}} \times 100$). In this equation the mental age is determined by standardized psychological testing although this is now infrequently carried out. The problem was that the IQ came to have too much influence in deciding on the capabilities of a given individual. For example, an IQ below an arbitrary level often meant that the individual had to remain in hospital for that reason alone. But, in practice, personality and social factors can be at least as important as the IQ in determining the capacity of the individual to manage in society. An IQ of 50–70 was regarded as mild handicap, 35–50 was of moderate degree. But, in reality, someone of relatively lower intellectual capacity might be helped to function at an effective level socially, perhaps because of a stable and sociable personality, while a person with a relatively higher intellectual level could remain dependent and of limited social function because of adverse personality factors and possible physical limitations. The contemporary trend is to help the individual to function at their highest possible level without attempting to predetermine that level by means of the merely mathematical number of the IQ.

With about one-third of handicapped people there is no apparent cause. In this group, those with moderately low levels of intellectual functions are likely to be without an abnormality and represent one end of the normal distribution of intelligence, just as the intellectually talented represent the other end. Some in this group, especially with more severely limited intelligence, will have unknown abnormalities. It is uncommon for a child in higher social classes (assessed by the parents' type of employment) to have a mild or moderate handicap because the inheritance predisposes to higher IQ levels. So in these higher social groups the handicap tends to be severe and related to organic pathology. Conversely, in lower social classes there are generally fewer with major central nervous system abnormalities. In these cases the handicap is mild to moderate as it relates more to an IQ inheritance at the lower end of normal and to social deprivation.

The commonest of the known abnormalities are Down's syndrome of chromosome 21 trisomy and other chromosomal abnormalities. These may involve other chromosomal trisomies and abnormalities of structure such as deletions, ring formation, inversions and translocations. Some are sex chromosome abnormalities but not all are associated with mental handicap (Turner's syndrome is not).

The group of primary genetic disorders involving inborn errors of metabolism are fairly numerous among the remaining cases but there will also be cases of central nervous system damage and abnormal development, neurodegenerative disorders and cases with epilepsy.

Neurologists will be particularly concerned with four disorders which are likely to result in future problems. These include tuberous sclerosis (see p. 360), an autosomal dominant condition with 70 per cent having mental handicap; neurofibromatosis (*see* p. 359), an autosomal dominant condition with 10 per cent of cases being mentally handicapped; the Sturge-Weber syndrome (*see* p. 362), often associated with severe epilepsy and 50 per cent are mentally handicapped; and hydrocephalus (*see* p. 370).

Many individuals with mental handicap will need a neurological assessment at some time because of the frequency of associated organic pathology. The neurological examination of these cases is not always easy to carry out because of the patient's lack of cooperation, limited concentration, inability to understand and distractability. Observation then becomes nearly as important as physical signs. Patience is needed in quantity, and flexibility helps. The aim is to amuse the patient or involve him in play, judiciously mixed with the clinical examination, in the context of the neurologist as jester.

Further Reading and References

Chapters 1–3

Adams, R. D. and Victor, M. (1985). *Principles of Neurology*, 3rd edn. McGraw Hill Book Company, New York.

Benson, D. F. (1979). *Aphasia, alexia and agraphia*. Churchill Livingstone, London.

Bickerstaff, E. R. (1963). *Neurological Examination in Clinical Practice*. Blackwell Scientific Publications, Oxford.

Folstein, M. F., Folstein, S. E. and McHugh, P. R. (1975). Mini-mental state – a practical method for grading the cognitive state of patients for the clinician. *Journal of Psychiatric Research* **12**, 189–198.

Plum, F. and Posner, J. B. (1980). *Diagnosis of Stupor and Coma*. 3rd edn. F. A. Davis Company, Philadelphia.

Ross, R. T. (1983). *How to Examine the Nervous System*. Medical Examination Publishing Company, New York.

Teasdale, G. and Jennett, B. (1974). Assessment of Coma and impaired consciousness: a practical scale. *Lancet* ii, 81–84.

Walton, J. (1985). *Brain's Diseases of the Nervous System*, 9th edn. Oxford University Press, New York.

Chapter 4

Dubovitz, V. and Brooke, M. H. (1985). *Muscle Biopsy: a Modern Approach*, 2nd edn. W. B. Saunders Company Ltd, London.

Walton, J. (Ed). (1981). *Disorders of Voluntary Muscle*, 4th edn. Churchill Livingstone, Edinburgh.

Chapters 5–8

Asbury, A. K. and Gilliatt, R. W. (Eds). (1984). *Peripheral Nerve Disorders*. Butterworths, London.

Maurice-Williams, R. S. (1981). *Spinal Degenerative Disease*. J. Wright and Sons, Bristol.

Chapters 9-12

Cummings, J. C. and Benson, D. F. (1983). *Dementia. A Clinical Approach.* Butterworths, Boston.

Laidlaw, J., Richens, A. and Oxyley, J. G. (1988). *A Textbook of Epilepsy.* Churchill Livingstone, London.

Marsden, C. D. and Fahn, S. (Eds). (1982). *Movement Disorders.* Butterworths, London.

Marsden, C. D. and Fahn, S. (Eds). (1987). *Movement Disorders 2.* Butterworths, London.

Ounsted, C. (1971). *Recent Advances in Paediatrics* no. 4. Churchill Livingstone, London.

Pedley, T. A. and Meldrum, B. S. (Eds). (1983, 1985, 1986). *Recent Advances in Epilepsy*, vols 1, 2 and 3. Churchill Livingstone. London.

Porter, R. J. and Morselli, P. L. (1985). *The Epilepsies.* Butterworths, London.

Chapters 13-15

Briggs, M. *et al.* (1984). Guidelines for the initial management after head injury in adults. *British Medical Journal* **288**, 983–985.

Crockard, A., Hayward, R. and Hoff, J. J. (Eds). (1985). *Neurosurgery.* Blackwell Scientific Publications, London.

Henson, R. A. and Urich, H. (1982). *Cancer of the Nervous System.* Blackwell Scientific Publications, Oxford.

Jennett, B. and Galbraith, S. (1983). *An Introduction to Neurosurgery*, 4th edn. William Heinemann Medical Books Ltd, London.

Kennedy, P. G. E. and Johnson, R. T. (Eds). (1987). *Infections of the Nervous System.* Butterworths, London.

Northfield, D. W. C. (1973). *The Surgery of the Central Nervous System.* Blackwell Scientific Publications, Oxford.

Chapters 16-20

Allen, C. M. C., Harrison, M. J. C. and Wade, D. T. (1988). *The Management of Acute Stroke.* Castle House Publications, Tunbridge Wells.

Bundey, S. (1985). *Genetics and Neurology.* Churchill Livingstone, London.

Harding, A. A. (1984). *The Hereditary Ataxias and Related Disorders.* Clinical Neurology and Neurosurgery Monographs, no. 6. Churchill Livingstone. Edinburgh.

Marshall, J. (1976). *The Management of Cerebrovascular Disease.* Blackwell Scientific Publications, Oxford.

Matthews, W. B. (1985). *McAlpine's Multiple Sclerosis.* Churchill Livingstone, Edinburgh.

McDonald, W. I. and Silberberg, D. H. (Eds). (1986). *Multiple Sclerosis.* Butterworths, London.

Rosenberg, R. N. and Harding, A. E. (1988). *The Molecular Biology of Neurological Disease.* Butterworths, London.

Ross-Russell, R. W. (Ed). (1983). *Vascular Disease of the Central Nervous System.* Churchill Livingstone, London.

Victor, M., Adams, R. D. and Collins, G. H. (1971). *The Wernicke-Korsakoff Syndrome*. F. A. Davis Company, Philadelphia.

Chapter 21

Edwards, G., Grossman, M. M., Keller, M., Moser, J. and Room, H. (1977). *Alcohol Related Disabilities*. World Health Organization, Geneva.

Gelder, M., Gath, D. and Mayou, R. (1983). *Oxford Textbook of Psychiatry*. Oxford University Press, Oxford.

Kendell, R. E. (1976). The classification of depressions: a review of contemporary confusion. *British Journal of Psychiatry* **129**, 15–28.

Lishman, W. A. (1987). *Organic Psychiatry*, 2nd edn. Blackwell Scientific Publications, Oxford.

Slater, E. (1965). The diagnosis of hysteria. *British Medical Journal* **1**, 1359–1399.

Stafford-Clark, D. and Smith, A. C. (1983). *Psychiatry for Students*, 6th edn. George Allen and Unwin, London.

Steadman, J. H. and Graham, J. G. (1970). Head injuries: an analysis and follow-up study. *Proceedings of the Royal Society of Medicine*, **63**, 23–28.

Trimble, M. R. (1981). *Post-traumatic Neurosis*. John Wiley and Sons, Chichester.

Trimble, M. R. (1983). Pseudoseizures. *British Journal of Hospital Medicine* **29**, 326–333.

Tyrer, P. J. (Ed.) (1982). *Drugs in Psychiatric Practice*. Butterworths, London.

Walsh, F. (1965). Diagnosis of hysteria. *British Medical Journal* **2**, 1451–1454.

List of Drugs

Generic name	British name	American proprietary name
Acyclovir	Zovirax	Zovirax
Amantadine	Symmetrel	Symmetrel
Amitriptyline	Tryptizol, Lentizol	Elavil, Endep
Amphotericin-B	Fungizone	Fungizone
Ampicillin	Penbritin	Omnipen
Azathioprine	Imuran	Imuran
Baclofen	Lioresal	Lioresal
Benzathine penicillin	Penidural	Bicillin
Benzhexol	Artane	Artane
Benztropine	Cogentin	Cogentin
Benzyl penicillin	Crystapen, Penicillin G	Penicillin G
Betahistine	Serc	Betaserc, Serc, Vasomotal
Bromocriptine	Parlodel	Parlodel
Carbamazepine	Tegretol	Tegretol
Carbimazole	Neomercazole	n/a
Cefotaxime	Claforan	Claforan
Ceftazidime	Fortum	Fortaz, Tazicef, Tazidime
Cefuroxime	Zinacef	Kefurox, Zinacef
Chloramphenicol	Chloromycetin	Chloromycetin
Chlormethiazole	Heminevrin	n/a
Cinnarizine	Stugeron	n/a
Clonazepam	Rivotril	Klonopin
Clonidine	Dixarit	Catapres
Cotrimoxazole	Bactrim, Septrin	Bactrim
Cyclizine	Valoid	Marezine
Cyclophosphamide	Endoxana	Cytoxan, Neosar
Dantrolene sodium	Dantrium	Dantrium
Dexamethasone	Decadron, Oradexon	Decadron, Hexadrol
Dexamphetamine	Dexedrine	Dexedrine
Diazepam	Atensin, Diazemuls, Valium	T-Quil, Valium
Dimenhydrinate	Dramamine	Dramamine
Domperidone	Evoxin, Motilium	n/a
Dothiepin	Prothiaden	n/a
Edrophonium	Tensilon	Enlon, Tensilon
Ethambutol	Myambutol	Myambutol
Ethosuximide	Emeside, Zarotin	Zarontin
Flucytosine	Alcobon	Ancobon
Flupenthixol	Fluanxol	n/a
Frusemide	Aluzine, Diuresal, Lasix	Lasix
Gentamicin	Genticin	G-myticin, Garamycin, Gentafair
Haloperidol	Haldol, Serenace	Haldol
Hydroxocobalamin	Neocytamen	alphaRedisol

Generic name	British name	American proprietary name
Indomethacin	Indocid	Indocin
Iohexol	Omnipaque	Omnipaque
Isoniazid	Rimifon	INH, Laniazid, Rifamate
Levodopa + benserazide	Madopar	n/a
Levodopa + carbidopa	Sinemet	Sinemet
Lithium carbonate	Camcolit, Priadel	Eskalith, Lithane, Lithobid
Lofepramine	Gamanil	n/a
Mefenamic acid	Ponstan	Ponstel
Methylphenidate	Ritalin	Ritalin
Methysergide	Deseril	Sansert
Metoclopramide	Maxolon	Octamide, Reglan
Metronidazole	Flagyl	Flagyl, Metric 21, Protostat
Naproxen	Naprosyn	Naprosyn
Neostigmine	Prostigmin	Prostigmin
Orphenadrine	Disipal	Myotrol, Norflex
Penicillamine	Distamine	Cuprimine, Depen
Phenobarbitone	Gardenal, Luminal	Antrocol, Belladenal, Donnatal
Phenytoin	Epanutin	Dilantin
Pimozide	Orap	Orap
Pizotifen	Sanomigran	n/a
Praziquantel	Biltricide	Biltricide
Primidone	Mysoline	Mysoline
Procainamide	Pronestyl	Procan, Pronestyl
Prochlorperazine	Stemetil	Compazine
Promazine	Sparine	Sparine
Pyrazinamide	Zinamide	n/a
Pyridostigmine	Mestinon	Mestinon, Regonol
Pyrimethamine	Daraprim	Daraprim, Fansidar
Rifampicin	Rifadin	Rifadin, Rifamate, Rimactane
Selegiline	Eldepryl	n/a
Sodium valproate	Epilim	n/a
Sulpiride	Dolmatil	n/a
Tetrabenazine	Nitoman	n/a
Thiopentone sodium	Intraval, Pentothal	Pentothal
Thioridazine	Melleril	Mellaril
Thyroxine	Eltroxin	Choloxin, Euthroid, Levothroid
Trimipramine	Surmontil	Surmontil
Vancomycin	Vancocin	Vancocin, Vancoled
Vincristine	Oncovin	Oncovin, Vincasar

n/a, the drug in question is not available in the US.

Index

Abetalipoproteinaemia   140, 358
Abdominal reflexes   60
Abducens nerve   53
   palsy   75, 162
Abscess
   fungal   338
   intracranial   317
      investigation   319
      symptoms and signs   318
      treatment   320
   spinal   191
Abstinence syndromes   409
Accessory nerve   57
Accommodation   53
Acoustic neuroma   313
Acromegaly   303, 414
Action tremor   46
Acuity, visual   52
Acute confusional states   440
Addison's disease   416
Adenoma, pituitary   303, 414
Adenoma sebaceum   360
Adie's pupil (tonic)   69
Adrenal disturbances   415
Adrenoleucodystrophy   351
Adult-onset ataxia   357
Aerocele   288
Affective disorders   431, 435, 439
Afferent pupillary defect   67
Agnosia   51, 66
AIDS   20, 337, 338, 367
Akathisia   203, 222, 435
Akinetic rigid states   200, 207
Alcoholic
   damage   410
   dependence   444
   hallucinosis   445
   myopathy   112
   neuropathy   134
Alcoholism
   abstinence syndromes   409
   acute intoxication   409
   dementia   445
   head injury   283
algorithm
   acute encephalitis   335
   acute meningitis   324–5
alpha-fetoprotein   375
Alzheimer's disease   48, 233
Amantadine   205

Amaurosis fugax   34, 389
Amblyopia   33
   toxic   408
   tropical   408
Aminoacidurias   366
Amnesia, transient global   31
Amnesic syndrome   48
Amniocentesis   375
Amphetamines   260, 423, 445
Amyloid
   angiopathy   386
   neuropathy   140
Amyotrophic lateral sclerosis   351
Amyotrophy
   diabetic   133
   neuralgic   37, 151
Anaemia, pernicious   135, 408
Anaesthesia
   dissociated   90, 196
   dolorosa   166
Anal reflex   155
Aneurysm   387, 401
Aneurysmal rupture   23, 387
Angiography   12
Angioma
   cerebral   385, 402
   spinal   190
Anomic aphasia   65
Anorexia nervosa   443
Anosmia   157
Anosognosia   66
Anoxia   412
Anterior cerebral artery infarction   396
Anti-cholinergic drugs   205
Anti-convulsant drugs   249
   therapeutic levels   252
Antidepressant drugs   125, 423, 438, 439
Antidiuretic hormone   388, 419
Antipsychotic drugs   435, 439, 442
Anton's syndrome   69
Anxiety states   425
Aphasia   64
Apneustic breathing   96
Appetite suppressants   439
Apraxia   52, 66
Arbovirus encephalitis   334
Arcuate fasciculus   65
Areflexic syncope   30
Argyll Robertson pupil   70, 342
Arnold–Chiari malformation   372

Arteriovenous malformation 388, 402
Arterides 402
Arteritis giant cell 23, 402
Arthritis, rheumatoid 138
Aseptic meningitis 339
Aspergillus infection 338
Asterixis 418
Astrocytoma
  cerebellar 310
  cerebral 298
  spinal 189
Ataxias 356
  adult-onset 357
  Friedreich's 356
  sensory 45
Ataxia telangiectasia 140, 358
Ataxic nystagmus 74
Athetosis 47, 212
Atlanto-axial subluxation 138, 375
Atrial myxoma 380
Atypical facial pain 27
Auditory nerve 56, 169
Auras 28, 243
Automatism, post-epileptic 29
Autonomic
  disturbances 128
  functions 61
  neuropathy 133
Autoregulation 384
Axillary freckles 60
Axonal degeneration 141

B 1, vitamin deficiency 134, 162, 407
B 12, vitamin deficiency 135, 408
Babinski reflex 60
Bacterial meningitis 323
Barber's chair sign 345
Barbiturates 250, 411, 423
Basal ganglia 45, 201
Basilar artery infarction 398
Basilar impression 374
Basilar migraine 265
Bassen–Kornzweig disease 140, 358
Becker's dystrophy 106
Becker's myotonic dystrophy 118
Behcet's disease 421
Belle indifférènce 428
Bell's palsy 166
Bends 413
Benign congenital hypotonia 117
Benign essential tremor 214
Benign intracranial hypertension 297
Benign positional vertigo 171
Benzodiazepines 43, 411, 423, 431, 445
Binswanger's disease 208
Biopsy
  brain 20
  muscle 20, 104
  nerve 20, 128
Bitemporal hemianopia 67
Bladder disturbance 61, 347, 350
Blepharoclonus 203
Blepharospasm 203, 221
Blood gases 43, 130
  respiratory failure 43, 95, 130
Bornholm disease 115
Borrelia burgdorferi 333
Botulinus toxin 221
Bourneville's disease 360
Bowel disturbances 61

Brachial
  neuritis 151
  plexus damage 149
Bradykinesia 203
Bradyphrenia 203
Brain abscess 317, 338
Brain injury 273
Brain stem
  demyelination 346
  infarction 398
Broca's aphasia 64
Bromocriptine 206, 305
Brown–Séquard syndrome 90
Bruits 61
Bulbar
  function 130
  palsy 84, 353
  polio 339
  progressive palsy 353
Bulimia 443

Café au lait spots 62, 359
Calcium metabolism 420
Caloric tests 79, 98
Candida infection 338
Carbamazepine 165, 173, 251, 252, 350, 440
Carbon dioxide tension 43, 102, 130
Carcinomatous
  meningitis 174
  neuropathy 124, 137
  non-metastatic complications 124
Cardiac syncope 91, 247
Carnitine deficiency 110
Carnitine palmityltransferase
  deficiency 110
Carpal tunnel syndrome 38, 142
Carriers – muscular dystrophy 106
Cataplexy 260
Catatonic stupor 434
  symptoms 434
Cauda equina claudicans 41
Cauda equina symptoms 42, 178
Caudate haemorrhage 394
Central core disease 116
Central neurogenic hyperventilation 96
Central pontine myelinolysis 410
Central retinal artery occlusion 160
Centronuclear myopathy 116
Cerebellar
  astrocytoma 310
  ataxia 45
  degeneration 44
  ectopia 373
  haemorrhage 395
  tumours 310
Cerebello-pontine angle tumours 313
Cerebral
  abscess 317
  atrophy 224
  blood flow 94
  blood flow and injury 278
  death 101
  embolism 382
  haemorrhage 385
  infarction 381
  lymphoma 308
  malaria 336
  metastases 306
  oedema 275, 384
  palsy 375

palsy 375
  steal 384
  thrombosis 381
  tumours 298
  venous thrombosis 388, 403
Cerebrospinal fluid 18
  gamma globulin 19, 348
  normal values 19
  meningitis 326
  rhinorrhoea 288
  syphilis 342
Cerebrovascular disease 378
  classification 379
  clinical features 389
  pathology 379
  risk factors 378
Ceruloplasmin 210
Cervical
  myelopathy 152, 177
  radiculopathy 36, 38
  root problems 151
  spondylosis 25, 38, 152, 193
Chamberlain's line 375
Charcot 429
Charcot–Bouchard aneurysm 385
Charcot's joints 128, 342
Charcot–Marie–Tooth disease 139
Cheyne Stokes respiration 96, 418
Chiari malformation 372
Chiasmal compression 67, 303
Childhood
  hydrocephalus 296
  migraine 265
Chloramphenicol 328
Chlormethiazole 285
Chlorpromazine 423, 439, 445
Chorda tympani 56, 167
Chordoma 317
Chorea 46
  causes 212
  gravidarum 216
  Huntington's 217
  oral contraceptive pill 216
  Sydenham's 216
Chromophobe adenoma 303
Chronic
  headache 24
  inflammatory demyelinating
    neuropathy 131
  paroxysmal hemicrania 267, 296
  spinal muscular atrophy 355
Chvostek's sign 420
Ciliospinal reflex 97
Classical migraine 262
Clonazepam 251, 257
Clonus 60, 79
Clouding of consciousness 441
Cloward's procedure 153, 187
'Cluster' headache 266
Cocaine 445
Coma 92
  assessment 96
  causes 93
  investigation 101
  pathophysiology 94
  scale 93
Common migraine 263
Common symptoms in neurology 22
Communicating hydrocephalus 371
Compensation neurosis 425, 430

Completed strokes 381
  management 398
Compulsion 427
Computerized tomography (CT) 7
Concussion 272
Cones 95
  foramen magnum 294
  subfalcine 293
  transtentorial 293
Confabulation 441
Confusional states 440
Congenital, fibre type disproportion 116
Congenital myopathies 116
Conjugate eye movements 71
Connective tissue disorders 137
Conn's syndrome 420
Consciousness, episodic loss 31
Constructional apraxia 66
Continuing stroke 384
Conversion symptoms 427
Co-ordination 58
Copper 209
Cord compression, causes 188
Corneal reflex 55
Cortical blindness 69
Cough syncope 30
Cramps 40
Cranial arteritis *see* Giant cell 402
Cranial dystonia 221
Cranial nerve syndromes 157
Craniopharyngioma 302
Creatine kinase 104
Cremasteric reflex 60
Creutzfeldt–Jakob disease 49, 237
Cryptococcal meningitis 237, 332
Cushing's syndrome 111, 124, 415
Cutaneous nerves 86
Cysticercosis 321
Cysts, parasitic 320

Deafness 56, 169
Decerebrate rigidity 99
Decorticate rigidity 99
Decompression sickness 413
Déjérine–Sottas 127
Delirium 424, 441
Delirium tremens 410, 444
Delusions 424, 432, 442
Dementia 47, 63, 221
  assessment 227
  causes 49, 225
  cerebrovascular 225
  dialysis 418
  epidemiology 226
  head injury 235
  investigation 229
  metabolic 238
  multi-infarct 226
  pugilistica 236
  senile 224
  subcortical 236
  treatment 240
  types 233
Demyelinating disease 344
Depressive
  headache 24
  neurosis 425
  stupor 436
Dermatomyositis 113
Dermoid cyst 375

Desensitisation   431
Deteriorating stroke   384
Developmental disorders   367
Devic's disease   352
Dexamethasone   96, 300
Diabetes insipidus   414
Diabetic
 amyotrophy   40, 133
 autonomic neuropathy   133
 cranial neuropathy   133
 hyperosmolar coma   417
 keto-acidosis   417
 neuropathies   132
Dialysis dementia   238, 418
Diastematomyelia   368, 375
Diazepam
 in spasticity   350
 in status epilepticus   257
Diffuse brain disease   208
Diffuse cerebral sclerosis   351
Digital subtraction angiography   380
Diphtheritic neuropathy   136
Diplopia   71, 162
Discs, prolapsed   192
 cervical   193
 lumbar   194
 thoracic   194
Disorders of emotion   434
Disseminated encephalomyelitis   351
Disseminated intravascular coagulopathy   328
Disseminated sclerosis see Multiple sclerosis   344
Dissociated sensory loss   90
Doll's head manoeuvre   97
Dopa   201, 205
Dopamine receptor   435
Dopaminergic neurones   202
Down's syndrome   367, 447
Dressing apraxia   66
Drop attacks   389
Drug dependence   445
 induced movement disorders   221
  pseudoparkinsonism   207
Duchenne dystrophy   104
Dysarthria   3, 51
Dysequilibrium syndrome   419
Dyskinesias   45, 46, 211
Dyslexia   65
Dysmetria   58
Dysphasia   2, 48, 51, 64
Dysphonia   3, 51
Dysraphism   367
Dysthyroid eye disease   163, 415
Dystonia   47
Dystonic reactions   222
Dystonic writer's cramp   221
Dystrophia myotonica   119
Dystrophies see Muscular dystrophy   104

E, vitamin deficiency   136, 358
Edrophonium (Tensilon) Test   121
Ekbom's syndrome   41
Electric shock   413
Electrocardiography   61
 Duchenne dystrophy   105
 Friedreich's ataxia   356
Electroconvulsive therapy (ECT)   427, 438
Electroencephalography (EEG)   13
Electromyography (EMG)   16, 104, 128
Electroretinography (ERG)   363
Embolism   381

Emotion   424
Emotional disorders   434
Emotional lability   85, 347, 354, 398
Empty sella   414
Empyema, subdural   317
Encephalitis   333
 algorithm   335
 arbovirus   334
 herpes simplex   334
 lethargica   45, 207
 periaxalis diffusa   351
 SSPE   237, 336
Encephalopathy
 AIDS   238
 hypertensive   403
 lead   411
 progressive multifocal   238, 338
 Wernicke's   407
Endocrine disturbances
 adrenal   415
 pituitary function   414
 thyroid   415
Endocrine myopathies   111
Endogenous depression   425, 426, 436, 437
Enterovirus infections   333
Enuresis   369
Ependymoma
 cerebral   310
 spinal   189
Epilepsy   284
 classification   244
 complex partial seizures   243
 diagnosis   245
 driving and   256
 grand mal, tonic clonic   28, 244
 hystero-epilepsy   32, 429
 investigation   247
 myoclonic   46, 218, 244
 petit mal   29, 244
 pregnancy   255
 simple partial seizures   243
 post-traumatic   284
 temporal lobe   29, 243
 treatment – starting   248
 treatment – stopping   254
Epileptic status   256
Epiloia   360
Episodic vertigo   171
Ergotamine   269
Escherichia coli infections   329
Ethosuximide   251, 252
Evoked potentials
 auditory brain stem   15
 somatosensory   16
 visual   14
Exophthalmic ophthalmoplegia   111
Extradural haematoma   274, 285
Eye movements
 testing   53, 55
 volitional control   76

Fabry's disease   140, 364
Facial
 hemi-atrophy   169
 migraine   266
 myokymia   169
 nerve   56
 pain   26
 paralysis (Bell's palsy)   166
Facio-scapulo-humeral dystrophy   106

Faints, syncope   28, 30, 247
False localising signs   292, 294
Familial periodic paralysis   109
Fat embolism   285
Faun's tail   368
Femoral nerve   148
    stretch test   155
Femoral neuropathy   133
Finger–nose test   58
Finger print inclusion myopathy   116
Fits *see* Epilepsy   284
Five-hydroxytryptamine   267, 423
Flights of ideas   439
Focal cortical syndromes   48
Focal (partial) seizures   28, 243
Fog's test   376
Foot drop   40
Foramen magnum cone   95, 294
Foramina
    of Luschka   295, 370
    of Magendie   295, 370
Freud   423
Friedreich's ataxia   356
Frontal lobe syndromes   48
Frozen shoulder   37
Fugue   428
Fungal infections   387
    cryptococcal   332
    others   338
F wave   17

Gag reflex   57, 98
Gait disorders   41
Galen, vein of, aneurysm   308
Gangliosidosis   364
Gargoylism   363
Gaucher's disease   364
Gegenhalten   59
General paralysis of the insane (GPI)   342
Germinoma   308
Geniculate zoster   167
Giant cell arteritis   23, 402
Giddiness   34, 77, 170
Gilles de la Tourette syndrome   219
Glasgow coma scale   93, 280
Glioblastoma multiforme   298
Gliomas   298
Global aphasia   64
Glomus jugulare tumour   173
Glossopharyngeal nerve   57
    neuralgia   27, 173
Glycogen storage diseases   110
Gram-negative bacillary infections   330
Grand mal, tonic clonic seizures   28, 244
Granuloma
    orbital   163
    Wegener's   403
Granulomatous myositis   115
Grief   426
Group B streptococcal infections   329
Guillain–Barré syndrome   129
Gumma   341
Guyon's canal   145

Haemangioblastoma   312
Haematoma
    acute subdural   274
    chronic subdural   287
    extradural   285, 274
    intracerebral   274

Haemophilus influenzae meningitis   329
Haemorrhage
    caudate   394
    cerebellar   395
    cerebral   385
    lobar   394
    pontine   394
    putaminal   394
    subarachnoid   23, 387, 400
    thalamic   394
Hallucinations   433, 444, 445
Haloperidol   220, 439
Hartnup disease   366
Headache
    acute   23
    chronic   24
    'cluster'   266
    migrainous   24, 362
    raised intracranial pressure   24, 290
    subacute   23
    tension   25
    uncommon causes   25
Head injuries   272, 427
    complications   288
    conscious level   280
    intracranial pressure   275
    local effects   272
    management   278
    motor function   281
    pupils, effect on   281
Hearing   56, 169
Heat stroke   413
Heavy metal poisoning   411
Hemianopia   33, 53, 68
Hemiballism   218
Hemifacial spasm   168
Hemiplegia   3
Hemiplegic migraine   264
Hepatic failure   417
Hereditary ataxias   356
Hereditary spastic paraplegia   359
Herniations   293
Herpes simplex encephalitis   334
Herpes zoster infection   167, 352
    neuralgia   26, 27
Holmes–Adie syndrome   69
Holmes ataxia   357
Homocystinuria   366
Horner's syndrome   71, 150, 397
Human T lymphotropic virus   352
Hunter's mucopolysaccharidosis   363, 365
Huntington's chorea/disease   217, 236
Hurler's mucopolysaccharidosis   365
Hydatid cyst   320
Hydrocephalus   295, 369, 370
    in childhood   296
    communicating   371
    diagnosis   296
    meningitis   325
    normal pressure   296, 371
    obstructive   32, 371
    treatment   297
Hypercalcaemia   420
Hyperglycaemia   416
Hyperkalaemia   109
Hyperosmolar coma   417
Hyperpyrexia   111
Hypersomnia   261
Hypertension   378
Hypertensive encephalopathy   403

Hyperventilation   32
Hypnagogic hallucinations   259
Hypocalcaemia   420
Hypoglossal nerve   57
Hypoglycaemia   31, 247, 416
Hypokalaemia   109, 420
Hypomania   438
Hyponatraemia   419
Hypopituitary function   414
Hypothermia   413
Hypothyroidism   111, 415
Hysteria   427
Hysterical
    dissociation   428
    fugue   428
    personality   428
Hystero-epilepsy   428–9

Ideomotor apraxia   66
Illusions   433
Imipramine   423
Immune-depressed infections   332, 337
Impotence   61
Inappropriate antidiuretic hormone
    secretion   125, 388, 419
Inattention, visual   53
Incontinence   61
    multiple sclerosis   346, 347
Infantile hemiplegia   376
Infarction, cerebral   381
Infection
    bacterial   327
    fungal   332, 338
    immuno-compromised   337
    meningeal   323
    meningococcal   327
    pneumococcal   328
    spinal   192
    syphilitic   341
    tuberculous   331
    viral   333
Infranuclear lesions, eye movements   71
Innervation of muscles   82, 83
Insulinomas   416
Intelligence quotient (IQ)   446
Intelligence tests   63, 228
Intention tremor   46
Internuclear lesions, eye movements   74
Internuclear ophthalmoplegia   74
Intracerebral haematoma   274
Intracranial-extracranial anastomosis   391
Intracranial
    hypertension, benign   297
    pressure   291, 292
    reduction of   95
Intradural-extramedullary spinal tumours   189
Intramedullary spinal tumours   189
Involuntary movements   45
    dyskinesias   211
Iproniazid   423
Ischaemic papillitis   160
Ischaemic, transient cerebral attacks   379, 389
Isoniazid   134, 332

Jacksonian epilepsy   243
Jakob–Creutzfeldt (see Creutzfeldt-J.)   49, 237
Jaw jerk   56
Jaw winking   167
Jekyll and Hyde   433

Joint position sense   60
Jugular foramen syndrome   172
Juvenile parkinsonism   209

Kayser–Fleischer rings   210
Kearns–Sayre syndrome   116
Kernig's sign   62, 262, 322
Kernohan's notch effect   293
Keto-acidosis, diabetic   417
Klippel–Feil syndrome   374
Korsakoff's psychosis   407, 441
Krabbe's leucodystrophy   363
Kveim's test   422
Kyphoscoliosis   356

Labyrinthine function   77
Lactate, cerebrospinal fluid   19
Lacunar infarct   398
Lacunar stroke   391
Lacunes   383
Lambert–Eaton syndrome   42
Laminectomy   153, 196
Language dominance   64
Latent syphilis   341
Lateral cutaneous nerve, of thigh   148
Lateral popliteal nerve palsy   146
Lead poisoning   411, 134
Leber's optic atrophy   161
Leprosy   136
Leptospiral infections   333
Leucodystrophies   351
Leukaemia   137
Levodopa *see* Dopa   201, 205
Lewy bodies   45, 201
Lhermitte's phenomenon   345
Lightning pains   342
Limb-girdle dystrophy   108
Lipidoses   363
Lipoma   375
Lisch's nodules   360
Listeria monocytogenes meningitis   329, 330
Lithium
    in mania   440
    in migrainous neuralgia   270
Little's disease   376
Liver failure   417
Liver function tests   417, 418, 444
Lobar haemorrhage   394
Locked-in syndrome   93
Locomotor ataxia *see* Tabes dorsalis   342
Louis-Bar syndrome   358
Lumbar puncture   18
Lumbar root lesions   153
Lupus anticoagulant   380
Lupus erythematosus, systemic (SLE)   138
Lyme disease   333
Lymphocytic meningitis   331
Lymphoma, cerebral   308
Lymphoma, neuropathy   137
Lysergic acid diethylamide (LSD)   445

Macroglobulinaemia   137
Magnetic resonance imaging (MRI)   10
Main d'accoucheur   420
Major epilepsy (grand mal)   28, 244
Major strokes   393
Malabsorption   136
Malaria, cerebral   336

Malformations
  anticonvulsants 255
  congenital 367
Malignant disease
  neurological complications 124
  polymyositis 114
Malignant hyperpyrexia 111
Malignant neuroleptic syndrome 411
Malignant spinal tumours 187
Malingering 430
Mania 438
Manic-depressive disease 435
Marche á petits pas 235
Marchiafava–Bignami disease 239, 410
Marcus Gunn phenomenon 67
Mean corpuscular volume (MCV) 445
Measles
  and encephalomyelitis 351
  and SSPE 237, 336
Median longitudinal bundle (fasciculus) 71, 74, 398
Median nerve 142
Medulloblastoma 310
Ménière's disease 170
Meningeal syphilis 342
Meningioma
  cerebral 301
  sites 301
  spinal 189
Meningitis 322
  aetiology 323
  bacterial 323
  causes 323
  cerebrospinal fluid changes 326
  cryptococcal 332
  diagnosis 326
  haemophilus influenzae 329
  listeriosis 330
  meningococcal 327
  neonatal 329
  partially treated 331
  pneumococcal 328
  tuberculous 331
  viral 333
Meningofacial angiomatosis 362
Meningocoele 368
Meningovascular syphilis 403
Mental handicap 446
Metabolic myopathies 109
Metachromatic leucodystrophy 140, 351, 364
Metastases 306
Methyl phenyl tetrahydropyridine (MPTP) 202
Methysergide 270
Metoclopramide 269
Microglioma 308
Micturition syncope 30
Migraine 24, 262
  basilar 265
  causes 267
  childhood 265
  classical 262
  common 263
  equivalents 265
  facial 266
  hemiplegic 264
  lower half headache 266
  ophthalmoplegic 264
  precipitants 263
  prevention 269

  retinal 265
  treatment 269
Migrainous neuralgia 27, 266
Miller Fisher variant polyneuropathy 131
Mini-mental state examination 63
Mitochondrial myopathies 116
Mongolism *see* Down's syndrome 367, 447
Monoamine oxidase inhibtors 431
Mononeuritis multiplex 42, 126, 132, 138, 403
Morquio–Brailsford disease 365
Motor neurone disease 353
Mountain sickness 414
Movement disorders 45, 200
Mucopolysaccharidoses 365
Multi-infarct dementia 405
Multiple sclerosis (disseminated sclerosis) 344
  aetiology 344
  causes 347
  investigation 348
  optic neuritis 158, 345
  paroxysmal brain stem disorders 346
  pathology 345
  relapses 347
  spasticity 347
  symptoms and signs 345
  treatment 349
Multiple system atrophies 208
Mumps
Muscle
  biopsy 104
  power 59
  wasting 79
  weakness 79
Muscular dystrophy 104
  Becker variant 106
  carrier detection 106
  diagnosis 103
  Duchenne 104
  facio-scapulo-humeral 106
  limb-girdle 108
  ocular 108
  pseudohypertrophic (Duchenne) 104
  X-linked 104
Myasthenia gravis 72, 121, 164
  diagnosis 121
  treatment 123
Myasthenic syndrome 123
Myelitis, transverse 351
Myelodysplasia 375
Myelography 13
Myelomeningocoele 369
Myoclonic seizures 363
Myoclonus 212, 213
  action 218
  focal 219
  generalized 218
  palatal 219
  post-anoxic 218
  reflex 218
  spinal 219
Myopathy
  congenital 116
  endocrine 111
  inflammatory 112
  metabolic 108
  ocular 108
  toxic 112
Myopia 32
Myositis

granulomatous   115
  tropical   115
  viral   115
Myotonia congenita   117
Myotonic dystrophy   119
Myxoedema   415

Narco-analysis   431
Narcolepsy   259
Nasopharyngeal carcinoma   173
Neck, stiffness   62, 152, 322
Neisseria meningitis (meningococcal)   327
  complications   328
  treatment   328
Nemaline myopathy   116
Neonatal
  meningitis   329
  myasthenia   123
Nerve
  abducens (CN 6)   53
  accessory (CN 11)   57
  auditory (CN 8)   56
  biopsy   20, 128
  conduction   16
  facial (CN 7)   56
  femoral   148
  glossopharyngeal (CN 9)   57
  hypoglossal (CN 12)   57
  lateral cutaneous of thigh   148
  lateral popliteal   146
  median   142
  oculomotor (CN 3)   53
  olfactory (CN 1)   52
  optic (CN 2)   52
  sciatic   145
  trigeminal (CN 5)   55
  trochlear (CN 4)   53
  ulnar   143
  vagal (CN 10)   57
Neuralgia
  glossopharyngeal   27, 173
  migrainous   27, 266
  post-herpetic   26, 27
  Raeder's   27
  trigeminal   27, 164
Neuralgic amyotrophy   50, 151
Neurofibroma, spinal   189
Neurofibromatosis   359, 447
Neurological
  examination   50
  symptoms   21
Neuroma
  acoustic   313
  plexiform   360
Neuromyelitis optica (Devic's)   352
Neuropathy
  alcoholic   134
  autonomic   128, 133
  carcinomatous   124
  causes   127
  chronic inflammatory demyelinating   131
  connective tissue disorders   137
  diabetic   132
  hereditary   139
  infective   136
  investigations   128
  malignancy   137
  pathogenesis   126
  protein disturbances   137
  symptoms and signs   127

  post-infective (Guillain–Barré)   129
  tropical   408
  toxic   134
  unknown   140
  uraemic   135
  vitamin B12 deficiency   135
Neuroradiology   7
Neuroses   424
  treatment   430
Neurosyphilis   341
Nicotinic acid (niacin)   408
Niemann–Pick disease   364
Nocardial infections   338
Noradrenaline   423
Normal pressure hydrocephalus   296, 371
Nutritional
  amblyopia   408
  neuropathy   409
Nystagmus   55
  ataxic   74
  downbeat   373
  positional   171

Obscurations of vision   33
Obsessional neurosis   427, 437
Obstructive hydrocephalus   32, 371
Obstructive sleep apnoea   260
Ocular motor palsies   161
Ocular movements   71
Ocular myopathy   108
Oculocephalic reflexes   76, 93, 97
Oculogyric crises   207
Oculomotor nerve   53
Oculomotor palsy   73, 162
Oculovestibular reflexes   98
Olfactory nerve   52
Oligodendroglioma   298
One-and-a-half syndrome   76
Ophthalmoplegic migraine   264
Opisthotonus   340
Opportunistic pathogens   337
Optic atrophy   160
  causes   160
Optic fundi   53
Optic nerve   52
Optic neuritis   158
  signs   159
  treatment   159, 349
Optic radiation   68
Oral contraceptive pill   216, 264, 297, 388, 403
Organic psychosis   433
Orthostatic syncope   247
Oscillopsia   74, 346, 373
Osmolality   419
Otolith apparatus   77
Overbreathing   32
Oxygen, hyperbaric   350
Oxygen tension   43, 130

Paget's disease   374
Pain
  arm   36
  face   26
  leg   39
  referred   26
Palatal myoclonus   219
Papilloedema   157, 323
  causes   158
Paraldehyde   258
Parameningeal suppuration   333

Paramyotonia 118
Paraneoplastic syndromes 124
Paraphasia 65
Paraplegia, acute 43
Parasitic cysts 320
Parasomnias 261
Parinaud's syndrome 70, 308
Parkinson's disease
  aetiology 201
  clinical features 202, 203
  diagnosis 204
  pathogenesis 201
  treatment 205
Paroxysmal hemicrania, chronic 267
Patterns of sensory loss 89, 90, 91
Pellagra 408
Pelvic carcinoma 40
Penicillamine 112, 211
Penicillin 328, 343
Periodic migrainous neuralgia 266
Periodic paralysis 109
Peripheral neuropathy *see* Neuropathy
Pernicious anaemia 135, 408
Personality 424
Petechial rash 328
Petit mal (absences) 29, 244
Phakomatoses 359
Phenobarbitone 250, 252
Phenylketonuria 366
Phenytoin 121, 165, 250, 252
Pheochromocytoma 246
Phobic anxiety 425, 437
Pick's disease 234
Pineal region tumours 308
Pineoblastoma 308
Pineocytoma 308
Pituitary adenoma 303, 414
Pituitary apoplexy 414
Pituitary tumours 302
Pizotifen 270
Plantar responses 60
Pneumococcal meningitis 328
Poliomyelitis 338
Polyarteritis nodosa 138, 402
Polycythaemia 391
Polymyalgia rheumatica 37, 402
Polymyositis 112
Polyneuritis cranialis 173
Polyradiculoneuropathy 129
Pontine haemorrhage 395
Pontine paramedian centre 76
Porphyria 135
Portosystemic encephalopathy 417
Positional vertigo 171
Posterior cerebral artery infarct 396
Posterior communicating artery, aneurysm 401
Post-concussional syndrome 289, 429
Post-herpetic neuralgia 27
Post-traumatic epilepsy 289
Post-traumatic syndrome 24
Pressure palsies 141
Prevention of migraine 269
Primary generalized dystonia 220
Primidone 216, 250, 252
Progressive bulbar palsy 353
Progressive external ophthalmoplegia 72
Progressive multifocal leucoencephalopathy 338
Progressive muscular atrophy 353
Prolactin secreting tumours 303, 414
Propranolol 216, 270

Prosopagnosia 66
Pseudoathetosis 58
Pseudodementia 47
Pseudohypertrophic muscular dystrophy 104
Pseudoseizures 32, 246
Psychoses 424, 432
Pupillary abnormalities 69
Pupils
  Adie's (tonic) 69
  afferent defect 67
  Argyll Robertson 70, 342
  Horner's (sympathetic) 71
  light-near dissociation 70
  pontine 97
Purpuric rash 328
Pursuit eye movements 55, 76
Putaminal haemorrhage 394
Pyrazinamide 332
Pyridostigmine 123

Quadriplegia, acute 43
Quinine 121, 336

Rabies 334
Rachischisis 367
Radiation fibrosis 151
Radicular syndromes
  cervical 152, 176
  lumbar 154, 178
Radiology 7
Radionuclide scans 12
Radiotherapy 299, 303, 307, 309, 312
Raeder's neuralgia 27
Raised intracranial pressure 291
  symptoms and signs 24, 292
Ramsay Hunt syndrome 167
Ramsay Hunt ataxia 219
Raven's progressive matrices 63
Raynaud's phenomenon 149
Reactive depression 425
Red cell transketolase 407
Reducing body myopathy 116
Rectal biopsy 363
Reflexes 60
  cutaneous 60
  plantar 60
  tendon 60
Reflex, vaso-vagal syncope 30, 247
Refsum's disease 140, 363
Rehabilitation after stroke 405
Relapses in multiple sclerosis 347
Relaxation 431
Renal failure 418
Respiration
  apneustic 96
  ataxic 96
  central neurogenic hyperventilation 96
  Cheyne–Stokes 96
Respiratory failure 43, 130, 412
Respiratory function 130
Restless legs 41
Retention of urine 178
Retinal artery occlusion 160
Retinal migraine 265
Retinitis pigmentosa 363
Retrocollis 221
Reversible ischaemic neurological deficit
  (RIND) 383
Reye's syndrome 418
Rheumatoid arthritis 138

Rifampicin 332, 328
Rigidity 59
  cogwheel 202
Rinne's test 57
Romberg's sign 58
Root tension signs 155
Roots, avulsion of 149
Roussy–Levy syndrome 140
Rum fits 409
Ruminations 426

Saccadic eye movements 55, 76
Sacral sensation 155
Sanfilippo disease 365
Sanger–Brown's ataxia 357
Sarcoidosis 421
Saturday night paralysis 142
Scalloped vertebrae 360
Scans
  computerized tomographic (CT) 7
  magnetic resonance imaging (MRI) 10
  radionuclide (isotope) 12
Scapulo-peroneal atrophy 356
Schilder's disease 351
Schilling test 136, 408
Schizophrenia 423, 433, 439
  catatonic symptoms 434
  delusions and hallucinations 434
  disorders of emotion 434
  disorders of thinking 434
  treatment 434
Sciatica 39
Sciatic nerve lesions 145
Seeligmuller's spastic paraplegia 359
Senile dementia 224, 438
Sensory ataxia 356
Sensory loss
  cortical 92
  dissociated 90
  suspended 91
  thalamic 92
Serological tests, syphilis 342
Serum angiotensin converting enzyme (SACE) 422
Shagreen patch 360
Shakes, alcoholic 409
Shifts *see* Herniations 293
Shunt associated meningitis 330
Shunts 297, 372
Shy-Drager syndrome 208
Sinusitis 26, 318
Sjögren's syndrome 114
Sleep disorders 259
Sodium valproate 251, 252
Spasmodic torticollis 221
Spastic diplegia 375
Spasticity 59
  treatment 372
Spastic paraparesis 44
Spastic weakness of one leg 44
Spina bifida 367
  cystica 369
  occulta 367
Spinal cord
  compression 177
  investigation 179
Spinal degeneration
  cervical 193
  lumbar 194
  thoracic 194

Spinal disease
  surgical treatment 186
  symptoms and signs 175
Spinal infection 191
Spinal tumours 187
Spinal muscular atrophy 355
Spirochaetal infections 333, 341
Squint 71
Status epilepticus 256
  management 257
Steele–Richardson–Olszewski's syndrome 207
Stereognosis 92
Steroid myopathy 112
Stokes Adams attacks 31
Stroke
  in evolution 384
  rehabilitation 405
  risks 378
Strumpell's spastic paraplegia 359
Sturge–Weber syndrome 362
Subacute bacterial endocarditis 318
Subacute combined degeneration 135, 408
Subacute sclerosing panencephalitis (SSPE) 336
Subarachnoid haemorrhage 387, 400
Subdural
  effusions 329
  empyema 318
  haematoma 274, 287
Subfalcine herniation 293
Subungual fibroma 360
Suicide 426, 436, 438
Superior oblique palsy 74
Supranuclear lesions, eye movements 75
Supratentorial tumours, investigation 305
Sydenham's chorea 216
Symptomatic migraine 268
Syncope 30
  cardiac 31
  cough 30
  micturition 30
  orthostatic 247
  paralytic 30
  reflex 30
  vasovagal 30
Syphilis 341
  course of 341
  general paralysis of the insane (GPI) 342
  gumma 341
  meningitis, chronic 342
  serological tests for 342
  tabes dorsalis 342
  treatment 343
Syringomyelia 196, 373
Systemic lupus erythematosus (SLE) 138

Tabes dorsalis 342
Tangier disease 140
Tapeto-retinal degeneration 363
Tardive dyskinesia 222, 411, 435
Tarsal tunnel 148
Taste 52, 56, 167
Tay-Sachs disease 364
Temporal arteritis *see* Giant cell 23, 402
Temporo-mandibular joint, pain 26
Tendon reflexes 60
Tensilon (edrophonium) test 121
Tension headache 25
Tentorial herniation 293